TREATMENT OF METABOLIC BONE DISEASE:
MANAGEMENT STRATEGY AND DRUG THERAPY

This book is to be returned on or ᴧ
the last date stamped b᷅ ᴧw.

TREATMENT OF METABOLIC BONE DISEASE: MANAGEMENT STRATEGY AND DRUG THERAPY

Edited by

DAVID HOSKING MD FRCP
Consultant Physician and Professor
Division of Mineral Metabolism
Nottingham City Hospital
Nottingham
UK

JOHANN RINGE MD
Head of Department of Internal Medicine 4
Klinikum Leverkusen
Akademisches Lehrkrankenhaus der
Universität zu Köln
Leverkusen
Germany

MARTIN DUNITZ

© Martin Dunitz Ltd 2000

First published in the United Kingdom in 2000
Martin Dunitz Ltd
The Livery House
7–9 Pratt Street
London NW1 0AE

A CIP catalogue record for this book is available from the British Library

ISBN 1-85317-755-5

Distributed in the United States by:
Blackwell Science Inc.
Commerce Place, 350 Main Street
Malden MA 02148, USA
Tel: 1-800-215-1000

Distributed in Canada by:
Login Brothers Book Company
324 Salteaux Crescent
Winnipeg, Manitoba R3J 3T2
Canada
Tel: 1-204-224-4068

Distributed in Brazil by:
Ernesto Reichmann Distribuidora de Livros, Ltda
Rua Coronel Marques 335, Tatuape 03440-000
Sao Paulo,
Brazil

Composition by Wearset, Boldon, Tyne and Wear
Printed and bound in Spain by Grafos S.A. Arte sobre papel

Contents

Contributors

Nina Bjarnason
Center for Clinical and Basic Research
Ballerup Byjev 222
DK-2750 Ballerup
Denmark

Henry Bone
Michigan Bone and Mineral Clinic PC
22201 Moross Road, Suite 260
Detroit
MI 48236
USA

Peter Burckhardt
Department de Medicin Interne
CHUV
CH-1011 Lausanne
Switzerland

Juliet Compston
University of Cambridge
Department of Medicine
Box 157
Addenbrooke's Hospital
Hills Road
Cambridge CB2 2QQ
UK

Tim Cundy
Department of Medicine
University of Auckland
Private Bag 92019
Auckland
New Zealand

Michael Davies
Department of Medicine
Manchester Royal Infirmary
Manchester
M13 9WL
UK

Roger Francis
MSU Department
Freeman Hospital
High Heaton
Newcastle-upon-Tyne
NE7 7DN
UK

David Hosking
Division of Mineral Metabolism
Nottingham City Hospital
Hucknall Road
Nottingham NG5 1PB
UK

Badri Lamichhane
Medizin. Univ. Klinik
Abt. Nephrologie
Bergheimer Strasse 58
D69115 Heidelberg
Germany

Cornelle Parker
Division of Mineral Metabolism
Nottingham City Hospital
Hucknall Road
Nottingham NG5 1PB
UK

Pernille Ravn
Center for Clinical and Basic Research
Ballerup Byjev 222
DK-2750 Ballerup
Denmark

Ian Reid
Department of Medicine
University of Auckland
Private Bag 92019
Auckland
New Zealand

Johann Ringe
Leitender Arzt der Med. Klinik 4
Klinikum Leverkusen
Akademisches Lehrkrankenhaus der
Universität zu Köln
Dhunnberg 60
D 51375 Leverkusen
Germany

Eberhard Ritz
Medizin. Univ. Klinik
Abt. Nephrologie
Bergheimer Strasse 58
D 69115 Heidelberg
Germany

Michael Schömig
Medizin. Univ. Klinik
Abt. Nephrologie
Bergheimer Strasse 58
D69115 Heidelberg
Germany

Nicholas Shaw
The Birmingham Children's Hospital
Steelhouse Lane
Birmingham B4 6NH
UK

Roger Smith
Nuffield Orthopaedic Centre
Windmill Road
Headington
Oxford
OX3 7LD
UK

Reinhardt Ziegler
Medizin. Univ. Klinik
Med. Klinik 1
Bergheimer Strasse 58
D 69115 Heidelberg
Germany

Preface

The skeleton has a limited potential to show pathological change, and abnormality is generally detected through biochemical alterations in calcium homeostasis or bone turnover, reflected by characteristic radiographic features. For most clinicians who see patients with metabolic bone disease the problem is not usually one of diagnosis, but one of choice of the most appropriate and effective treatment. This is particularly so because metabolic bone disease often presents to general physicians, endocrinologists or rheumatologists who may not have extensive experience in this field. This problem is compounded because many textbooks often deal in detail with pathogenesis, clinical features and diagnosis, but fairly briefly with treatment.

We feel there is a need for a different approach, which starts from the premise that the diagnosis is known and what the reader needs is an authoritative account of the practical aspects of management. This should be broadly based to cover those clinical features or investigations that are needed to monitor the effects of treatment as well as all aspects of drug therapy. In order to achieve this aim, we have invited our friends and colleagues who have a particular interest in metabolic bone disease to write a chapter in a field of their particular expertise. The requirement was that this should provide all the necessary information to treat the majority of patients effectively and safely; drug treatments should be described in terms of their action on the skeleton, the methods of monitoring their effectiveness, the identification of adverse events and their beneficial clinical end-points.

The book is divided into two sections. The first covers the common types of metabolic bone disease – osteomalacia, hypoparathyroidism, primary hyperparathyroidism, malignancy, Paget's disease, renal osteodystrophy and post-transplant bone disease. Each chapter is self-contained and is set out with major headings for easier reference.

The second section covers the topic of osteoporosis. Primary prevention is considered separately from treatment of the established condition, followed by a detailed review of the drugs available for treating all types of osteoporosis. Secondary osteoporosis is then considered and includes glucocorticoid-induced osteoporosis and separate chapters on osteoporosis in men and children. The final chapter describes the management of osteogenesis imperfecta and other types of inherited bone disease; although rare, these conditions present sufficiently often for physicians to need to have a general idea of management.

As editors, we have tried to maintain consistency of style in each chapter, but have also tried to avoid being proscriptive. All our chosen authors have extensive experience in their field, and we wanted this to be apparent in their contributions. This often means that different approaches to similar problems are offered, particularly in the management of osteoporosis.

This is important because it illustrates that often there is a range of treatment options that are equally valid.

We hope that this book will be of value to everyone who treats patients with metabolic bone disease. It is particularly aimed at the non-specialist who we hope will find the contributions helpful and will become confident in managing these conditions. If they come to share our enthusiasm and pleasure at effectively treating patients with metabolic bone disease, then this will have been an added bonus.

David Hosking
Johann Ringe

1

Treatment of Osteomalacia

Michael Davies

The physiology of vitamin D and the parathyroid glands • Vitamin D deficiency • Intestinal malabsorption • Post-gastrectomy osteomalacia • Coeliac disease • Pancreatic disease • Chronic liver disease • Drug-induced osteomalacia • Vitamin D dependency • Hypophosphataemic osteomalacia • Pharmacology of vitamin D and its metabolites • 25-hydroxyvitamin D_3 • Calcitriol • 1-hydroxycholecalciferol (alphacalcidol)

Osteomalacia is not a diagnosis, but a state of the skeleton arising from a disorder in the physiological process of bone turnover in which the mineralization phase of remodelling is impaired. There is a variety of conditions that may ultimately produce osteomalacia, but the majority arise as a result of disturbances to the supply and metabolism of vitamin D or from disturbances of phosphorus metabolism. The successful treatment of osteomalacia is achieved by delineating the aetiology and instituting appropriate treatment. Because the majority of cases of osteomalacia arise from derangement of vitamin D metabolism it is necessary to have at least a working knowledge of the physiology of vitamin D and parathyroid hormone.

THE PHYSIOLOGY OF VITAMIN D AND THE PARATHYROID GLANDS

Two sources of vitamin D are available to humans. The most important and only true physiological source is the production of vitamin D_3 in the skin by the photochemical conversion of its provitamin, 7-dehydrocholesterol.

In temperate climates this conversion can only occur during summer sunlight exposure and is impeded by clothing and glass. Dietary vitamin D is of secondary importance and, in the UK, the supply of vitamin D in the diet is insufficient to protect against vitamin D deficiency in the absence of solar exposure.[1]

Both vitamin D_3 (cholecalciferol) and vitamin D_2 (ergocalciferol) are present in small amounts in the diet. Although there are minor differences in the further metabolism of these sterols, these differences are of no importance clinically. The term calciferol(s) will be used to denote vitamin D_2 or vitamin D_3 where specification is not necessary.

Both endogenously produced vitamin D_3 and diet-derived calciferols undergo metabolism in the body before acquiring biological activity. Both sources of vitamin D undergo hydroxylation in the liver to 25-hydroxyvitamin D (25(OH)D), and this is the main circulating storage metabolite of vitamin D, showing seasonal changes that reflect summer solar exposure.[2]

A proportion of 25(OH)D is next converted in the kidney to the active metabolite of vitamin D, 1,25 dihydroxyvitamin D (calcitriol or ergocalcitriol, depending upon the source of the precursor). This renal metabolic step is tightly regulated, being enhanced by the presence of parathyroid hormone (PTH), hypocalcaemia and hypophosphataemia, and suppressed by hypercalcaemia, hyperphosphataemia and impaired renal function. The hepatic hydroxylation is not under strict control, so that supraphysiological amounts of 25(OH)D can occur in subjects chronically dosed with large oral doses of vitamin D, as one sees with the daily use of strong calciferol (1.25 mg) in the management of hypoparathyroidism and other vitamin D-resistant states.

It is important to recognize that derangements of these metabolic pathways are rare and negligible when compared with inadequate supplies of vitamin D itself; the sole exception to this is the decline in renal 1-hydroxylase activity that accompanies renal insufficiency. The vitamin D endocrine system is inherently inefficient, with about 70% of calciferol and 25(OH)D normally being converted to metabolically inactive and more polar metabolites that are excreted in the bile and faeces.[3] As a result less than 10% of vitamin D produced daily is converted to calcitriol.

During states of vitamin D insufficiency more vitamin D is converted into active metabolites, especially if there is a degree of secondary hyperparathyroidism. In states of calcium deficiency (low calcium intake or malabsorption), which lead to secondary hyperparathyroidism and an increase in the circulating concentration of calcitriol, the serum half life of 25(OH)D is reduced, and thus the requirement for native precursor vitamin D is increased.[4] The mechanism surrounding this phenomenon is not understood, but may involve accelerated catabolism of 25(OH)D by the liver.[5]

PTH maintains a normal plasma concentration of ionized calcium, and any change in the latter leads to reciprocal changes in hormone secretion, increasing renal 1-hydroxylase activity, bone turnover and osteoclasis, and the renal excretion of phosphate during times of calcium insufficiency.

Most conditions leading to osteomalacia will be due to vitamin D deficiency and will be accompanied by a degree of secondary hyperparathyroidism, with an increase in serum PTH. Occasionally, particularly in adolescents, the PTH response to vitamin D deficiency is blunted, and the biochemistry may resemble that of hypoparathyroidism.[6]

VITAMIN D DEFICIENCY

Vitamin D deficiency and osteomalacia are associated with a variety of clinical disorders, which are presented in Table 1.1.

The term nutritional or privational osteomalacia should be reserved for patients in whom there is no underlying disorder of intestinal, pancreatic, hepatic or renal function, no evidence of primary hyperparathyroidism, and no history of drug therapy known to affect calcium or vitamin D metabolism. A diagnosis of nutritional osteomalacia is therefore made by the exclusion of other associated abnormalities. Nutritional osteomalacia is extremely uncommon in the white UK population, being virtually confined to elderly and infirm subjects. It is however relatively common in the Asian population, and results from a suboptimal supply of vitamin D from diet and solar exposure; it is cured using small doses of vitamin D daily. In a recent review Dunnigan et al. present a very

Table 1.1 Associations between vitamin D deficiency and osteomalacia.
Asian immigrants
Vegetarian lifestyle
Elderly and infirm
Partial gastrectomy
Intestinal malabsorption
Chronic cholestatic liver disease
Alcoholic liver disease
Anticonvulsant medication
Primary hyperparathyroidism
Chronic renal insufficiency

strong case for a vegetarian diet as being a strong risk factor for the development of nutritional osteomalacia in Asians.[7] Dietary phytate, long known to be an anticalcifying agent, was at most only a weak risk factor for vitamin D deficiency in these subjects. Since many of these Asians were lactovegetarians, calcium insufficiency did not appear to be a risk factor.[7] Subjects suffering from nutritional osteomalacia need lifelong supplementation with additional vitamin D to cure the osteomalacia and prevent recurrence. Unless lifestyle and diet can be altered vitamin D deficiency will recur if supplementation is withdrawn. The osteomalacic component may not improve clinically until several weeks have elapsed from the start of treatment, and the bone disease may take many months to heal histologically. There is no place for the use of vitamin D metabolites in this clinical situation. The use of vitamin D itself permits its further metabolism according to the needs of the body for calcitriol. Because of the background secondary hyperparathyroidism that accompanies this type of osteomalacia, supraphysiological amounts of calcitrol are produced[8] and continue to be formed until the secondary hyperparathyroidism becomes suppressed as the bone disease heals. Thereafter vitamin D metabolism returns to the normal state, with small amounts of calcitriol being formed as necessary to maintain normal calcium homeostasis. Small doses of one alpha or calcitriol (1 mcg / day) do not achieve supranormal serum concentrations of calcitriol, delay the healing process unnecessarily and, if used in larger amounts beyond the phase of healing of the osteomalacia, may produce hypercalcaemia. Finally, the cost of native vitamin D is significantly less than that of vitamin D analogues.

Vitamin D in a dose of 400–800 IU/day orally will heal nutritional osteomalacia and prevent its recurrence. If there is a problem with compliance periodic dosing with much larger oral doses will achieve the same result. There is no need to use parenteral vitamin D in this situation. A single dose of 15 mg (600 000 IU) is effective and produces favourable changes in plasma biochemistry and evidence of radiological healing of rickets within 2 weeks of dosing.[9] Such treatment, while curative of the bone disease, should be followed by maintenance treatment of 400–800 IU/day or by further single doses (up to 300 000 IU) every 6–12 months. In the elderly, oral calciferol 100 000 units every 6 months keeps the serum 25(OH)D concentration above the level recommended to protect against osteomalacia,[10] but this may not be sufficient to protect against secondary hyperparathyroidism seen in the elderly. If one can ensure compliance with treatment there is no need for regular biochemical or radiological monitoring. Evidence for radiological healing of rickets should be sought 4–6 weeks after starting treatment and Looser's zones, if present, should be healing by 3 months.

Changes in serum biochemistry occur much sooner, with a rise in serum phosphate and a fall in serum PTH. Sometimes there is a paradoxical rise in serum alkaline phosphatase as the earliest sign of response to treatment, occurring within days of instituting vitamin D.

Although there is no need for additional calcium supplements, patients who have a habitual low intake of calcium (< 0.5 g/day) would benefit from a 500–1000 mg calcium supplement to facilitate bone healing. In patients with symptomatic hypocalcaemia, which is most likely to occur in adolescents,[6] calcium supplementation is mandatory.

Occasionally a patient with a normal serum calcium concentration at diagnosis becomes overtly hypercalcaemic on vitamin D treatment (Figure 1.1). Provided treatment has been initiated as outlined above this represents primary hyperparathyroidism masked by vitamin D deficiency. The hypercalcaemia occurs within a few weeks of starting treatment with vitamin D. Such patients should continue treatment with vitamin D until their bone disease has healed, i.e. until the serum alkaline phosphatase has returned to normal. Once the clinical and biochemical signs of bone disease have resolved, parathyroidectomy can be performed if it is considered appropriate clinically. It is exceptional for such patients to develop severe symptomatic hypercalcaemia; the norm is for the biochemistry to deteriorate (worsening hypercalcaemia), while the patient's clinical state (bone pain, muscle weakness) improves.

In summary, nutritional osteomalacia can be managed by daily doses of vitamin D (400–800 IU/day), with additional calcium supplements if necessary, or by giving large oral doses intermittently (200 000–600 000 IU every 3–6 months) in cases where compliance may be a problem. Unless lifestyle (diet and solar exposure) is modified the regimes described above will be required for life to prevent recurrence. Biochemical monitoring is not mandatory, but repeat measurement of serum calcium phosphate and alkaline phosphatase may be performed 2 weeks, 12 weeks and 26 weeks after starting treatment to confirm correction of the bone disease and thus compliance with treatment. In difficult cases, which can only mean poor compliance, measurements of serum 25(OH)D, calcitriol and PTH can be undertaken, and these will show no change, despite the patient apparently taking treatment. In such situations I give the patient 200 000 IU vitamin D orally, in my presence, monthly, for 3 months, to everyone's benefit.

INTESTINAL MALABSORPTION

Osteomalacia in patients with disturbed function of the liver, intestine or pancreas is due to vitamin D deficiency, correction of which results in cure of the osteomalacia. Osteoporosis is a more common and more difficult bone problem to manage in patients with gut disease. Minor aberrations of 25(OH)D synthesis may occur in chronic alcoholic liver disease,[11] but osteomalacia is cured by providing the native vitamin in adequate amounts. Steatorrhoea results in varying degrees of malabsorption of vitamin D[12] (Figure 1.2). The major factor producing vitamin D deficiency is the increased catabolism of 25(OH)D due to secondary hyperparathyroidism induced by calcium malabsorption.[4,13,14] This phenomenon has even been observed in patients with partial gastrectomy, when there may be no evidence of fat malabsorption.[14] An earlier claim that 25(OH)D and perhaps other vitamin D metabo-

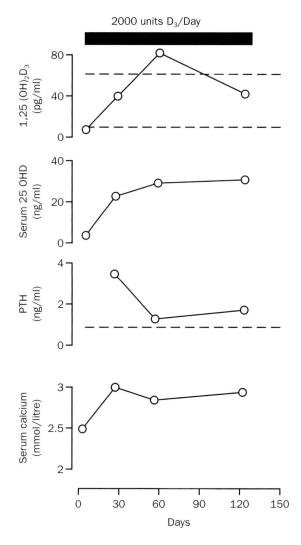

Figure 1.1 Hypercalcaemic primary hyperparathyroidism produced from correcting an underlying vitamin D deficiency. Note: serum 25(OHD) becomes stable at 20–30 ng/ml.

lites undergo a conservative enterohepatic circulation[15] has been reassessed and found to be wanting.[16] In patients with biliary obstruction water-soluble vitamin D metabolites appear in large amounts in the urine,[17] but it is doubtful if this represents a loss of 'vitamin D' from the body, as these metabolites would normally appear in the gut and be excreted in the faeces.

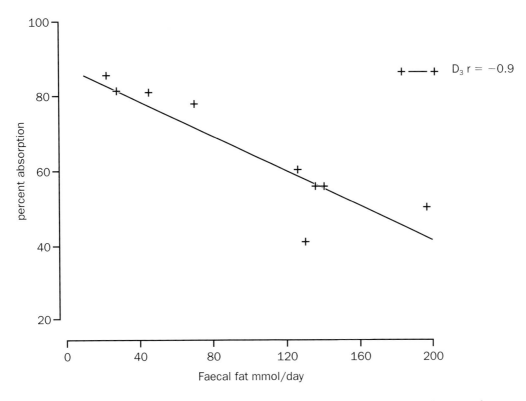

Figure 1.2 Percentage absorption of vitamin D (1000 IU) given to patients with varying degrees of steatorrhoea.

The sole manifestation of coeliac disease may be osteomalacia, so that white subjects with vitamin D deficiency and no obvious cause should be screened for gluten enteropathy by the measurement of endomyseal antibodies. Because coeliac disease affects primarily the duodenum and jejunum, malabsorption of calcium and vitamin D is common in this condition.[18,19]

Pancreatic insufficiency is not normally associated with osteomalacia unless it is complicated by other conditions such as cystic fibrosis or alcoholism.

Management of osteomalacia accompanying intestinal malabsorption is similar to that of nutritional osteomalacia, using either small daily doses of the native vitamin, larger doses given daily or at intervals, or parenteral vitamin D. The main difficulty in managing bone disease in this heterogeneous group of conditions is knowing whether vitamin D is being absorbed sufficiently to achieve cure of osteomalacia or whether the dose of vitamin D being used is likely to prove toxic in the medium to long term. As a result, biochemical monitoring is much more important and useful than in the management of uncomplicated nutritional osteomalacia.

POST-GASTRECTOMY OSTEOMALACIA

This responds to physiological amounts of vitamin D unless there is an accompanying steatorrhoea. In the absence of fat malabsorption it should be managed as outlined in the section on nutritional osteomalacia. The aetiology of post-gastrectomy osteomalacia appears to be related to increased catabolism of 25(OH)D.[14] Additional calcium supplementation should be given to suppress any tendency to continuing secondary hyperparathyroidism because of presumed calcium malabsorption once the osteomalacia has healed. It is, therefore, important to measure serum PTH in addition to routine biochemistry once the bone disease has healed and to titrate the dose of calcium supplementation to achieve normal concentrations of serum PTH. Vitamin D supplements (400–800 IU/day) should be continued indefinitely as this will guarantee freedom from recurrence of osteomalacia, even if it is not possible fully to suppress background secondary hyperparathyroidism.

Where post-gastrectomy steatorrhoea is present and concomitant coeliac disease has been excluded, larger doses of vitamin D will be necessary. Initially, 50 000 IU daily as strong calciferol can be used orally, and the response can be assessed biochemically by measuring alkaline phosphatase activity, PTH and serum 25(OH)D. These parameters can be measured on initiation of treatment and at one month. It is most unlikely that this dose of vitamin D will be ineffective; but if at one month the serum 25(OH)D is less than 10 ng/ml then the dose should be doubled to 100 000 IU (2.5 mg/day). It is however much more unlikely that the serum 25(OH)D will be above 10 ng/ml, and one should repeat this measurement monthly to ensure that the serum 25(OH)D is not continuing to rise.

If the first or any subsequent value is in excess of 80 ng/ml the dose of vitamin D will need to be reduced to 50 000 units on alternate days or once per week. The dose should be adjusted to ensure a serum 25(OH)D between 20 and 40 ng/ml but not getting perturbed at any stable level of 25(OH)D between 40 and 80 ng/ml. Once patients have been cured of their bone disease, a holiday at more southerly latitudes will increase the cutaneous synthesis of vitamin D. An increase in serum 25(OH)D following such a holiday does not demand a reduction in vitamin D dose. Calcium supplementation will also be necessary to facilitate bone healing and to protect against background secondary hyperparathyroidism. An alternative to larger oral doses of vitamin D would be to give 100 000 IU of the vitamin every month by intramuscular injection. It is important not to give injections subcutaneously, as most of the administered vitamin D would then stay in the fat. It is almost impossible to poison patients with parenteral vitamin D: a single injection of 100 000 IU vitamin D might increase serum 25(OH)D by up to 10 ng/ml in 2–3 months, but the effects show individual variability.[20] Once the patient is stable then the injections can be reduced to 100 000 IU every 2 months, reverting to monthly dosing if serum 25(OH)D concentrations fall below 15–20 ng/ml.

In subjects with steatorrhoea, calcidiol (25-hydroxyvitamin D_3) has been shown to be absorbed better than vitamin D itself.[12] It is an alternative to oral vitamin D. The dose should be adjusted to achieve 25(OH)D values of 20–40 ng/ml. A preparation is available in the US, but not in the UK, but has no major clinical benefits over native vitamin D.

COELIAC DISEASE

The provision of a gluten-free diet alone will eventually cure any associated osteomalacia as the gut morphology and physiology return to normal. Additional calcium and vitamin D should be given to hasten the healing process. Initially, because of the possibility of malabsorption of vitamin D, larger oral doses can be given: 50 000 units daily for one month should be sufficient to achieve healing of the bone disease. Continuing beyond this time in a patient adhering to gluten exclusion will make vitamin D intoxication a distinct possibility, because absorption of the vitamin will be normal and catabolism will be reduced. The safest policy is to start using smaller doses after the first month (400–800 IU/day), maintaining this until the biochemistry has returned to normal. There is no need to monitor serum 25(OH)D, but checking endomyseal antibodies will reveal any covert ingestion of gluten. As with post-gastrectomy syndromes, calcium supplementation facilitates bone healing and will suppress any continuing secondary hyperparathyroidism in those patients who do not adhere strictly to a gluten-free diet. Regular measurements of PTH should be taken to ensure that calcium supplementation is adequate. A number of treated coeliac patients show evidence of continuing secondary hyperparathyroidism,[21] presumably from calcium malabsorption, which can be helped by additional calcium supplements. Since many patients with coeliac disease have a reduced bone mass compared with age-matched controls, supplementation with 1 g calcium and 800 IU vitamin D per day will aid bone health, prevent vitamin D deficiency, compensate for any tendency to malabsorb calcium and suppress secondary hyperparathyroidism.

PANCREATIC DISEASE

Osteomalacia is rare in patients with pancreatic disease. It will respond to oral vitamin D and, if steatorrhoea is controlled by pancreatic extracts, no more than 400–800 IU/day will be necessary. If, however, steatorrhoea remains a problem, larger oral doses may be necessary. Serum 25(OH)D levels should be monitored monthly if daily doses in excess of 10 000 IU/day (0.25 mg) are used. An alternative means of giving the vitamin without requiring biochemical monitoring is to resort to monthly doses of vitamin D 100 000 IU by intramuscular injection.

CHRONIC LIVER DISEASE

Primary biliary cirrhosis may be complicated by osteomalacia, although osteoporosis is much more common. The use of bile sequestrants for itching contributes to malabsorption of vitamin D, the metabolism of which is normal. Osteomalacia responds to vitamin D, the only problem being the propensity to malabsorb vitamin D as jaundice increases. Thus an oral dose of vitamin that was adequate to maintain normal vitamin D nutrition may be insufficient as the disease progresses, jaundice deepens and fat absorption deteriorates. Although there have been reports that hepatic osteomalacia is resistant to vitamin D, the consensus of opinion is that it responds to either oral or parenteral vitamin D. The oral dose requires adjustment to compensate for malabsorption. Prevention of

osteomalacia can be achieved by oral doses of vitamin D or parenteral administration. Measurement of serum 25(OH)D is necessary to monitor response to oral vitamin D in this situation. Vitamin D delivered in tablet or capsules is less well absorbed than vitamin D in a solution with alcohol.

In practical terms, once the patient is jaundiced oral vitamin D should be tried in a dose of 10 000 IU per day, and if the serum 25(OH)D does not rise towards 20 ng/ml the dose should be doubled each month until the serum 25(OH)D becomes 20–40 ng/ml. Once stability is achieved serum 25(OH)D will need measuring every 3 months and, as jaundice progresses, the dose of vitamin D may have to be increased. Alternatively, monthly or 3-monthly injections of 100 000–300 000 IU of vitamin can be used and the response can be assessed by measuring serum 25(OH)D. As mentioned previously, the peak 25(OH)D response from a single intramuscular injection of vitamin D may take 2–3 months to develop.[20]

Osteomalacia arising in other forms of cholestatic liver disease and alcoholic liver disease can be managed in the same way. All patients with steatorrhoea will malabsorb dietary calcium to a greater or lesser extent and should, therefore, receive additional calcium supplements of 1–2 g/day, depending upon the degree of steatorrhea. A good guide as to the adequacy of any supplement is the absence of secondary hyperparathyroidism manifested by a normal serum PTH concentration.

DRUG-INDUCED OSTEOMALACIA

There is an association between the use of anticonvulsants and osteomalacia, especially with the use of phenytoin and phenobarbitone, which induce liver enzymes and increase the metabolism and clearance of vitamin D.[22] Additionally, these drugs reduce calcium absorption but well-nourished patients with adequate solar exposure avoid osteomalacia. Patients with anticonvulsant-associated osteomalacia respond adequately to additional vitamin D, but occasionally require up to

4000 IU/day. Treatment should be continued, as relapse is likely once vitamin D treatment is withdrawn, unless medication is changed to non-enzyme inducing anticonvulsants, such as sodium valproate. Correction of osteomalacia will be achieved using doses of vitamin D ranging from 800 to 4000 units/day.[23] Improvement in plasma biochemistry will be apparent within a few weeks of initiating treatment. The dose of vitamin D can be increased every 4–6 weeks until a response is seen, with a rise in calcium and phosphate and a fall in PTH and alkaline phosphatase. A dose in excess of 4000 IU/day should not be necessary, and so intoxication with these doses is most unlikely.

Rifampicin may also accelerate vitamin D catabolism, but its use is short-lived (up to 9 months) and unlikely to produce symptomatic osteomalacia. However, since TB is commoner in those racial groups prone to vitamin D deficiency one needs to be attentive to the possible precipitation of clinical bone disease in these circumstances. Fortunately, the bone disease that arises from a mixture of nutritional vitamin D deficiency and enzyme induction responds to treatment along the lines already discussed in the section on nutritional osteomalacia.

Aluminium hydroxide can lead to hypophosphataemic osteomalacia by binding phosphate in the gut. The urine is virtually free from phosphorus, and there is hypercalciuria. The bone disease heals on withdrawing the aluminium-containing antacid.

Etidronate if used for periods in excess of 3–6 months at a dose of 20 mg/kg can lead to an osteomalacic syndrome. When treatment is withdrawn the process of healing begins, and may be helped by supplemental calcium and vitamin D. Unlike what happens in other forms of osteomalacia, the serum phosphate concentration is elevated owing to changes in the tubular reabsorption of phosphorus.

VITAMIN D DEPENDENCY

Vitamin D dependency type I, also known as vitamin D pseudodeficiency, is inherited as an autosomal recessive condition resulting from mutations in the gene for the 1-hydroxylase enzyme.[24] As a result, the kidney cannot synthesize calcitriol appropriately and children present with rickets in infancy with serum biochemistry compatible with nutritional rickets. However, if measured, serum 25(OH)D concentrations are normal and serum calcitriol levels are subnormal and remain so despite treatment with conventional doses of vitamin D. Serum biochemistry is unaffected by this treatment. Large oral doses of vitamin D (20 000–40 000 IU daily) produce healing of the rickets and correction of the abnormal biochemistry but it is easier to use physiological doses of calcitriol. Initially, the dose of calcitriol can be 1–3 mcg/day until rickets is healed, with a maintenance dose of 0.25–1.0 mcg/day depending upon the age of the child. Adults require 0.5–1.0 mcg/day. Cessation of treatment is followed by early biochemical relapse, of which an increase in serum PTH is the earliest sign. Patients in receipt of treatment require regular biochemical monitoring, at least every 3 months. This involves assessing adequacy of treatment by measuring serum PTH, ensuring a normal serum creatinine, maintaining the urinary calcium/creatinine ratio below 1.0 mmol/mmol and performing renal ultrasound perhaps annually, to ensure that there is no nephrocalcinosis. Over-treatment can produce hypercalciuria, hypercalcaemia with renal damage.[25] During the initial stages of treatment, when there is active rickets, calcium supplements in addition to calcitriol, can be given to ensure a total intake of calcium of around 1 g. The amount of supplementary calcium should be reduced to avoid hypercalciuria as the healing of the bone disease progresses and the urinary calcium/creatinine ratio approaches 1.0 mmol/mmol.

Type II vitamin D-dependent rickets, also known as hereditary 1,25 dihydroxyvitamin D-resistant rickets, is a rare genetic disorder resulting from defects in the gene for the vitamin D receptor.[26] Early-onset rickets is the hallmark of the disease, with biochemistry similar to that of nutritional vitamin D deficiency. Additionally, many affected children have hair loss, some with alopecia totalis. If measured, serum levels of calcitriol are increased, and the rickets is resistant to pharmacological doses of calcitriol, up to 20 mcg daily being necessary to heal the bone disease.[27] Patients with alopecia totalis appear more resistant to calcitriol than others, and the use of large oral doses of calcium (up to 4 g/day) or daily intravenous infusions of calcium is of benefit.[28,29] It has to be emphasized that this condition is exceedingly rare and that treatment with calcitriol and calcium supplements demands close biochemical and radiological monitoring.

HYPOPHOSPHATAEMIC OSTEOMALACIA

This results from either a genetically determined or an acquired renal tubular defect, resulting in phosphate wasting coupled with disturbances of the renal production of calcitriol. The commoner form is the genetically determined X-linked vitamin D-resistant hypophosphataemic rickets and osteomalacia (XLH).

X-linked hypophosphataemic osteomalacia

Children present with rickets in infancy, but myopathy is not a feature of the disease. Occasionally adults may present with osteomalacia or the extraosseous manifestation of the disease without a past history of rickets. Although the disease is inherited as an X-linked dominant condition spontaneous mutations do occur, so that children may have unaffected parents.

Management of this form of rickets and osteomalacia is difficult because it is almost impossible to restore the skeleton to normal. In children, deformity of the legs will correct with growth and treatment with vitamin D and phosphate supplements. Occasionally epiphyseal stapling may be necessary to aid straightening of the limb. After growth has ceased and the epiphyses have fused, corrective osteotomies may be necessary. In addition to osteomalacia with its attendant bone pains and propensity to fracture the clinician may have to manage adult patients who become increas-

ingly incapacitated by the extraosseous complications of the disease.[30]

The aim of treatment is to maintain the level of serum phosphate close to normal for the greater part of the day. This involves the use of phosphate supplements (up to 1–4 g of elemental phosphorus) given orally in four to six divided doses. The medication is unpleasant and prone to produce flatulent diarrhoea, with its attendant embarrassment. As a result compliance is poor in both children and adults. Within a few hours of the administration of a dose of phosphate supplement the serum phosphate concentration will return to its subnormal value. Phosphate supplements alone can improve the radiographic appearance of XLH, but induce secondary hyperparathyroidism because of small reductions in serum calcium that follow phosphate loading. The tendency to secondary hyperparathyroidism is exacerbated by reduced responsiveness of the renal 1-hydroxylase to PTH. This has been shown by a smaller increase in serum calcitriol compared to normal controls following infusion of exogenous PTH.[31] The management is therefore to provide phosphate supplements to facilitate mineralization and sufficient vitamin D to promote calcium absorption and prevent secondary hyperparathyroidism. In children the dose of native vitamin varies from 20 000 to 100 000 IU/day; adults require 50 000 to 100 000 IU per day. Calcitriol or 1α-hydroxyvitamin D_3 are the favoured means of delivering vitamin D.

There are theoretical grounds for believing that outcomes may be improved. No double-blind cross-over studies have been performed to show superiority of calcitriol compared to pharmacologic doses of vitamin D. If intoxication occurs it is less prolonged using vitamin D analogues. Both regimens can, however, result in overdosage and hypercalcaemia, so that patients and parents of children should be warned about this complication, the symptoms that occur, and the need to stop medication and seek immediate medical help. Patients need biochemical assessment at least every three months, and sometimes more frequently if the clinical situation is unstable. In children calcitriol 30 ng/kg/day and phosphate supplements 1–2 g/day in divided doses should be given and evidence for the healing of rickets should be sought by serial radiography every 3–6 months. The dose of calcitriol should be increased if the child shows no response and up to 70 ng/kg/day of calcitriol may be required. Following each adjustment to dose, the serum biochemistry must be checked and a fasting urine sample taken for the calcium/creatinine ratio so that treatment can be reduced if hypercalciuria develops.[32] Nephrocalcinosis has been reported in subjects treated as outlined above,[33] and this has been shown to be due to depositioned calcium phosphate. The amount of calcitriol will need to be increased during the adolescent growth spurt, and sometimes deformity increases at this stage. It is difficult to predict the exact dose of calcitriol, but it should be increased by about 25% initially, monitoring the urine for hypercalciuria and serum biochemistry for calcium phosphate and creatinine. If osteotomies are required treatment should be stopped during periods of bed rest, since this results in a reduction in bone formation and accelerated bone resorption. Such changes are conducive to hypercalcaemia if treatment is continued. Once the patient is ambulant on crutches treatment is reintroduced. Not all children respond to medical treatment with improvements in growth velocity and for this reason growth hormone has been tried. The addition of human growth hormone 0.6 IU/kg/week to standard therapy had a positive effect on growth.[34]

In addition to routine serum and urine biochemical monitoring, serum PTH should be measured periodically, perhaps every six months. This is because phosphate therapy may induce secondary hyperparathyroidism. If the amount of vitamin D, 1α-hydroxyvitamin D or calcitriol is insufficient to counteract the hypocalcaemic effect of phosphate therapy, PTH values will rise and the parathyroid cell mass will increase. If this remains unchecked, there is the possibility that with parathyroid cell proliferation an alteration in either the PTH set point or the cell cycle or both will occur, resulting in a monoclonal proliferation of cells.[35] Even without treatment, there is some evidence

to suggest that secondary hyperparathyroidism may be inherent in XLH.[36] If PTH values begin to increase, phosphate treatment should be reduced or the dose of vitamin D or its analogue increased. Whenever the dose of vitamin D or its analogue is increased biochemical assessment needs to be performed more frequently (e.g. monthly) until one can be certain that toxic effects are being avoided and the desired effects upon PTH are being achieved.

If PTH exceeds the upper limit of normal all treatment should be stopped to see if the serum calcium remains normal. Phosphate supplements may suppress hypercalcaemia and, upon withdrawal, overt hypercalcaemia may result. This indicates tertiary hyperparathyroidism – i.e. monoclonal proliferation of parathyroid cells producing an adenoma against a background of secondary hyperparathyroidism. Such patients may require parathyroidectomy.

It is sometimes possible to discontinue medical treatment at skeletal maturity. Some adults relapse with bone pains from pseudofractures, which will however heal with the use of phosphate supplements 1–3 g/day and calcitriol 1–2 mcg/day. Biochemistry is monitored in the same way as in children but compliance with phosphate therapy is a major problem. If the patient and the physician are determined to persist with management even the most resistant pseudofractures will heal.

A common finding in adults over 40 years of age is a progressive stiffness in the back and major joints as a result of calcification at tendinous and ligamentous insertions into bone. This problem is progressive, unrelated to treatment, and a cause of considerable disability. As a result, adaptations to the home may be necessary, including the lowering of light switches and sinks and modifying toilets and bathrooms to allow patients to maintain personal hygiene.

Calcification and ossification of the ligamentum flavum can lead to spinal canal stenosis, and may cause neurological syndromes from nerve root involvement or spinal cord compression.[37] If patients also experience cochlear dysfunction[38] an erroneous diagnosis of demyelinating disease may be made.[37] At around the age of 40 all patients need to be assessed for evidence of spinal stenosis and, if this is present, followed to ensure that there are no symptoms or signs of developing cord compression. Decompressive laminectomy by an experienced neurosurgeon can prevent paralysis in affected individuals but the surgeon needs to understand the likelihood of abnormal bone formation with distorted anatomy before surgery. Patients who develop 'Ménières'-type illness can be treated conventionally with drugs such as betahistine to suppress labyrinthine dysfunction.

Acquired hypophosphataemic osteomalacia

Over 100 patients with acquired hypophosphataemic osteomalacia have been reported in whom a tumour has been implicated.[39] Removal of benign tumours, commonly mesenchymal in origin, results in cure of the condition. Malignant tumours include prostate cancer and mesenchymal sarcomas such as fibrosarcoma. Hypophosphataemic osteomalacia is also seen in neurofibromatosis and fibrous dysplasia. The aetiology is thought to be humoral factor(s) that produce a renal phosphate leak and inhibition of renal 1-hydroxylase. Experimental evidence exists to support this conclusion[40,41] but the nature of the factor(s) is unknown. Some of the benign mesenchymal tumours may be quite small. They may not be identified in some patients with acquired hypophosphataemic osteomalacia despite exhaustive searches, and the patients labelled idiopathic. In addition to bone pains these patients are profoundly myopathic, by contrast with XLH. Radiographs appear osteopenic, and Looser's zones can be hard to find. Isotope bone scans can be helpful in delineating pseudofractures through cortical bone, especially in ribs and the pelvis.

PTH values are normal, as are the serum concentrations of calcium and 25(OH)D. Hypophosphataemia and low calcitriol levels confirm the diagnosis. Serum alkaline phosphatase is usually increased, but may be normal.

If a tumour can be found and resected this disease is self-limiting. If no tumour is found, or resection is not possible, treatment with calcitriol and phosphate supplements can achieve improvement in the myopathy and osteomalacia. Some patients can be made asymptomatic and maintain a good quality of life on these two medications.

Regular monitoring of biochemistry (every 3 months) ensures compliance and safety. In a personal experience of three cases where no tumour was found the bone disease was healed clinically and radiologically using calcitriol 1 mcg/day and phosphate supplements 1–2 g/day (Figure 1.3).

The healing process can be expedited by using larger doses of calcitriol initially – up to 5 mcg/day to achieve supraphysiological concentrations of calcitriol such as one sees in the healing phase of nutritional osteomalacia. As the serum alkaline phosphatase falls to normal it is prudent to reduce the dose of calcitriol to 1–2 mcg/day. If the osteomalacia is accompanied by a normal alkaline phosphatase it is better to monitor the response to 1 mcg doses of calcitriol initially, only increasing the dose if there is no clinical improvement. Long-term monitoring is necessary, measuring serum PTH to ensure that there is no evidence of developing hyperparathyroidism. Tertiary hyperparathyroidism requiring parathyroidectomy may develop[42] if too much phosphate or too little calcitriol is used in management; hence the need for regular follow-up, including PTH measurements. In those cases deemed to be idiopathic careful re-examination for small tumours should be undertaken; but where a patient is easily managed medically, exhaustive reinvestigations looking for small benign lesions are not necessary.

PHARMACOLOGY OF VITAMIN D AND ITS METABOLITES

Vitamin D_2 is the most commonly used preparation of vitamin D; but vitamin D_3 is also used therapeutically and there is some evidence that their biological activities differ. Both are effective in clinical use, but they do have different meta-

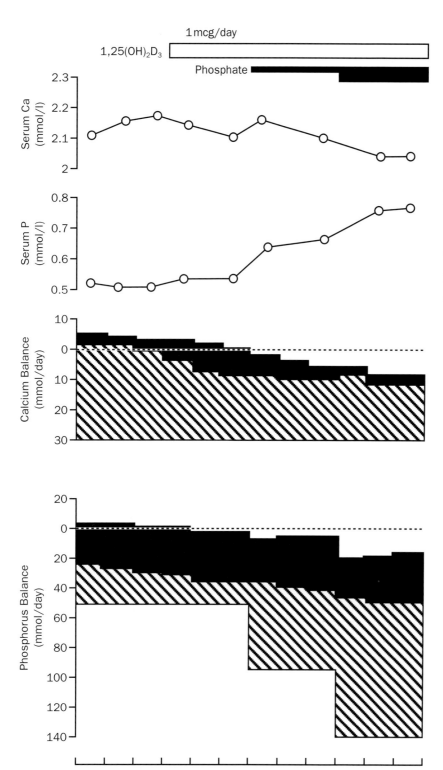

Figure 1.3 External mineral balance in acquired hypophosphataemic osteomalacia showing response to 1 mcg calcitriol and the benefits of 1 g and then 2 g of elemental phosphorus given as Sando-P.

Dietary intake is plotted down from zero line. From the intake line the figures for faeces (hatched) and urine (solid) are plotted back towards the zero line. An area above the zero line represents a negative balance and a gap below a positive balance.

bolic pathways. Not only is vitamin D_2 metabolized to $25(OH)D_2$, but a proportion is converted to 24-hydroxyvitamin D_2 $(24(OH)D_2)$.[43] This may account for some of the difference in the concentration of $25(OH)D$ achieved after equimolar dosing using both forms of the vitamin.[44] Because vitamin D is fat-soluble it accumulates in body fat, and if intoxication occurs it can last for several weeks after withdrawing treatment. It may take several months before vitamin D disappears from the serum.[45]

All the actions of calcitriol can be achieved using the native vitamin but its use should be limited to situations where renal 1-hydroxylase is intact. Thus the native vitamin orally or parenterally is best reserved for nutritional osteomalacia and osteomalacia arising from enzyme-inducing drugs or disease of the gastrointestinal tract.

25-HYDROXYVITAMIN D_3

This preparation is not available in the UK. It is better absorbed than vitamin D, reaching a peak serum value at 4–8 hours after dosing (vitamin D: 12–24 hours).[12] It has an estimated serum half life of 20 days,[46] making it less toxic than vitamin D with respect to the duration of any induced hypercalcaemia. There are no good reasons to use $25(OH)D_3$ in preference to the native vitamins.

CALCITRIOL

This is the agent of choice where there is an abnormality of vitamin D metabolism. In addition to those conditions discussed in this chapter, calcitriol is useful in renal insufficiency and hypoparathyroid states. Calcium absorption is increased within a few hours of oral administration. The peak serum concentration of calcitriol occurs 4–8 hours after dosing, and usually returns to baseline at 24 hours.[47] The serum half life of calcitriol is a few hours, but its biological half life is several days,[48] and so twice-daily dosing is unnecessary. Intravenous administration increases the peak serum concentration four-fold when compared to oral dosing.[47] This is because when given orally a proportion of calcitriol binds to its receptor in the gut to stimulate calcium absorption. Since calcitriol also stimulates tissue 24-hydroxylase to degrade calcitriol to its trihydroxymetabolite as part of its degradation to calcitroic acid, a proportion of orally administered calcitriol will also be metabolized in the intestinal mucosa. This intravenous route is less calcaemic than oral administration, and offers a better chance of controlling parathyroid overactivity in renal failure by a direct non-calcaemic effect on parathyroid cells. Intravenous calcitriol, available as Calcijex 1–2 mcg/ml, is useful in renal failure. For all other vitamin D-resistant conditions the oral route is preferable, with a dose of 0.5–1.0 mcg/day sufficient for most situations. All patients in receipt of calcitriol require regular biochemical monitoring every 2–4 weeks upon initiation of treatment and at least every 3 months when stable.

1-HYDROXYCHOLECALCIFEROL (ALPHACALCIDOL)

This metabolite requires 25-hydroxylation by the liver to produce calcitriol, and has a potency about half that of calcitriol. Because it requires metabolism by the liver its calcaemic effect is slower in onset than that of calcitriol, but the biological half life is also slightly longer. It has no advantages over calcitriol other than cost; but since twice the amount is required compared to calcitriol the cost advantage is minimal. It should be used with the same precautions as for calcitriol, but has no role in managing renal hyperparathyroidism.

REFERENCES

1. Stanbury SW, Mawer EB, Lumb GA et al. (1971). Some aspects of vitamin D metabolism in man. *Endocrinology* (London) 1971: 487–499.
2. Poskitt EME, Cole TJ, Lawson DEM (1979). Diet, sunlight and 25 hydroxyvitamin D in healthy

children and adults. *BMJ 1:* 221–223.

3. Stanbury SW, Mawer EB (1990). Metabolic disturbances in acquired osteomalacia. In: *The metabolic and molecular basis of acquired disease*, eds RD Cohen, B Lewis, KGMM Allerti, AM Deman, pp. 1717–1782. Baillière Tindall, London.

4. Clements MR, Johnson L, Fraser DR (1987). A new mechanism for induced vitamin D deficiency in calcium deprivation. *Nature 325:* 62–65.

5. Clements MR, Davies M, Fraser DR et al. (1987). Metabolic inactivation of vitamin D is enhanced in primary hyperparathyroidism. *Clin Sci 73:* 659–664.

6. Large DM, Mawer EB, Davies M (1984). Dystrophic calcification, cataracts and enamel hypoplasia due to long standing, privational vitamin D deficiency. *Metab Bone Dis Rel Res 5:* 215–218.

7. Dunnigan MG, Henderson JB (1997). An epidemiological model of privational rickets and osteomalacia. *Proc Nutr Soc 56:* 939–956.

8. Stanbury SW, Taylor CM, Lumb GA et al. (1981). Formation of vitamin D metabolites following correction of human vitamin D deficiency. *Miner Electrolyte Metab 5:* 212–227.

9. Shah BR, Finberg L (1994). Single day therapy for nutritional vitamin D deficiency rickets: a preferred method. *J Pediatr 125:* 487–490.

10. Davies M, Mawer EB, Hann JT et al. (1985). Vitamin D prophylaxis in the elderly: a simple effective method suitable for large populations. *Age and Ageing 14:* 349–354.

11. Mawer EB, Klass HJ, Warnes TW et al. (1985). Metabolism of vitamin D in patients with primary biliary cirrhosis and alcoholic liver disease. *Clin Sci 69:* 561–570.

12. Davies M, Mawer EB, Krawitt EL (1980). Comparative absorption of vitamin D_3 and 25-hydroxyvitamin D_3 in intestinal disease. *Gut 21:* 287–292.

13. Clements MR, Davies M, Hayes ME et al. (1992). The role of 1,25 dihydroxyvitamin D in the mechanism of acquired vitamin D deficiency. *Clin Endocrinol 37:* 17–27.

14. Davies M, Heys SE, Selby PL et al. (1997). Increased catabolism of 25 hydroxyvitamin D in patients with partial gastrectomy and elevated 1,25 dihydroxyvitamin D levels. Implications for metabolic bone disease. *J Clin Endocrinol Metab 82:* 209–212.

15. Arnaud SB, Goldsmith RS, Lambert PW, Go VLW (1975). 25 hydroxyvitamin D_3. Evidence of an enterohepatic circulation in man. *Proc Soc Exp Biol 149:* 570–572.

16. Clements MR, Chalmers TM, Fraser DR (1984). Enterohepatic circulation of vitamin D: a reappraisal of the hypothesis. *Lancet 1:* 1376–1379.

17. Krawitt EL, Grundman MJ, Mawer EB (1977). Absorption hydroxylation and excretion of vitamin D_3 in primary biliary cirrhosis. *Lancet 2:* 1246–1249.

18. Thompson GR, Lewis B, Booth CC (1966). Absorption of vitamin D_3-^{3}H in control subjects and patients with intestinal malabsorption. *J Clin Invest 45:* 94–102.

19. Melvin KEW, Hepner GW, Bordier P et al. (1970). Calcium metabolism and bone pathology in adult coeliac disease. *Q J Med 39:* 83–113.

20. Davies M, Mawer EB (1979). The absorption and metabolism of vitamin D_3 from parenteral injection sites. In: *Vitamin D, basic research and its clinical application*, eds AW Norman, K Schaefer, pp. 609–612. De Gruyter, Berlin and New York.

21. Selby PL, Davies M, Warnes TW et al. (1995). Bone metabolism in celiac disease. *J Bone Miner Res 10* (suppl 1): S507.

22. Hahn TJ, Birge SJ, Scharp CR, Avioli LV (1972). Phenobarbitol induced alterations in vitamin D metabolism. *J Clin Invest 51:* 741–748.

23. Collins N, Mather J, Cole M et al. (1991). A prospective study to evaluate the dose of vitamin D required to correct low 25 hydroxyvitamin D levels, calcium and alkaline phosphatase in patients at risk of developing antiepileptic drug induced osteomalacia. *Q J Med 286:* 113–122.

24. Fu GK, Lin D, Zhang MYH et al. (1997). Cloning of human 25 hydroxyvitamin D-1 hydroxylase and mutations causing vitamin D dependent rickets type I. *Mol Endocrinol 11:* 1961–1970.

25. Glorieux FH (1990). Calcitriol treatment in vitamin D dependent and vitamin D resistant rickets. *Metabolism 39* (suppl 1): 10–12.

26. Hughes MR, Molloy PJ, Kieback D et al. (1988). Point mutations in the human vitamin D receptor gene associated with hypocalcaemic rickets. *Science 242:* 1702–1705.

27. Marx SJ, Spiegal AM, Brown EM et al. (1978). A familial syndrome of decreased sensitivity to 1,25 dihydroxyvitamin D. *J Clin Endocrinol Metab 47:* 1303–1310.

28. Sakati N, Woodhouse NJY, Niles N et al. (1986). Hereditary resistance to 1,25 dihydroxyvitamin D: clinical and radiological improvement during high dose calcium therapy. *Horm Res 24:* 280–287.

29. Balsan S, Garabedian M, Larchet M et al. (1986). Long term nocturnal calcium infusions can cure rickets and promote normal mineralisation in hereditary resistance to 1,25 dihydroxyvitamin D. *J Clin Invest 77:* 1661–1667.

30. Davies M, Stanbury SW (1981). The rheumatic manifestations of metabolic bone disease. *Clin Rheum Dis 7:* 595–646.

31. Lyles KW, Drezner MK (1982). Parathyroid hormone effects on serum 1,25 dihydroxyvitamin D levels in patients with X-linked hypophosphatemic rickets. Evidence for abnormal 25 hydroxyvitamin D-I-hydroxylase activity. *J Clin Endocrinol Metab 54:* 638–644.

32. Harrell RM, Lyles KW, Harrelson JM et al. (1985). Healing of bone disease in X-linked hypophosphatemic rickets/osteomalacia. *J Clin Invest 75:* 1858–1868.

33. Goodyer PR, Kronick JB, Jequier S et al. (1982). Nephrocalcinosis and its relationship to treatment of hereditary rickets. *J Pediatr 111:* 700–704.

34. Saggese G, Baroncelli GI, Bertelloni S, Perri G (1995). Long term growth hormone treatment in children with hypophosphatemic rickets: effects on growth, mineral metabolism and bone density. *J Pediatr 127:* 395–402.

35. Davies M (1995). Hyperparathyroidism in X-linked hypophosphataemic osteomalacia. *Clin Endocrinol 42:* 205–206.

36. Carpenter TO, Mitnick MA, Ellison A et al. (1994). Nocturnal hyperparathyroidism: a frequent feature of X-linked hypophosphatemia. *J Clin Endocrinol Metab 78:* 1378–1383.

37. Adams JE, Davies M (1986). Intraspinal new bone formation and spinal cord compression in familial hypophosphataemic vitamin D resistant osteomalacia. *Q J Med 61:* 117–129.

38. Davies M, Kane R, Valentine J (1984). Impaired hearing in X-linked hypophosphataemic (vitamin D resistant) osteomalacia. *Ann Intern Med 100:* 230–232.

39. Drezner M (1996). Tumor-induced rickets and osteomalacia. In: *Primer on the metabolic bone diseases and disorders of mineral metabolism*, ed. MJ Favus, 3rd edition, pp. 319–325. Lippincott-Raven, Philadelphia and New York.

40. Aschinberg LC, Soloman LM, Zeis PM et al. (1977). Vitamin D resistant rickets induced with epidermal nevus syndrome: demonstration of a phosphaturic substance in the dermal lesions. *J Pediatr 91:* 56–60.

41. Miyauchi A, Fukase M, Tsutsumi M, Fujita T (1988). Hemangiopericytoma induced osteomalacia: tumor transplantation in nude mice causes hypophosphatemia and tumor extracts inhibit renal 25 hydroxyvitamin D-1-hydroxylase activity. *J Clin Endocrinol Metab 67:* 46–53.

42. Reid IR, Tietelbaum SL, Dusso A, Whyte MP (1987). Hypercalcemic hyperparathyroidism complicating oncogenic osteomalacia: effect of successful tumor resection on mineral homeostasis. *Am J Med 83:* 350–354.

43. Mawer EB, Jones G, Davies M et al. (1998). Unique 24 hydroxylated metabolites represent a significant pathway of metabolism of vitamin D_2 in humans: 24 hydroxyvitamin D_2 and 1,24 dihydroxyvitamin D_2 detectable in human serum. *J Clin Endocrinol Metab 83:* 2156–2166.

44. Serbert JL, Garabedian M, de Chasteigner C, Defrance D (1991). Comparative effects of equal doses of vitamin D_2 and vitamin D_3 for the correction of vitamin D deficiency in the elderly. In: *Vitamin D gene regulation structure-function analysis and clinical application*, eds AW Norman, R Bouillon, M Thomasset, pp. 764–765. De Gruyter, Berlin and New York.

45. Akasnes L, Aarskog D (1980). Vitamin D metabolites in serum from hypoparathyroid patients treated with vitamin D_2 and 1-hydroxyvitamin D_3. *J Clin Endocrinol Metab 51:* 823–829.

46. Haddad JG, Royanasathit S (1976). Acute administration of 25 hydroxycholecalciferol in man. *J Clin Endocrinol Metab 42:* 284–290.

47. Mawer EB, Backhouse J, Davies M et al. (1976). Metabolic fate of administered 1,25 dihydroxycholecalciferol in controls and patients with hypoparathyroidism. *Lancet 1:* 1203–1206.

48. Brickman AS, Coburn JW, Massry SG, Norman AW (1974). 1,25 dihydroxyvitamin D_3 in normal men and patients with renal failure. *Ann Intern Med 80:* 161–168.

2

Hypoparathyroidism

Tim Cundy

Introduction • Pathophysiology of hypoparathyroidism • Causes of hypoparathyroidism • Clinical features • Laboratory investigations • Surgical techniques to prevent hypoparathyroidism • Aims of treatment of hypoparathyroidism • Treatment of acute hypoparathyroidism • Treatment of chronic hypoparathyroidism • Alternative therapies

INTRODUCTION

Hypoparathyroidism is a disorder characterized by insufficiency of, or resistance to the action of, parathyroid hormone (PTH). In patients with normal renal function this is accompanied by hypocalcaemia and hyperphosphataemia. The clinical symptoms associated with hypoparathyroidism may be severe. They seem to be related to the resultant hypocalcaemia rather than directly to the PTH deficiency, since they reverse irrespective of the method used to raise plasma calcium. Perhaps because of this, and because it is a rare disorder (population surveys estimate the prevalence of undiagnosed hypoparathyroidism at around 1 per 100 000) there have been very few controlled trials comparing different therapies, and most reports in the literature describe small numbers of patients. A literature search for the years 1966 to 1998, using Embase and Medline databases, revealed only three randomized controlled trials of treatment or prevention of hypoparathyroidism.

Hypoparathyroidism can be permanent or transient, complete or partial, acquired or of genetic origin. Considering the rarity of the dis-

order an extraordinary range of genetic defects have been identified, and insights from these discoveries have highlighted the clinical heterogeneity of hypoparathyroidism and had an impact on treatment strategies. The aetiology of the hypoparathyroid disorders is best explained in terms of the anatomy and physiology of the parathyroids, which are therefore reviewed briefly.

PATHOPHYSIOLOGY OF HYPOPARATHYROIDISM

The parathyroid glands are derived embryologically from the third branchial arch (which because of caudual migration forms the lower parathyroid glands) and the fourth branchial arch (which forms the upper glands). Parathyroid tissue is present in the fetus from about 5 weeks' gestation. Amongst other structures, the third branchial arch also contributes to the development of the thymus.

In adult life the primary function of the parathyroids is the regulation of extracellular ionized calcium concentration. In response to a reduction in plasma-ionized calcium the glands secrete PTH which in turn is inhibited by hypercalcaemia. The calcium-sensing receptor, a seven transmembrane domain receptor spanning the cell membrane of the parathyroid cells, is responsible for sensing the ionized calcium concentration and transmitting the message to the nucleus of the parathyroid cells. PTH is synthesized as a 115 amino acid peptide (pre- pro-PTH) from which two N-terminal peptides are consecutively cleaved before the native hormone of 84 amino acids is secreted. A magnesium-dependent process is believed to be involved in the secretion of PTH.

The PTH receptor is also a seven transmembrane domain receptor. Interaction of PTH with its receptor triggers membrane-associated G proteins that activate signal effector systems that generating second messages, which include cAMP, inositol triphosphate, diacylglycerol and cytosolic calcium. The G protein system, which is utilized by a number of hormones, thus couples the PTH receptor to its second messenger. G proteins have a heterotrimeric structure comprising α, β and δ subunits. The Gα subunit is thought to confer functional specificity on each G protein.

PTH has two main target organs – bone and kidney. In bone, PTH stimulates osteoclastic bone resorption, which, in terms of mineral homeostasis, results in the release of both calcium and phosphate into the circulation. In the renal tubule PTH has three functions. First, it increases renal tubular reabsorption of filtered calcium – thus reducing urine calcium loss and raising plasma calcium. Secondly, it decreases the renal tubular reabsorption of filtered phosphate (TmP/GFR) – thus increasing urinary phosphate and lowering plasma phosphate. Thirdly, it acts to stimulate the conversion of the prohormone 25-hydroxyvitamin D (calcidiol) to its active form of 1,25 dihydroxyvitamin D (calcitriol). This is achieved through stimulating activity in the 1α hydroxylase enzyme. The other major stimulant to 1α hydroxylase activity is hypophosphataemia. Patients with hypoparathyroidism lacking PTH (or PTH activity) and with a high serum phosphate levels therefore have very low 1α hydroxylase activity, and very low serum calcitriol levels.

This suppression of 1α hydroxylase activity in hypoparathyroidism explains why the condition is 'vitamin D resistant', i.e. physiological doses of native vitamin D are ineffective in raising plasma calcium.

CAUSES OF HYPOPARATHYROIDISM

The major causes of hypoparathyroidism are listed in Table 2.1, and a more detailed description of the genetic syndromes associated with hypoparathyroidism is given in Table 2.2.

Post-surgical hypoparathyroidism

Hypoparathyroidism can result from various types of neck surgery, as a consequence of extirpation of, or damage to, the glands or damage to their blood supply. The risk of permanent hypoparathyroidism varies according to the extent of the surgery (for example, being higher after total thyroidectomy than after partial thyroidectomy) and with the skill and experience of the surgeon. Representative rates from the recent literature suggest a 1% to 3% incidence

---

Table 2.1   Causes of hypoparathyroidism.

Acquired
   Post-surgical
   Hypomagnesaemia
   Iron overload (thalassaemia)
   Rare associations (post I[131], lupus,
      systemic sclerosis, Wilson's disease,
      metastatic disease)
   Transient hypocalcaemia in neonates

Idiopathic

Genetic syndromes
   pseudohypoparathyroidism and
   hypomagnesaemic syndromes

Table 2.2 Genetic causes of hypoparathyroidism.

MIM*	Syndrome	Clinical features	Mechanism	Genetic locus	Inheritance
188400	Di George syndrome (neonatal hypocalcaemia, thymic hypoplasia, cardiac malformation, dysmorphic faces)	Neonatal hypocalcaemia, may resolve in childhood	Parathyroid hypoplasia	22q11 deletions (also 10p deletions)	AD
307700	X-linked hypoparathyroidism	Neonatal onset	Parathyroid agenesis	Xq 26–27	X
241400 146255	Hypoparathyroidism, sensorineural deafness, renal dysplasia		?	10p13 deletions	AR
247410	Lymphoedema – hypoparathyroidism	Progressive renal failure	?	Not known	AR or X
241410	Hypoparathyroidism, short stature, mental retardation, seizures	Low birthweight, dysmorphic features	?	Not known	AR
168450	Familial isolated hypoparathyroidism	No other systems involved	• Mutation in pre-pro-sequence of PTH gene; defective processing • Mutation in intron 2 of PTH gene; exon skipping	11p15	AD, AR
601199	Autosomal dominant hypocalcaemia with hypercalciuria	Detectable PTH, hypomagnesaemia often asymptomatic	Activating mutations in calcium-sensing receptor	3q13	AD
127000 244460	Kenney–Caffey syndrome (dwarfism, cortical thickening of tubular bones, hypocalcaemia)	Hypocalcaemic convulsions in infancy	?	Not known	AD, AR, X
240300	Autoimmune polyendocrinopathy – candidiasis, ectodermal dysplasia (polyglandular autoimmune syndrome I)	Hypocalcaemia onset 7–10 years, other autoimmune diseases	Autoantibodies to calcium-sensing receptor mutations in autoimmune regulator (AIRE) gene mediated by	21q22	AR
530000	Kearns–Sayre syndrome (ophthalmoplegia, ptosis, heart block)		? altered signalling caused by ATP deficiency ? impaired processing or secretion of pro-PTH	Mitochondria deletions/ duplications	Maternal

*MIM: Mendelian inheritance in main reference number.

Table 2.2 Continued.

MIM	Syndrome	Clinical features	Mechanism	Genetic locus	Inheritance
300800	Pseudohypoparathyroidism – Albright hereditary osteodystrophy	AHO: short stature, brachydactylyl, mental retardation, subcutaneous ossification	Resistance to PTH action		
		Type IA AHO: other hormone resistance, hypocalcaemia develops around 8 years GSα activity reduced		20q13	AD
		Type IB AHO rare, other hormone resistance absent, normal GSα activity	?	?	?
		Type II Normal urine cAMP response to PTH, normal GSα activity, hypocalcaemia onset in childhood	?	?	?
602014	Familial hypomagnesaemia (hypomagnesaemia with secondary hypocalcaemia)	Neonatal seizures	Impaired PTH secretion (and action)	9q12–q22 mutations	AR
248250	Defect in renal tubular transport of magnesium	Neonatal seizures	Impaired PTH secretion (and action)	?	?

Hypoparathyroidism has also been described with other mitochondria disorders (MELAS and trifunctional protein deficiency).
Reduced urine phosphate and cAMP response to exogenous PTH.

of hypoparathyroidism after surgery for thyroid cancer, multinodular goitre or Graves' disease. Some centres report higher rates in children with thyroid cancer and <1% for first operations for primary hyperparathyroidism and for head and neck cancer. The highest rates of post-surgical hypoparathyroidism follow re-exploration of the neck for hyperparathyroidism, when rates averaging 14% are reported. Higher rates of post-surgical hypoparathyroidism are also reported after procedures for multiple endocrine neoplasia 1 (parathyroidectomy) and, in some series, multiple endocrine neoplasia 2A (thyroidectomy for medullary carcinoma).

Transient hypocalcaemia following thyroid surgery (particularly for Graves' disease) is common,[1] but the majority of cases do not progress to permanent hypoparathyroidism. Although support with calcium and/or vitamin D supplements may be required, the majority of patients can discontinue these within 4 months. If hypocalcaemia persists 12 months after surgery it is generally regarded as permanent, although there are occasional cases where recovery has occurred beyond this time. Cases of post-surgical hypoparathyroidism with the onset of symptoms apparently delayed for many years after surgery are also recognized, but why this phenomenon occurs is poorly understood.

Hypomagnesaemia

Severe magnesium depletion (plasma magnesium <0.5 mmol L^{-1}) can result in impaired secretion of PTH and can thus cause a reversible form of hypoparathyroidism. In addition there is evidence of target organ resistance, since the administration of PTH to magnesium-deficient subjects does not correct hypocalcaemia. The common causes of hypomagnesaemia are listed in Table 2.3.

Iron overload

Hypoparathyroidism is a rare but recognized complication of iron overload. In adolescents

---

Table 2.3   Causes of hypomagnesaemia.

Inadequate intake
  Alcoholism
  Protein calorie malnutrition
  Prolonged infusion or ingestion of low Mg solutions or diet

Malabsorption
  Inflammatory bowel disease
  Gluten enteropathy
  Intestinal bypass
  Radiation enteritis
  Familial hypomagnesaemia*

Renal tubular dysfunction
  Alcoholism
  Hyperaldosteronism
  Bartter's syndrome
  Post-renal obstruction
  Post-renal transplant
  Nephrotoxic drugs
  Potassium depletion
  Diuretics (non-K^+-sparing)
Osmotic diuresis
Defective renal tubular transport of magnesium*

Intracellular shift
Post-myocardial infarction
Post-parathyroidectomy
Recovery from diabetic ketoacidosis
Recovery from starvation
Acute pancreatitis

*Genetic conditions.

---

with thalassaemia major who are transfusion-dependent, hypoparathyroidism occurs in 3% to 4% of subjects around the age of 18. All also have other significant organ damage from iron loading.[2]

Idiopathic hypoparathyroidism

This term refers to hypoparathyroidism which is not due to acquired causes and is not caused by a recognized genetic defect. Some cases have a clear familial occurrence and are thus likely to have a genetic basis. With the expansion of knowledge of genetic causes of hypoparathyroidism it is probable that the proportion of hypoparathyroid cases designated as 'idiopathic' will decline. Idiopathic hypoparathyroidism can be subdivided into those cases where it is the sole finding (isolated hypoparathyroidism) and those where it occurs in association with other abnormalities.

Genetic disorders

The main recognized genetic syndromes associated with hypoparathyroidism are listed in Table 2.2. Although much remains to be learnt, it is apparent that numerous defects can result in hypoparathyroidism, with at least 10 different genetic loci already identified. In some instances the mechanism whereby hypoparathyroidism arises is more or less understood.[3,4]

The Di George syndrome, which like the closely related velocardiofacial syndrome, is associated with deletions at a 22q11 locus, is thought to result from abnormal development of the parathyroids. Although the hypoparathyroidism can be mild and a lesser component of the syndrome, patients have been described in whom hypoparathyroidism dominates the clinical picture.

Familial isolated hypoparathyroidism has been described with mutations in the pre- pro-PTH gene, resulting in both autosomal dominant and autosomal recessive forms.

The recently defined syndrome of autosomal dominant hypercalciuric hypocalcaemia (ADHH) results from activating mutations in the calcium-sensing receptor. This means that the parathyroids 'read' plasma-ionized calcium level as being higher than it really is: thus PTH secretion is inappropriately low for any given plasma calcium. The calcium-sensing receptor

may also be the target of autoantibodies in the autoimmune polyendocrinopathy-candidiasis ectodermal dysplasia (APCED) syndrome, which is characterized by the presence of multiple autoimmune phenomena.[5]

The pseudohypoparathyroidism syndromes are marked by resistance to PTH action. In only one form (IA) is the mechanism well understood, with the majority of cases being associated with reductions in Gsα activity within the receptor complex.

Table 2.4 Clinical features of hypoparathyroidism.

Severe
  Carpopedal spasm
  Laryngospasm
  Seizures (focal or generalized)
  Heart failure

Mild
  Hyper-irritability, fatigue
  Anxiety
  Perioral numbness
  Paraesthesiae
  Muscle cramps

Delayed dentition, enamel hypoplasia (if onset <5 years)

Skin changes

Cataract

Movement disorders
  Extrapyramidal
    Chorea
    Athetosis
    Tremor
    Hemiballismus
  Cerebellar

Organic brain syndromes
  Dementia
  Psychosis

CLINICAL FEATURES

The symptoms of hypocalcaemia (listed in Table 2.4) may be non-specific, particularly if the hypocalcaemia is mild. More severe hypocalcaemia is characterized by recurrent tetany (carpopedal spasm), laryngospasm and laryngeal stridor, and seizures, which may be refractory to anticonvulsant treatment. The Chvostek and Trousseau signs are most likely to be positive in these patients. A rare occurrence, described in both children and adults, is heart failure. This may occur in people with pre-existing heart disease. There are well-documented instances where there has been no obvious underlying cardiac disease, and where there is apparent reversibility of the cardiac dysfunction on restoration of normocalcaemia.

Chronic hypoparathyroidism can be associated with changes in other systems. Delayed dentition, caries and enamel hypoplasia are common in the teeth of children with hypoparathyroidism if the onset of their disease was before the age of five. Since similar problems are encountered in children with vitamin D-dependent rickets (but not in children with X-linked hypophosphataemic rickets), it seems probable that this is directly related to hypocalcaemia.[6] Cataract is also a recognized finding in patients with chronic hypoparathyroidism, although of course hypoparathyroidism accounts for only a tiny proportion of all cataracts. Cataract can be produced in animal models by inducing hypocalcaemia, and is associated with a reduced calcium content in the aqueous humour. Chronic hypocalcaemia is thus a probable precipitant or accelerant of cataract formation.

In addition to seizures, a variety of other neurological problems have been described in hypoparathyroidism, including extrapyramidal symptoms (athetosis, chorea, tremor, hemiballismus), cerebellar symptoms, dementia and psychosis. These are uncommon but important, as the symptoms may reverse with the restoration of normocalcaemia. Some skin diseases, particularly psoriasis, may be exacerbated by hypoparathyroidism. The reason is not clear, but in this case it may be due to the secondary deficiency of calcitriol rather than to hypocalcaemia *per se*. Topically applied calcitriol derivatives are effective treatments for psoriasis.

LABORATORY INVESTIGATIONS

Hypoparathyroidism is characterized by hypocalcaemia of varying degree, and by hyperphosphataemia. This combination can also be seen in patients with chronic renal failure when the glomerular filtration rate is below 30 ml/min and so it is always important to measure the plasma creatinine. If there is uncertainty about the total plasma calcium level because of a co-existing acid base disorder or hypoalbuminaemia, then an ionized calcium level can be helpful.

PTH assay is of course important, and can help to distinguish hypoparathyroidism (inadequate hormone secretion and low plasma PTH) from pseudohypoparathyroidism (end organ resistance and high plasma PTH). Measurement of plasma magnesium is also important in order to distinguish hypoparathyroidism due to hypomagnesaemia. Magnesium levels below 0.5 mmol L^{-1} are usually necessary to cause hypoparathyroidism. Mild hypomagnesaemia (0.5 to 0.7) is common, but probably not of pathophysiological importance, in autosomal dominant hypercalciuric hypocalcaemia (ADHH).

The 24-hour urine calcium excretion tends to be low in all subjects with hypoparathyroidism and pseudohypoparathyroidism, because the filtered load is low. However, because of the lack of PTH action on the renal tubule (normally stimulating calcium reabsorption) in hypoparathyroidism the calcium excretion is increased in relation to the plasma calcium level, when the former is expressed per litre of glomerular filtrate. Urine calcium excretion is inappropriately high in patients with ADHH, and a fasting urine calcium/creatinine ratio of ≥0.30 m mol/m mol in the presence of hypocalcaemia is very suggestive of this diagnosis. In idiopathic hypoparathyroidism this ratio is usually <0.33, and in ADHH the mean is 0.45.[7]

SURGICAL TECHNIQUES TO PREVENT HYPOPARATHYROIDISM

Post-surgical hypoparathyroidism remains an important cause of the syndrome, and there is a substantial surgical literature on methods of dissecting the neck to avoid damaging the parathyroids. Wide variations in the incidence of permanent hypoparathyroidism after thyroid or parathyroid surgery or radical neck dissection suggest that surgical technique is highly important. Surgical reviews stress the importance of accurately identifying the parathyroid glands during surgery, care in the use of suction, and avoiding devascularization.[8] Some 80% of all parathyroid glands derive their blood supply from the inferior thyroid artery, and the practice of avoiding ligation of the main trunk and instead ligating branches of the artery close to the thyroid capsule has also been stressed. However, one of the few controlled trials in this field, which compared the prevalence of hypoparathyroidism following thyroidectomy in two groups of subjects who either had ligation of the inferior thyroid artery or close dissection (50 in each group), failed to show any difference in the prevalence of permanent hypoparathyroidism.[9]

The technique of parathyroid autotransplantation, when the macroscopic appearance of a gland at surgery suggests that it has been devascularized, has also had strong support in the surgical literature.[10] Such glands may be cryopreserved and transplanted at a later date if hypoparathyroidism does develop, or autotransplanted in diced form at the time of the initial surgery – either into the sternomastoid muscle or the forearm. The most frequently cited work in support of this approach is the non-randomized study of Paloyan et al., in which 2 out of 64 patients undergoing total thyroidectomy developed hypoparathyroidism compared to 0 out of 54 undergoing the same procedure plus parathyroid autotransplantation.[11] This difference is not, of course, statistically significant ($P = 0.55$, χ^2 test). A similar, non-randomized comparison of the incidence of hypoparathyroidism in patients undergoing total or near-total thyroidectomy with or without autotransplantation also showed no significant difference.[12] Only 1 out of 75 patients having autotransplantation developed permanent hypoparathyroidism, compared with 3 out of 101 not having autotransplantation. Combining the results of these studies would seem to suggest that the prevalence of hypoparathyroidism after thyroidectomy with autotransplantation of the parathryoids is about a third less common than it would be after thyroidectomy without this additional procedure; but even this is not statistically significant. This illustrates the difficulty of evaluating treatments to improve outcomes in conditions where the outcome is usually good. Assuming this degree of effectiveness (a two-thirds reduction), it would take a randomized controlled trial with a minimum of 500 patients in each arm to prove statistically that the procedure worked. Such a study seems unlikely to be done; surgeons argue that the procedure is in any case safe, and adds little to the operating time.

Another difficulty in evaluating the procedure is the variation in surgeons' perceptions of the necessity for undertaking autotransplantation. Table 2.5 illustrates three recently reported series of adult patients undergoing bilateral or total thyroidectomy.[13–15] Despite the rate of autotransplantation ranging from 0 to 66%, the reported incidence of hypoparathyroidism, although very low in the patients from the group with the most aggressive autotransplantation policy, did not differ significantly between the groups ($P = 0.445$, χ^2 test). There is thus considerable subjectivity in determining which patients 'need' autotransplantation.

The value of parathyroid autotransplantation for patients undergoing surgery for parathyroid hyperplasia or recurrent primary hyperparathyroidism is similarly far from conclusive. Brunt and Sicard, using data from a non-randomized series of patients with non-familial parathyroid hyperplasia, compared those having subtotal ($3\frac{1}{2}$ gland) parathyroidectomy with those having total thyroidectomy with immediate autotransplantation.[10] Hypoparathyroidism developed in 12/71 (17%) of the former, compared to 3/57 (5%) of the latter ($P = 0.07$, χ^2 test). This contrasts with the findings in mul-

Table 2.5 Surgical studies of parathyroid autotransplantation.

Reference	13	14	15
Year of publication	1994	1990	1997
Number of subjects	393	301	62
Number 'requiring' autotransplantation	261 (66%)	44 (15%)	0 (0%)
Permanent hypoparathyroidism	2 (0.5%)	4 (1.3%)	1 (1.6%)

tiple endocrine neoplasia type 1 by Hellman et al., who compared 34 patients having subtotal parathyroidectomy with 23 having total parathyroidectomy with autotransplantation.[16] At follow-up (after a mean of 9 years) there was a significant difference ($P = 0.01$) in the proportions of patients with either hypoparathyroidism, euparathyroidism or recurrent hyperparathyroidism ($n = 4$, 9, 21 vs 7, 11, 5 respectively). Thus the total parathyroidectomy autotransplantation group had a lower rate of recurrent disease but more hypoparathyroidism.

The alternative approach, of cryopreserving parathyroid glands at the time of surgery and only reimplanting them if hypoparathyroidism develops, has been explored by Herrera et al. in patients undergoing neck exploration for recurrent hyperparathyroidism.[17] At an average 5 years' follow-up, 10 out of 18 patients having immediate autotransplantation were able to maintain normocalcaemia, compared to only 2 out of 12 having delayed transplantation of cryopreserved glands ($P - 0.08$). Other series have also reported that cryopreserved glands may be less effective. Clearly there is scope for proper randomized trials with adequate statistical power to clarify the problem of the prevention of surgical hypoparathyroidism.

Very few of the surgical trials have been adequately controlled, so it is difficult to draw firm conclusions about the value of parathyroid autotransplantation. For thyroid surgery it is certainly not clear how often the procedure is justified or whether it makes a significant difference to the rate of permanent hypoparathyroidism. The incidence of hypoparathyroidism is substantially higher for repeat parathyroidectomy and for parathyroidectomy in Multiple Endocrine Neoplasia type 1, when there is a good chance of removing all parathyroid tissue. In these circumstances a clear benefit from autotransplantation may be demonstrable, but delayed implantation of cryopreserved material may be less effective than immediate transplantation. In Multiple Endocrine Neoplasia type 1, as with parathyroid autotransplantation in renal failure, there is a substantial risk of recurrent hyperparathyroidism from the graft.

AIMS OF TREATMENT OF HYPOPARATHYROIDISM

It is important to remember that severe hypoparathyroidism is a life-threatening disorder, and that its symptoms are highly unpleasant. Before vitamin D became available in the 1930s there was no effective treatment available, and deaths from tetany and seizures occurred. All the severe features of hypoparathyroidism are due to hypocalcaemia, and so the primary aim of treatment is to raise the plasma calcium to a level that will alleviate those symptoms. The expectation is of definite improvement in tetany, seizure control, paraesthesiae, muscle cramps and tiredness. There may also be improvement in movement disorders, depression and heart failure. The hope is that treatment of patients with chronic hypoparathyroidism will also be able to slow or prevent cataract formation, although unsurprisingly there is no proof that this can be achieved.

TREATMENT OF ACUTE HYPOPARATHYROIDISM

Acute hypoparathyroidism can present either following surgery or as a manifestation of hypomagnesaemia or in the neonatal period.

Post-surgical hypoparathyroidism

Hypocalcaemia following thyroid or parathyroid surgery is common, although not all patients are symptomatic. One recent survey suggested that about a third of patients under-going total thyroidectomy needed some form of support for plasma calcium post-operatively, but the prevalence of permanent hypoparathyroidism (persisting for 12 months or more after surgery) was much lower (about 1.5%).[15] There are no controlled trials of treatment, but there are published guides (Table 2.6).[18]

Monitoring of plasma calcium, albumin and magnesium post-operatively is important. Calcium may need to be measured twice daily in the early post-operative period. If there is doubt about the measurements (for example, because of hypoalbuminaemia) then ionized calcium should be measured. The published guides agree that most patients are symptomatic once total calcium level is <1.75 mmol L^{-1} (ionized calcium 0.88 mmol L^{-1}), and the aim of early management is to keep it above this level, in order to avoid laryngospasm and seizures.

If treatment is required then it can be initiated by the use of intravenous calcium gluconate, which can be followed by giving oral calcium. If

---

Table 2.6   Management of early post-surgical hypoparathyroidism in adults.

Early post-operative period (patient unable to swallow), acute symptoms:
- 10–20 ml 10% calcium gluconate iv every 5–10 minutes*

Followed by:
- Continuous iv infusion of 9–18 mmol calcium every 24 hours in 2 L fluid

When patient able to swallow, start:
- Oral calcium 0.5 g four times daily

Persistent hypocalcaemia (patient able to swallow) despite oral calcium:
- Short-acting preparations of vitamin D

Short-acting vitamin D dosages:

	Dihydrotachysterol	Alfacalcidol	Calcitriol
Days 1–2	4 mcg	8 mcg	4 mcg
Days 3–4	2 mcg	4 mcg	2 mcg
Day 5	1 mcg	1–3 mcg	0.5–1.5 mcg

*10 ml 10% calcium gluconate solution provides 2.25 mmol calcium.

the patient remains unable to swallow and hypocalcaemia recurs, then a continuous intravenous infusion of calcium gluconate should be established. Careful monitoring of plasma calcium should of course continue in this period.

Patients who, after the early post-operative period, have persistent hypocalcaemia (<1.75 mmol L^{-1}) despite oral calcium, should be prescribed vitamin D. The short-acting preparations of dihydrotachysterol (DHT), alfacalcidol or calcitriol are preferred in this circumstance, as their short half life permits a rapid subsequent assessment later on as to whether treatment needs to be continued. If normocalcaemia (2.15 to 2.35 mmol L^{-1}) is maintained satisfactorily with the use of these agents then gradual withdrawal of therapy with vitamin D and calcium should be attempted, as it also should be if hypercalcaemia or high normal plasma calcium levels develop.

Plasma calcium should be monitored following complete withdrawal to see if hypocalcaemia recurs. If hypoparathyroidism persists, hypocalcaemia will recur within a week of discontinuing alfacalcidol or calcitriol, and within two weeks of discontinuing dihydrotachysterol.

About half the patients with hypocalcaemia early after operation recover by one month, and 75% by 4 months.[10]

Children and neonates

The treatment of neonatal tetany due to hypoparathyroidism in children requires special consideration.[19] A number of congenital forms of hypoparathyroidism can present as neonatal tetany. Symptomatic hypocalcaemia in infants may lead, through convulsions, laryngeal spasm and arrhythmias, to cerebral damage and sudden death. Initial therapy should be prompt, with intravenous calcium gluconate solution. Tetany and muscle spasms usually stop at once, but convulsions may persist for several days, requiring anticonvulsant therapy. Oral calcium supplements should be given as well as ergocalciferol therapy (Table 2.7).

The hypocalcaemia may be transient, allowing intravenous therapy to be stopped within a week. If it persists for longer, then vitamin D should be added. The requirements are proportional to body weight, and the newer 1α hydroxylated metabolites are preferable.

Table 2.7   Management of neonatal tetany.

Initial therapy
- I/v calcium gluconate diluted to a 2% solution (0.9 mmol calcium in 20 ml) at 0.1 mmol calcium/kg body weight/hr
  (adjust infusion rate every 4 hours depending on plasma calcium level)
- Oral calcium 2.5 mmol/kg/day of elemental calcium in 3 or 4 divided doses
- Ergocalciferol 10 mcg per day

Persistent hypocalcaemia

	Calcitriol (ng/kg per day)	**OR**	Alfacalcidol (ng/kg per day)	**OR**	Dihydrotachysterol (mcg/kg per day)	**OR**	Ergocalciferol (mcg/kg per day)
First 4 days	0.1–0.15		0.2–0.3		100–150		150–300*
Maintenance	0.01–0.05		0.02–0.1		20–50		25–100

*For first two weeks.

Therapy can be started at higher than maintenance doses for the first three to four days and then reduced. The advantage of using the short-acting metabolites in this situation is that upon withdrawal it becomes evident within a week whether or not hypocalcaemia has been transient and whether treatment needs to be prolonged.

Hypoparathyroidism due to hypomagnesaemia

Hypomagnesaemia may arise through inadequate absorption (or intake), by excessive urinary losses or by redistribution of magnesium from extracellular to intracellular compartments. There are two rare familial disorders (one characterized by a specific defect in intestinal absorption, the other by a specific defect in renal tubular reabsorption) – both of which present in neonates – hypomagnesaemia is an acquired condition. The major causes are listed in Table 2.3.

Hypoparathyroidism secondary to hypomagnesaemia is difficult to correct even with short-acting vitamin D metabolites, unless the magnesium deficiency is corrected first. There are no particular clinical features of hypoparathyroidism due to hypomagnesaemia that distinguish it from other forms of hypoparathyroidism. The key to its correct identification remains thinking of it as a possible diagnosis, and requesting a plasma magnesium estimation.

There are no controlled clinical studies of magnesium replacement, but most texts suggest that symptomatic deficiency is best treated by the intravenous route. Adults with good renal function should be given 12–15 mmol (in the form of magnesium sulphate in saline and dextrose) over 2 to 3 hours, and a further 12–15 mmol infused slowly over the following 24 hours. This regimen may need to be repeated over several days, as the tissue magnesium deficit takes longer to correct than the plasma level. If the plasma levels are raised too high then urinary magnesium losses increase. In infants and children, replacement is given in a similar manner, but with the dosage reduced to 0.2 to 0.3 mmol kg^{-1}. Plasma magnesium levels need to be monitored during and after replacement therapy. The intramuscular route may also be used for replacement but the injections are painful.

Where feasible, magnesium supplements may also be given orally (5–10 mmol per day, in divided doses). Suitable preparations include magnesium oxide, magnesium sulphate and magnesium carbonate, which are available as antacids or purgatives. Higher doses may cause diarrhoea.

The rare neonatal syndrome of familial hypomagnesaemia presents at two to three weeks of life with hypomagnesaemia and secondary hypocalcaemia. This can be managed initially by intramuscular or intravenous magnesium sulphate, 0.5–0.75 mmol kg^{-1} per day in 2 or 3 divided doses, followed by long-term oral magnesium salts.[19]

Autosomal dominant hypercalciuric hypocalcaemia (ADHH)

This syndrome, which, as explained above, results from activating mutations in the calcium-sensing receptor, is important to distinguish from other forms of hypoparathyroidism. The diagnosis is suggested by the presence of a family history suggestive of autosomal dominant inheritance, mild hypomagnesaemia, relative hypercalciuria, and low but detectable parathyroid hormone levels. Although patients with this syndrome may be symptomatic, many are not. Treatment with vitamin D or its metabolites typically produces little change in plasma calcium, but a dramatic increase in urine calcium excretion and a subsequent risk of nephrocalcinosis and renal impairment. Thus asymptomatic patients are best left untreated, and vitamin D should only be given to patients with definite hypocalcaemic symptoms (such as recurrent seizures), with the aim of alleviating symptoms rather than correcting the plasma calcium.[7]

TREATMENT OF CHRONIC HYPOPARATHYROIDISM

Aims of therapy

Most patients with chronic symptomatic hypocalcaemia will need vitamin D treatment in order to support their plasma calcium and relieve symptoms. In patients with milder degrees of hypocalcaemia, the use of calcium supplements and/or thiazide diuretics may raise plasma calcium concentrations without the use of vitamin D. However the rationale for this approach is not clear, since such patients are usually asymptomatic.[20]

The major aim of treatment of chronic hypoparathyroidism is to relieve symptoms of hypocalcaemia. This can usually be achieved by bringing plasma concentrations to the lower end of the normal range. The major complication of vitamin D therapy is disequilibrium hypercalcaemia, and the risk of this occurring is substantially increased if the plasma calcium levels run in the upper half of the normal range. The target range of 2.0–2.3 mmol L^{-1} is accepted by most authorities as providing the greatest benefit with the lowest risk. This should permit a plasma calcium $\times$ plasma phosphate product of <5 molar units. The precise plasma calcium level needed to reduce the risk of cataract is not clear.

The main difficulty encountered with vitamin D treatment is the narrow therapeutic range between inadequate treatment and overdosage. Since the object of treatment is only to relieve symptoms, it follows that mild asymptomatic hypoparathyroidism detected by biochemical screening does not necessarily need treatment. Such patients should have an accurate diagnosis made, should be reviewed from time to time to see if symptoms are occurring, and should be aware that certain drugs may precipitate more severe hypocalcaemia (see below).

Vitamin D treatment

All the available forms of vitamin D are effective in hypoparathyroidism but, because of the suppressed activity of the renal 1α hydroxylase, ergocalciferol (vitamin D_2) and calcidiol (25OH vitamin D), which require 1α hydroxylation, need to be given in supraphysiological doses. Maintenance dose ranges for the various compounds are given in Table 2.8. There are data to suggest that patients with pseudohypoparathyroidism are slightly more sensitive to vitamin D metabolites than patients with idiopathic

Table 2.8 Vitamin D treatment of hypoparathyroidism.

Vitamin D type	Ergocalciferol* (D_2)	Calcidiol (25 OHD_3)	Dihydrotachysterol (DHT)	Alfacalcidol (1α OHD_3)	Calcitriol (1,25$(OH)_2D_3$)
Maintenance dose range (mcg)	1000–5000	75–225	300–1000	1–3	0.75 2.25
Time to restore normocalcaemia (weeks)	4–8	2–4	1–2	1–2	0.5–1.0
Persistence of hypercalcaemia after cessation of treatment (weeks)	6–18	4–12	1–3	1–2	0.5–1.0

*1 mg = 40 international units.

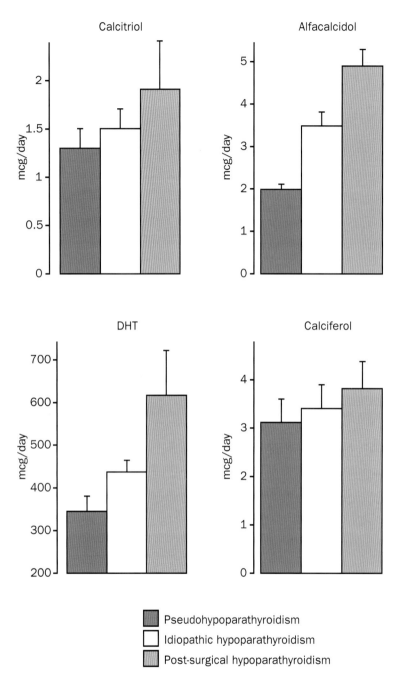

Figure 2.1 Maintenance doses of various vitamin D preparations in subjects with various forms of hypoparathyroidism. The doses were adjusted to maintain plasma calcium in the 2.3–2.4 mmol/l range. The relative potency of the four preparations is evident, plus the suggestion that dose requirements may differ according to aetiology. *(Reproduced from Reference 21, with permission.)*

hypoparathyroidism, and that patients with surgical hypoparathyroidism demonstrate the most marked resistance, and thus need higher doses.[21]

To speed the initial response some clinicians suggest giving 'loading doses' from the top end of these ranges for the early part of therapy, in the expectation that this will need reduction as plasma calcium normalizes. A more cautious approach, when serious symptoms requiring urgent relief are not present, is to start at a dose at the lower end of these ranges and to increase it by increments of 20% to 25%, until the desired response is reached. Doses may need to be changed every two to three days with the short-acting compounds, but no more frequently than 2 weeks with ergocalciferol. In the early phases of therapy several dose adjustments may be necessary – an average of 5 per patient in one study using ergocalciferol.[22]

The main difference between metabolites, apart from their potency, is the speed of onset and offset of action, which is very much more rapid for the analogues that are already 1α hydroxylated (DHT, alfacalcidol and calcitriol) than for ergocalciferol or calcidiol. Thus with ergocalciferol the response to dose change is slow, and the reversibility of hypercalcaemia, should it occur, is also prolonged.

Monitoring

Hypercalcaemic episodes are most likely to occur early in the course of therapy, and once a stable plasma calcium in the lower half of the normal range has been achieved there is usually little need to change the dose of vitamin D. All patients on vitamin D therapy, of whatever type, require monitoring of plasma calcium. Monitoring needs to be frequent in the early stages (initially every two to three days if short-acting agents are used, or weekly if long-acting agents are used). Once a stable dosage is reached frequency of monitoring can be gradually reduced, ultimately to three- to six-monthly. It does need to be continued, in order to try to detect incipient vitamin D toxicity. Disequilibrium hypercalcaemia can arise with any type of vitamin D treatment, particularly when plasma calcium has been allowed to rise into the upper half of the normal range.

Monitoring of 24-hour urine calcium excretion is advocated by many authorities.[23] The aim is to keep urine calcium excretion (in adults) below 8 mmol/day in order to minimize the risk of nephrolithiasis and nephrocalcinosis, and to detect incipient vitamin D toxicity. There is, however, no evidence that

this approach actually reduces the risk of these complications. In practice the vagaries of 24-hour urine collections mean that they are probably not an adequate surrogate for plasma calcium measurements upon which most clinical decisions should be based.

Children

In children dose requirements are proportional to body weight, and are increased during phases of rapid growth, and reduced as growth slows, paralleling the changes in endogenous calcitriol production. Because of these changes in requirement for vitamin D, children need careful monitoring of the plasma calcium, and may need more frequent dose adjustments.[24] Hypocalcaemia may develop during intercurrent febrile illness.

Drugs affecting hypoparathyroidism and its treatment

A number of recognized drug interactions can disturb apparently stable plasma calcium levels or precipitate symptomatic hypoparathyroidism in patients who were previously asymptomatic.

Loop diuretics
Frusemide can lower plasma calcium, through increases in urinary calcium excretion, necessitating increases in vitamin D dosages in patients with hypoparathyroidism. There have also been cases of tetany being precipitated by frusemide in patients with latent, previously unrecognized, hypoparathyroidism.[25]

Thiazide diuretics
Thiazides have the opposite effects to loop diuretics, in that they enhance renal tubular calcium reabsorption, and can precipitate hypercalcaemia in vitamin D-treated hypoparathyroidism. Use has been made of this property in the management of mild or partial hypoparathyroidism, in conjunction with calcium supplements.[20] However, as was dis-

cussed earlier, the majority of the patients in whom plasma calcium can be maintained with this regimen are actually asymptomatic, so that the value of this treatment is questionable.

Sex steroids
Sex steroids can have a profound effect on hypoparathyroidism. Oestrogen administration can precipitate overt hypocalcaemia in post-menopausal women with mild or partial hypoparathyroidism. In those with established hypoparathyroidism treated with vitamin D the addition of oestrogen prescription can precipitate hypocalcaemia. Withdrawal of oestrogen in women with hypoparathyroidism who have a stable plasma calcium on vitamin D therapy can precipitate hypercalcaemia,[26] as can prescription of the antioestrogen, danazol, in pre-menopausal women.[27] Hypocalcaemia can also be precipitated by the use of oestrogen in men with carcinoma of the prostate. These interactions are presumably the results of the anti-resorptive properties of oestrogens.

Glucocorticoids
Glucocorticoids have similar effects to sex steroids, although the mechanism may differ. In patients treated with vitamin D, prescription of glucocorticoids can precipitate hypocalcaemia.[28] In patients with the APCED syndrome, in whom the various endocrine manifestations do not always arise simultaneously, a well-recognized phenomenon can occur in patients with vitamin D-treated hypoparathyroidism, in whom the first manifestation of developing adrenal insufficiency may be the occurrence of severe hypercalcaemia.[29]

Anticonvulsants
Cases have been reported of patients with hypoparathyroidism taking anticonvulsants who were unresponsive to vitamin D, or required higher doses than usual to maintain plasma calcium levels.[30] The mechanism appears to operate through excessive hepatic catabolism of vitamin D, a result of enzyme induction. This phenomenon has been observed in patients taking 1α hydroxylated forms of vitamin D, as well as ergocalciferol and calcidiol.

The converse effect – hypercalcaemia after withdrawal of anticonvulsants in vitamin D-treated patients – is also recognized.

Pregnancy and lactation

Pregnancy represents a period of increased calcium demand for the mother, and several (but not all) reports of pregnancy in women with hypoparathyroidism treated with vitamin D have suggested that increased doses of vitamin D are required in the final trimester.[31,32] Postpartum hypercalcaemia is very liable to occur within two weeks of delivery unless the dose of vitamin D is reduced. The mechanism is not entirely certain, but there is clear evidence that endogenous calcitriol synthesis is substantially enhanced, meaning that there is a reduced need for exogenous vitamin D.[33]

Choice of vitamin D

There are very few studies comparing directly the different forms of vitamin D in the treatment of hypoparathyroidism, so the choice of therapy is informed by other considerations. There are a number of situations where the rapidly acting 1α hydroxylated metabolites might have advantages over the long-acting agents. These include the management of acute severe hypoparathyroidism, where rapid onset action is clearly desirable; use in children and neonates; and use in pregnancy and lactation, when changes in vitamin D dosage are expected.

In the management of chronic hypoparathyroidism in adults Parfitt has suggested that the variability in attained plasma calcium (representing the best estimate of precision of control) is better or no different for ergocalciferol than for the short-acting vitamin D derivates. The lower cost of the former therefore makes it the drug of choice.[18] Balanced against this is the much more rapid rate of reversal of hypercalcaemia, should it occur, and the stable formulation of the newer products, alfacalcidol and calcitriol. Many commercially available ergocalciferol formulations have had serious variabil-

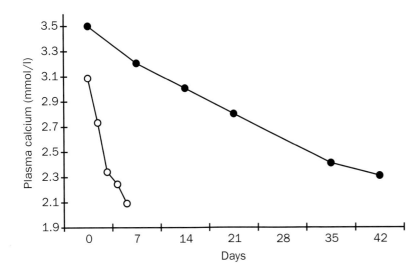

Figure 2.2 Changes in plasma calcium and calcitriol after withdrawal of calcitriol therapy in a woman with post-surgical hypoparathyroidism, following two episodes of hypercalcaemia. The open circles were when she was not pregnant or lactating, the closed circles show data shortly after delivery of a healthy child. In the latter instance, the plasma calcium declined slowly, presumably because of endogenous calcitriol production. *(Data from Reference 33, with permission.)*

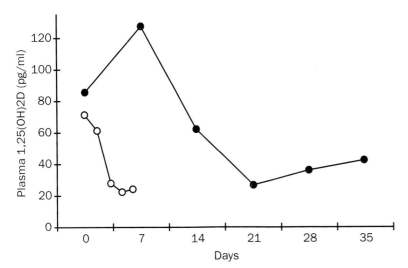

ity in their actual vitamin D content.[34] Long-term experience with alfacalcidol has confirmed that stability and low variance in plasma calcium can be achieved in hypoparathyroidism, with a very low rate of hypercalcaemia.[35] The only trial directly comparing vitamin D compounds was of short duration and did not report the incidence of hypercalcaemia.[21] Despite their short duration of action, alfacalcidol and calcitriol are usually effective in once-daily dosage.

The availability of products and physicians'

familiarity with them, also informs choice. In Germany, for example, most physicians use DHT for the treatment of hypoparathyroidism,[36] whereas in Japan, alfacalcidol (a product unavailable in the United States) is the product most commonly used.

Calcium supplements

In some cases plasma calcium can be normalized by the use of calcium supplements alone –

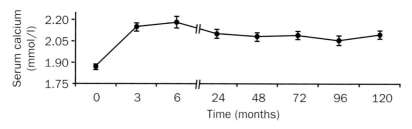

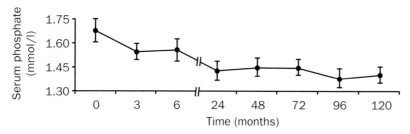

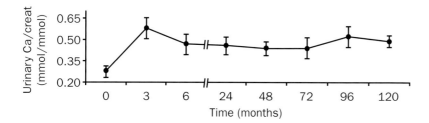

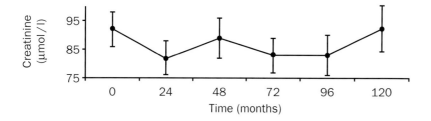

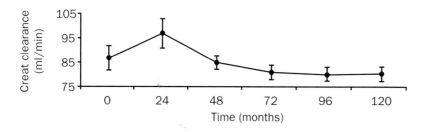

Figure 2.3 Long-term follow-up of 17 patients with hypoparathyroidism treated with alfacalcidol, with the aim of maintaining plasma calcium around 2.10 mmol/l. Note that calcium excretion increased markedly, but renal function remained stable.
(Reproduced from Reference 35, with permission.)

but these patients are generally asymptomatic or only mildly symptomatic. More severely hypocalcaemic patients may need massive doses of calcium salts (3–9 g per day) in order to reach a normal plasma calcium. Tolerance of this level of supplementation is poor, so that vitamin D treatment is usually required.

Many standard texts recommend that, in

addition to vitamin D, hypoparathyroid patients take calcium supplements to increase their daily calcium intake to 1–2 g.[23] The rationale for this is to minimize the vitamin D dose and the daily fluctuation in dietary calcium intake. The logic behind the former is presumably financial (saving on the cost of vitamin D) rather than physiological, since plasma calcium can be modulated successfully by adjusting the vitamin D dosage. The second point – that supplementing the diet will smooth out dietary fluctuations in daily calcium intake – does have more logic. However, there have been no studies comparing the precision of control with and without calcium supplements, and the advantage of taking them remains unproven. Certainly a number of patients treated long term with alfacalcidol in the study of Halabe et al. were able to discontinue calcium supplements without ill effect.[35] Adherence to therapy can be a problem with the prescription of more than one medication to treat the same condition, and irregular consumption of calcium supplements could be worse than taking none. A potential benefit of oral calcium supplements – that of acting as a phosphate binder – has not been explored in the literature.

Biochemical changes on vitamin D treatment

The low bone turnover of hypoparathyroid patients is not affected by vitamin D treatment, so formation and resorption markers remain substantially lower than in controls. The rise in bone turnover seen after the menopause is significantly attenuated in women with treated hypoparathyroidism.[37]

In patients with vitamin D treated hypoparathyroidism, calcium excretion (mmol/litre GF) rises, partly because the filtered load of calcium increases, and partly because the renal leak of calcium resulting from deficient PTH action is not corrected by vitamin D. In pseudohypoparathyroidism the increment in urine calcium is smaller.[38] Serum phosphate levels fall on vitamin D treatment, but remain substantially above normal – typically in the 1.6–1.8 mmol L^{-1} range, when calcium is main-

tained at 2.0–2.2 mmol L^{-1}. This is because vitamin D treatment does not correct the high TmP/GFR resulting from loss of PTH action. Concern over persisting high phosphate levels while plasma calcium is raised with vitamin D has led to some suggestions that phosphate should be lowered with oral phosphate-binding agents, in order to reduce the risk of metastatic calcification. However, there are no long-term data to support the use of phosphate binders in vitamin D-treated hypoparathyroidism.

Because of the high calcium excretion and hyperphosphataemia there have been concerns about the long-term impact of treatment on renal function. One study of eight children and adolescents with hypoparathyroidism or pseudohypoparathyroidism treated with calcitriol for a mean of $4\frac{1}{2}$ years showed ultrasonic evidence of nephrocalcinosis in six (75%). Nephrocalcinosis was more severe in those treated from infancy, but was not related to the duration of treatment. It was most severe in those who used higher calcitriol doses, and these patients also had higher rates of urine calcium excretion and were more likely to have a plasma calcium × plasma phosphate product of >5 molar units. This study is important in that it emphasizes the dangers of overtreatment, particularly in children.[39] In adults, long-term studies using alfacalcidol have shown that if the target levels for plasma calcium are adhered to, then there is no accelerated decline in renal function.[35]

The suggestion has been made that the risk of hypercalciuria may be reduced by the co-prescription of thiazide diuretics,[40] but there are no long-term data supporting their use.

Toxicity due to vitamin D

Hypercalcaemia is the greatest danger to patients treated with vitamin D. As indicated earlier, this may be precipitated by the co-prescription or withdrawal of certain drugs, or by lactation; but often no reason is identified. Patients are more liable to develop hypercalcaemia if they become volume-depleted or if the plasma calcium has been allowed to run in the upper part of the normal range. Detecting the latter is the main point of monitoring plasma calcium on treatment. Hypercalcaemia may present in a disequilibrium phase, of rapidly escalating plasma calcium because of volume depletion and falling GFR. The initial treatment should be with intravenous fluids and withdrawal of vitamin D and calcium supplements. Plasma calcium falls with a half time that varies according to the type of vitamin D

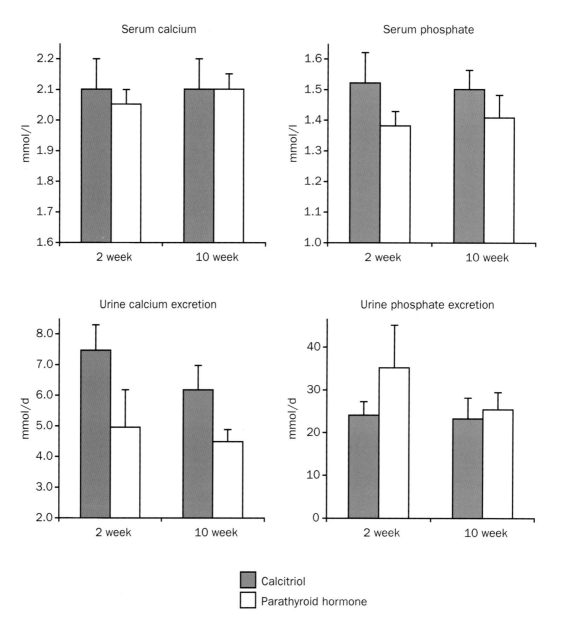

Figure 2.4 Fasting plasma calcium and phosphate and 24-hour urine calcium and phosphate excretion in 10 patients with hypoparathyroidism treated in a cross-over trial with calcitriol and synthetic PTH1-34. With PTH, plasma phosphate was lower, urine phosphate higher, and urine calcium lower.
(Reproduced from Reference 43, with permission.)

used, being shortest for calcitriol and increasing (in order) through alfacalcidol, DHT, calcidiol and ergocalciferol.

Hypercalcaemia can be very prolonged, lasting weeks or months, in patients made toxic through ergocalciferol use, and additional methods of reducing hypercalcaemia have been proposed. These include corticosteroids and intravenous bisphosphonates,[41,42] though the effectiveness of these interventions is debatable. Hypercalcaemia associated with ergocalciferol toxicity is associated with very high plasma ergocalciferol and calcidiol levels, but plasma calcitriol levels are not elevated.

ALTERNATIVE THERAPIES

Parathyroid hormone replacement

PTH replacement is the most logical way of treating hypoparathyroidism. Early efforts using bovine PTH failed because of the development of anti-PTH antibodies, causing resistance. A recent study has described the successful use of biosynthetic PTH 1-34 peptide (the bioactive N-terminal end of the PTH molecule). In one of the very few randomized trials in hypoparathyroidism, 10 adult patients were compared, in a cross-over design, whilst taking either twice daily calcitriol plus calcium or a once daily morning subcutaneous injection of 0.5–3.0 mg/kg per day of PTH 1-34 (Figure 2.4). This single dose, averaging 0.6 mg/kg per day after 10 weeks' treatment, was able to maintain plasma calcium at the lower end of the normal range, comparable to 0.5 mg a day of calcitriol (with calcium). Plasma calcium peaked at around 2.3 mmol L^{-1} some four to ten hours after the PTH 1-34 injection. Plasma phosphate levels were significantly reduced because of increased urine phosphate excretion. Markers of bone turnover also increased.[43] This study demonstrates that PTH replacement therapy using the 1-34 peptide is now feasible. Whether the product will be commercially available and at what cost compared to vitamin D treatment, as well as its long-term safety and acceptability to patients, are as yet unknown. Winer et al.

found that long-term treatment continued for up to two years in a smaller group of patients was without adverse events or loss of efficacy.[43]

Parathyroid gland allotransplantation

Parathyroid gland allotransplantation was considered as a potential treatment for hypoparathyroidism as far back as 1890, but earlier attempts were unsuccessful, presumably because of rejection. The Marburg group have recently attempted allotransplantation of microencapsulated parathyroid cells from ABO-matched donors into two patients with surgical hypoparathyroidism of 2 and 27 years' duration. The cells were passaged and cultured to deplete them of MHC-bearing cells and microencapsulated with sodium alginate. The microencapsulated cells were implanted into the forearm. No immunosuppression was used. In both cases graft function was evident for at least twelve weeks and, although neither patient was able to discontinue vitamin D, the dosage was halved.[44] Possibly vitamin D-independence could have been achieved by transplanting a greater quantity of cells. Although clearly experimental, and requiring considerably more research, this study does demonstrate that allotransplantation may become feasible in the future.

Co-enzyme Q and Kearns–Sayre syndrome

An uncommon association of hypoparathyroidism is with the Kearns–Sayre syndrome. This is a genetic disorder caused by deletions, rearrangements or duplications in mitochondrial DNA. The predominant manifestations of the Kearns–Sayre syndrome are progressive external ophthalmoplegia, and heart block or cardiomyopathy. The defect is believed to be in the enzymes regulating electron transfer in the mitochondrial respiratory chain. Why patients with Kearns–Sayre syndrome (and occasionally other mitochondrial disorders) get hypoparathyroidism is not known.

There are case reports describing beneficial

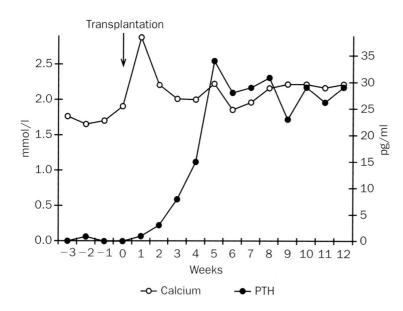

Figure 2.5 Plasma calcium and parathyroid hormone concentrations after allotransplantation of microencapsulated parathyroid cells in a patient with post-surgical hypoparathyroidism. *(Reproduced from Reference 44, with permission.)*

effects of co-enzyme Q10 treatment in some of the mitochondrial myopathies (co-enzyme Q10 transfers electrons on complexes I and II of the respiratory chain to complex III). A curious report from Greece described two patients with Kearns–Sayre syndrome with hypoparathyroidism, who having previously had stable calcaemia for a long period with alfacalcidol, both developed hypercalcaemia within two months of starting co-enzyme Q10 treatment. The patients remained normocalcaemic when alfacalcidol treatment was stopped, but hypocalcaemia returned when co-enzyme Q10 was replaced by placebo.[45] Since this remarkable phenomenon took place without apparent change in plasma PTH the mechanism remains mysterious; but it reminds us there is still much to learn about hypoparathyroidism and its treatment.

REFERENCES

1. Yamashita H, Noguchi S, Tahara K et al. (1997). Postoperative tetany in patients with Graves' disease: a risk factor analysis. *Clin Endocrinol 47:* 71–77.
2. De Santis V, Pintor C, Gamberini MR, Ughi M et al. (1995). Multicentre study on prevalence of endocrine complications in thalassaemia major. *Clin Endocrinol 42:* 581–586.
3. *On line Mendelian Inheritance in Man (OMIM)* (1998). Center for Medical genetics, Johns Hopkins University (Baltimore MD) and National Center for Biotechnology Information, National Library of Medicine (Bethesda, MD). http://www.ncbi.nlm.nih.gov./omim/
4. Bilezikian JP, Thakker RV (1997). Hypoparathyroidism. *Curr Opin Endocrinol Diabet 4:* 427–432.
5. Li Y, Song Y-H, Rais N, Connor E, Schatz D, Muir A, Maclaren N (1996). Autoantibodies to the extracellular domain of the calcium-sensing receptor in patients with acquired hypoparathyroidism. *J Clin Invest 97:* 910–914.
6. Nikiforuk G, Fraser D (1981). The etiology of enamel hypoplasia: a unifying concept. *J Pediatr 98:* 888–893.
7. Pearce SHS, Williamson C, Kifor O, Bai M et al. (1996). A familial syndrome of hypocalcemia with hypercalciuria due to mutations in the calcium-sensing receptor. *New Engl J Med 335:* 1115–1122.
8. Kahky MP, Weber RS (1993). Complications of surgery of the thyroid and parathyroid glands. *Surg Clin North Am 73:* 307–321.
9. Nies C, Sitter H, Zielke A, Bandorski T, Menze J,

Ehlenz K, Rothmund M (1994). Parathyroid function following ligation of the inferior thyroid arteries during bilateral subtotal thyroidectomy. *Br J Surg 81:* 1757–1759.

10. Brunt LM, Sicard GA (1990). Current status of parathyroid autotransplantation. *Semin Surg Oncol 6:* 115–121.

11. Paloyan E, Lawrence AM, Brooks MH, Pickelman JR (1976). Total thyroidectomy and parathyroid autotransplantation for radiation associated cancer. *Surgery 80:* 70–76.

12. Baldo Sierra C, Suárez Nieto C, Núñez Batalla F, Sota Eguizabel E, Pérez Vásquez P (1990). Parathyroid autotransplant in thyroid surgery. *Acta Otorrinolaringol Esp 41:* 239–242.

13. Walker RP, Paloyan E, Kelley TF, Gopalsami C, Jarosz H (1994). Parathyroid autotransplantation in patients undergoing a total thyroidectomy: a review of 261 patients. *Otolaryngol Head & Neck Surg 111:* 258–264.

14. Henry JF, Denizot A, Audiffret J (1990). Obligatory parathyroid autotransplantation in thyroid surgery. *Ann Chir 44:* 378–381.

15. Razack MS, Lore JM, Lippes HA, Schaeffer DP, Rassael H (1977). Total thyroidectomy for Graves' disease. *Head & Neck 19:* 378–383.

16. Hellman P, Skogseid B, Juhlin C, Akerstrom G, Rastad J (1992). Findings and long term results of parathyroid surgery in multiple endocrine neoplasia type 1. *World J Surg 16:* 718–722.

17. Herrera M, Grant C, Van Heerden JA, Fitzpatrick LA (1992). Parathyroid autotransplantation. *Arch Surg 127:* 825–830.

18. Parfitt AM (1989). Surgical, idiopathic and other varieties of parathyroid hormone-deficient hypoparathyroidism. In: *Endocrinology*, ed. LJ De Groot et al., pp. 1059–1061. Saunders, Philadelphia.

19. Daneman D, Kooh SW, Fraser D (1982). Hypoparathyroidism and pseudohypoparathyroidism in childhood. *Clin Endocrinol Metab 11:* 211–231.

20. Porter RH, Cox BG, Heaney D, Hostetter TH, Stinebaugh BJ, Suki WN (1978). Treatment of hypoparathyroid patients with chlorthalidone. *New Engl J Med 298:* 577–581.

21. Okano K, Furukawa Y, Morii H, Fujita T (1982). Comparative efficacy of various vitamin D metabolites in the treatment of various types of hypoparathyroidism. *J Clin Endocrinol Metab 55:* 238–243.

22. Sawicki A (1991). Post operative hypoparathyroidism: long term observation and therapy. *Pol Tyg Lek 46:* 811–813.

23. Fitzpatrick LA, Arnold A (1995). Hypoparathyroidism. In *Endocrinology*, ed. LJ De Groot et al., pp. 1123–1150. Saunders, Philadelphia.

24. Kind HP, Handysides A, Kooh SW, Fraser D (1977). Vitamin D therapy in hypoparathyroidism and pseudohypoparathyroidism: weight-related dosages for initiation of therapy and maintenance therapy. *J Paediatr 91:* 1006–1010.

25. Baskey A, NacNee W (1987). Tetany induced by frusemide in latent hypoparathyroidism. *BMJ 295:* 960–961.

26. Verbeelen D, Fuss M (1979). Hypercalcaemia induced by oestrogen withdrawal in vitamin D-treated hypoparathyroidism. *BMJ 1:* 522–523.

27. Hepburn NC, Abdul-Aziz LA, Whiteoak R (1989). Danazol-induced hypercalcaemia in alphacalcidol-treated hypoparathyroidism. *Postgrad Med J 65:* 849–850.

28. Vardi P, Benderly A, Etziani A, Levy J, Hochberg Z (1985). Hypocalcaemia induced by glucocorticoids in a child with hypoparathyroidism treated with 1α hydroxyvitamin D3. *Eur J Paediatr 144:* 280–282.

29. Walker DA, Davies M (1981). Addison's disease presenting as hypercalcaemic crisis in a patient with idiopathic hypoparathyroidism. *Clin Endocrinol 14:* 419–423.

30. Asherov J, Weinberger A, Pinkhas J (1977). Lack of response to vitamin D therapy in a patient with hypoparathyroidism under anticonvulsant drugs. *Helvet Paediatr Acta 32:* 369–373.

31. Caplan RH, Beguin EA (1990). Hypercalcemia in a calcitriol-treated hypoparathyroid woman during lactation. *Obstet Gynecol 76:* 485–489.

32. Cathebras P, Cartry O, Sassolas G, Rousset H (1996). Hypercalcemia induced by lactation in two patients with treated hypoparathyroidism. *Rev Med Interne 17:* 675–676.

33. Cundy T, Haining SA, Guilland-Cumming DF, Butler J, Kanis JA (1987). Remission of hypoparathyroidism during lactation: evidence for a physiological role for prolactin in the regulation of vitamin D metabolism. *Clin Endocrinol 26:* 667–674.

34. Parfitt AM (1968). A clinical comparison of two preparations of calciferol. *Australas Ann Med 17:* 56–62.

35. Halabe A, Arie R, Mimran D, Samuel R, Liberman UA (1994). Hypoparathyroidism: a long term follow-up experience with 1a vitamin D3 therapy. *Clin Endocrinol 40:* 303–307.

36. Schilling T, Ziegler R (1997). Current therapy of hypoparathyroidism: a survey of German endocrinology centres. *Exp Clin Endocrinol Diabet 105:* 237–241.

37. Fujiyama K, Kiriyama T, Ito M, Nakata K, Yamashita S, Yokoyama N, Nagataki S (1995). Abbreviation of postmenopausal high turnover bone loss in patients with hypoparathyroidism. *J Clin Endocrinol Metab 80:* 2135–2138.

38. Yamamoto M, Takawa Y, Masuko S, Ogata E (1988). Effects of endogenous and exogenous parathyroid hormone on tubular reabsorption of calcium in pseudohypoparathyroidism. *J Clin Endocrinol Metab 66:* 618–624.

39. Weber G, Cazzuffi MA, Frisone F, de Angelis M, Pasolini D, Tomaselli V, Chiumello G (1988–9). Nephrocalcinosis in children and adolescents: sonographic evaluation during long-term treatment with 1,25 dihydroxycholecalciferol. *Child Nephrol Urol 9:* 273–276.

40. Santos F, Smith MJ, Chan JC (1986). Hypercalciuria associated with long-term administration of calcitriol (1,25 dihydroxy vitamin D3). Action of hydrochlorthiazide. *Am J Dis Child 140:* 139–142.

41. Streck WF, Waterhouse C, Haddad JG (1979). Glucocorticoid effects in vitamin D intoxication. *Arch Int Med 139:* 974–977.

42. Rizzoli R, Stoermann C, Ammann P, Bonjour JP (1994). Hypercalcaemia and hyperosteolysis in vitamin D intoxication: effects of clodronate therapy. *Bone 15:* 193–198.

43. Winer KK, Yanovski JA, Cutler GB (1996). Synthetic human parathyroid hormone 1-34 vs calcitriol and calcium in the treatment of hypoparathyroidism. *JAMA 276:* 631–636.

44. Hasse C, Klock G, Schlosser A, Zimmermann OZ, Rothmund M (1997). Parathyroid allotransplantation without immunosuppression. *Lancet 350:* 1296–1297.

45. Papadimitriou A, Hadjigeorgiou GM, Divari R, Papagalonis N, Comi G, Bresolin N (1996). The influence of coenzyme Q10 on total serum calcium concentration in two patients with Kearns–Sayre syndrome and hypoparathyroidism. *Neuromusc Disord 6:* 49–53.

3

Primary Hyperparathyroidism

Reinhardt Ziegler

Introduction • The evaluation and diagnosis of primary hyperparathyroidism • Symptoms
• Indications for parathyroidectomy • Medical management

INTRODUCTION

Primary hyperparathyroidism is a relatively common condition, with an incidence of about 1 : 1000 depending on age. It is one of those diseases that have shown a distinct change in presentation since its original description over 50 years ago. Originally characterized by the features of 'stones, bones and abdominal groans', it gave the impression of an invariably symptomatic disease. Introduction of multi-channel analysers and the development of assays for intact PTH 1-84 showed that mild primary hyperparathyroidism was relatively common and that many patients appear to be asymptomatic.

In clinical practice we have come to separate the condition into two groups that require different approaches to management.[1] There are those with mild (biochemical) primary hyperparathyroidism who appear to have no symptoms and have a benign clinical course without treatment. The remainder have more severe hypercalcaemia, with symptoms that require parathyroidectomy to prevent long-term organ damage. However, debate continues about where the dividing line should be drawn

between these two approaches. It is also uncertain, in view of the recent data relating to late cardiovascular mortality in hyperparathyroidism,[2,3] whether even mild degrees of hyperparathyroidism are entirely benign.

THE EVALUATION AND DIAGNOSIS OF PRIMARY HYPERPARATHYROIDISM

The common causes of hypercalcaemia are shown in Table 3.1; but in both primary and secondary care malignancy and hyperparathyroidism together account for over 90% of cases.[4] The correct diagnosis can be usually established by a detailed history and careful physical examination supplemented by standard laboratory investigations (Table 3.1). In this respect the general availability of assays for intact PTH has greatly facilitated early diagnosis. Although establishment of the diagnosis of primary hyperparathyroidism is well within the competence of the generalist, the evaluation of hyperparathyroidism with respect to the need for surgery needs to be performed by a specialist with experience of this condition.

Table 3.1 Causes and pathogenesis of hypercalcaemia.

	Mechanism	Diagnostic features
Condition		
• primary hyperparathyroidism (pHPT)	increased intestinal Ca-absorption, renal Ca-reabsorption, osteolysis	Ca ↑, PTH ↑
• tertiary hyperparathyroidism	as above	history: sustained secondary hyperparathyroidism, Ca ↑, PTH ↑
• humoral hypercalcaemia of malignancy	secretion of osteolytic factors PTHrP, IL1, IL6, TNF, prostaglandins, calcitriol	evidence of primary tumour tumour markers ↑, PTHrP ↑ calcitriol ↑, PTH ↓
• immobilization with high turnover bone disease in young patients or Paget's disease	calcium release from skeleton due to immobilization	history, X-rays, exclusion of pHPT (PTH ↓)
• thyrotoxicosis	increase in bone turnover	T3 ↑, T4 ↑, TSH ↓, PTH ↓
• adrenal failure, Addison's disease,	lack of a 'PTH-antagonist'	short synacthen test, history, PTH ↓
• acute renal insufficiency	decrease in calcium excretion	history, renal function ↓
• dehydration	as above	history, renal function ↓
• familial hypocalciuric hypercalcaemia	decrease in calciuria due to calcium receptor defect	calciuria ↓, phosphaturia (normal) PTH n or ↑, Ca/creat <0.01
• hard water syndrome (haemodialysis)	calcium influx to ECF	control of dialysate calcium
• sarcoidosis	over-production of calcitriol	chest X-ray, ACE ↑, calcitriol ↑
• tuberculosis, histoplasmosis, leprosy	over-production of calcitriol	chest X-ray, TB isolates, serology, calcitriol ↑
• infantile idiopathic hypercalcaemia	(PTHrP ↑ ?)	age, exclusion of other causes, PTH ↓, PTHrP ↑
Drugs		
• vitamin D intoxication	calcium absorption ↑, osteolysis ↑	history, calcidiol ↑, PTH ↓
• vitamin A intoxication	osteolysis ↑	history
• thiazides (in conditions prone to hypercalcaemia)	calciuria ↓	history
• tamoxifen in metastatic breast cancer	'flare up' due to paradoxical receptor activation	history
• theophylline	?	history

Table 3.2 Symptoms of primary hyperparathyroidism that justify surgery.

Organ	Components of hypercalcaemic syndrome		Structural/functional manifestation
	Disturbance (reversible)	Resulting symptom or complication	
Kidney	Impaired water conservation hypercalciuria, sodium, potassium loss → hypokalaemia	Polyuria, polydipsia, dehydration, muscle weakness, arrhythmia	Nephrolithiasis (recurrent), nephrocalcinosis, oliguria, anuria azotaemia
Intestine	Increased gastric acid secretion, pancreatic enzyme secretion, delayed intestinal transport	Loss of appetite, nausea, vomiting, weight loss, abdominal pain, constipation	Peptic ulcer (recurrent), pancreatitis
Central nervous system	Psychological symptoms, EEG changes	Weakness, tiredness, loss of initiative, depression dizziness, loss of appetite	Somnolence, coma
Musculature	Increase in level of neuromuscular excitability	Muscle weakness	
Cardiovascular system	ECG: shortened QT-interval	Arrhythmia, hypertension	Cardiogenic shock, calcinosis (rare)
Skeleton	Increased bone turnover, negative remodelling balance	Bone pain, fracture	Osteoporosis, ostitis fibrosa cystica
Major joints	Calcification of joint cartilage	Joint pain	Chondrocalcinosis (pseudogout)

SYMPTOMS

General

It is relatively easy to identify the clinical features of hypercalcaemic organ damage, such as renal stones, bone disease or gastrointestinal upset (Table 3.3) that indicate the need for parathyroidectomy. Much more difficult is the evaluation of patients with mild hyperparathyroidism (serum calcium <3 mmol/l) who

appear to be asymptomatic. Merely because many of these patients will be detected by chance through multi-channel analyser screening[5], it does not necessarily follow that they are asymptomatic.

Hypercalcaemia from any cause is often accompanied by non-specific symptoms whose severity tends to be related to the degree of hypercalcaemia. These include loss of appetite, decreased muscle strength and psychological symptoms such as lassitude, fatigue, irritability, deteriorating mood and loss of initiative. What is currently unresolved, but is critical to management decisions, is whether these symptoms are specific to hyperparathyroidism and are reversed by parathyroidectomy.[6]

Bone disease

Overt hyperparathyroid bone disease occurs in <5% of patients, but many will have reduced bone mineral density (BMD).[7] Measurement of BMD by dual energy X-ray absorptiometry (DXA) is an essential part of the evaluation of patients with primary hyperparathyroidism even if they appear entirely asymptomatic. A BMD measurement at spine or hip >2.5 SD below the normal young adult mean (T-score) indicates the presence of osteoporosis (WHO criteria). It indicates that hyperparathyroidism is having a significant impact on the skeleton and is an indication for surgery. Lesser degrees of bone loss (osteopenia) are indications for future monitoring.

Renal involvement

Renal function must be carefully evaluated both biochemically and through imaging. Serum creatinine and urea are essential basic measurements and should be supplemented by estimation of creatinine clearance in the event of any significant degree of impairment. This is needed to provide a baseline for future management. Abdominal radiography may show evidence of renal calculi; but renal ultrasound is more sensitive at assessing the presence of nephrocalcinosis and excluding obstruction.

Cardiovascular disease

The importance of hypertension[8] and cardiac disease[2,3] to long-term survival has been increasingly recognized and must be assessed by standard means (electrocardiography, echocardiography or exercise testing where appropriate). The main concern is that the response to parathyroidectomy is uncertain, and long-term prognosis may be unmodified by surgical treatment.

INDICATIONS FOR PARATHYROIDECTOMY

Since many patients will be asymptomatic, guidelines for parathyroidectomy should include those features that predict long-term organ damage. Unfortunately we do not have the information to predict long-term complications, and the guidelines therefore embody a strong element of pragmatism (Table 3.3)

The level of serum calcium above which surgery should be advised ranges from about 2.85 to 3.0 mmol/l. The upper value may have at least an element of logic, since as the calcium increases above 3 mmol/l there may be a degree of nephrogenic diabetes insipidus, which may predispose to dehydration and disequilibrium hypercalcaemia. An episode of severe hypercalcaemia with renal impairment (even if this is reversible by treatment) is also an indication for parathyroidectomy.

Renal stones that are enlarging or multiplying, nephrocalcinosis or renal impairment are also strong pointers to the need for surgery. A urinary calcium of >10 mmol/24 hours is often included in this category, but its predictive value for future stone formation is poor. More secure indications of end organ damage include parathyroid bone disease or a BMD at hip or spine below a T score of −2.5. Pancreatitis may be a recurrent problem, even at modest degrees of hypercalcaemia, and may respond to restoration of normocalcaemia. Although there is doubt whether parathyroidectomy will prevent long-term cardiovascular morbidity and mortality, their medical management may be easier after hypercalcaemia is corrected.

Finally, patients may express a preference, and some may prefer surgical cure to long-term medical follow-up; and this may be particularly true for the younger patient. Equally, where patients fail to comply with conservative treatment the indication for surgery becomes more persuasive.

Pre-operative assessment

It is essential to control current systemic disease such as angina or hypertension, and to correct

Table 3.3 Indications for parathyroidectomy.

1. Serum calcium	i.	>3 mmol/l. Increased risk of nephrogenic diabetes insipidus and dehydration
	ii.	Single episode of severe disequilibrium hypercalcaemia
2. End organ damage	i.	Parathyroid bone disease or BMD T score below −2.5 at spine or hip
	ii.	Progressive recurrent renal stone disease ± urinary calcium >10 mmol/day
	iii.	Nephrocalcinosis or renal impairment
	iv.	Single episode of acute pancreatitis
	v.	Poor control of hypertension or cardiovascular disease
3. Monitoring	i.	Patient preference to avoid prolonged medical follow-up
	ii.	Young (<50 years) patients with greater lifetime risk of complications
	iii.	Inability or unwillingness to comply with conservative treatment

electrolyte imbalances such as hypokalaemia that may predispose to intra-operative cardiac arrhythmias. It is also important to confirm that renal function is stable and that the patient is well hydrated.

Disequilibrium hypercalcaemia
In most patients with primary hyperparathyroidism the serum calcium is stable with time,[9] but occasional patients are seen pre-operatively where the serum calcium is rising and is unstable. In some instances this may be because the diagnosis of primary hyperparathyroidism is incorrect, while in others the hyperparathyroidism has become destabilized, either by dehydration or through inappropriate medical therapy. Severe dehydration from any cause will lead to disequilibrium hypercalcaemia,[10] because the enhanced proximal tabular reabsorption of calcium (and sodium) cannot be offset as in normal subjects by parathyroid suppression with increased distal tubular excretion of calcium. Occasionally an unstable calcium may be produced by inappropriate drug therapy, such as calcium-containing antacids, particularly if combined with bicarbonate, or thiazide diuretics, which lead to dehydration

and enhanced distal tubular calcium reabsorption. These mechanisms must be corrected pre-operatively by saline rehydration and withdrawal of inappropriate medication.

Severe hypercalcaemia is a life-threatening condition,[11] and may have a diverse pathophysiology (Table 3.4). Although some clues may be observed from the clinical presentation, treatment should be started promptly without waiting for the completion of all investigations. However, since most cases of severe hypercalcaemia will respond to standard emergency treatment the risks from incomplete diagnosis are minimal.

The approach to the treatment of disequilibrium hypercalcaemia is either to increase renal excretion of calcium or to inhibit bone resorption and calcium release from the skeleton. Since nausea and vomiting are early features of severe hypercalcaemia the entry of calcium into the ECF from the gut is of marginal relevance and can be ignored. The exception is the milk alkali syndrome, where the consumption of antacid must be identified and stopped.

Correction of dehydration, which is an invariable feature of disequilibrium hypercalcaemia, is a mandatory first step.[11] Although in

Table 3.4 Measures for symptomatic treatment of hypercalcaemia.*

Type	Measure	Dosage	Specific indication	Mode of action	Side-effects, complications
Increased renal excretion of calcium	Increase oral fluids low in calcium, high in sodium	2 to 3 l/day	universal	restoration GFR†† increase in calcium excretion	limited by nausea or vomiting
	i.v. infusion of saline	4 to 6 l/day	universal	increase in calcium excretion (via natriuresis)	volume over-expansion, hypokalaemia hypomagnesaemia
	furosemide	20 to 500 mg/day	fluid overload	increase in calcium diuresis	hypokalaemia hypomagnesaemia
		100 mg/hr → 24 hrs	(not recommended)		Requires intensive care support to monitor fluid balance
Inhibition of bone resorption	*Bisphosphonates:* • clodronate	300 mg i.v. over 6 to 8 hrs for 2–6 days 400–3200 mg orally for days or weeks	universal (including HHM)[†]	inhibition of osteolysis	renal insufficiency with rapid administration (rarely gastrointestinal complaints)
	• pamidronate	15–90 mg i.v. over 4–6 hrs			as above occasionally feverish reaction
	• ibandronate	2–6 mg i.v. over 2 hrs			(none)
	Calcitonin	200–500 IU/day	weak inhibition of bone resorption	inhibition of osteolysis, promotion of urinary calcium excretion	nausea, vomiting not very effective
'extractive'	haemodialysis	Ca-free dialysate	hypercalcaemic crisis and renal insufficiency	dialysis of calcium from the circulation	dialysis-related
'antiabsorptive'	diet low in Ca and vitamin D	<100 mg Ca/day	universal	decrease in calcium supply and absorption	none
	prednisone	40–100 mg/day	vitamin D intoxication, sarcoidosis (rarely HHM)[†]	decrease in calcium absorption, increase in calciuria	iatrogenic Cushing's syndrome

* Contraindicated during hypercalcaemia: digitalis; hydrochlorothiazides.
† HHM – humoral hypercalcaemia of malignancy.
†† glomerular filtration rate.

the early stages it may be possible to rehydrate the patient with oral fluids, severe hypercalcaemia above 3 mmol/l requires intravenous saline. The usual approach is to give 3–6 litres of a 0.9% saline over the first 24 hours to restore ECF volume and then continue at an infusion rate that maintains a urine output of 2–3 litres per day.[12] Re-expansion of the ECF restores glomerular filtration rate and increases the filtered load of calcium. It also decreases the proximal tubular reabsorption of sodium, to which calcium reabsorption is linked, thereby delivering more calcium for excretion by the distal nephron. Attention must also be paid to the correction of hypokalaemia, which may be caused by associated nausea and vomiting and exacerbated by high urine flow rate and distal tubular sodium–potassium exchange.

Forced calcium diuresis with high-dose frusemide (100 mg per hour) plus high-volume saline infusion (up to 20 litres per 24 hours) has been described, but this requires intensive-care monitoring of ECF volume.[13] The potential of these infusion rates for causing pulmonary oedema in patients with impaired renal function is high, and this technique is unsuitable except for very specialized centres. It should be emphasized in this context that thiazide diuretics are absolutely contraindicated in hypercalcaemia because they reduce calcium excretion.

If rehydration fails to restore a stable serum calcium below 3 mmol/l then intravenous bisphosphonates should be given to inhibit bone resorption. Their excellent safety profile, particularly in relation to the risks of uncontrolled severe hypercalcaemia, allows their use irrespective of the cause of the hypercalcaemia.

The agents of first choice are pamidronate (15–90 mg over 4–6 hours), or ibandronate (2–6 mg over 2 hours), which are powerful osteoclast inhibitors producing rapid decreases in serum calcium with few side-effects.[14] Clodronate is less potent, and larger doses have to be given (300 mg over 6–8 hours repeated daily 2–6 times) but it has the potential for oral maintenance therapy. The first-generation bisphosphonate, etidronate, has been superseded by the more potent compounds. Amino-bisphosphonates may cause an acute phase

response with a febrile reaction, but this resolves spontaneously over a few days and does not recur with subsequent treatment. Repeated doses of pamidronate and ibandronate can be given after 72 hours if the serum calcium remains above 3 mmol/l but this is an unusual circumstance with currently presenting primary hyperparathyroidism.

Calcitonin has been replaced by the bisphosphonates as osteoclast inhibitors, but it may be used to inhibit distal renal tubular reabsorption of calcium. This may have an additive effect to that of the bisphosphonates in malignant hypercalcaemia,[15,16] but little additional benefit in primary hyperparathyroidism.

Haemodialysis against a calcium-free dialysate is the treatment of choice for severe hypercalcaemia (>4 mmol/l), which is usually accompanied by renal failure. These patients tend to be somnolent or comatose, with circulatory failure and the severe renal impairment limits the ability to promote a calcium diuresis. Removing calcium from the circulation by haemodialysis may improve both the clinical state and renal function within a period of hours. It should be combined with bisphosphonate therapy to inhibit skeletal calcium efflux. Doses should be reduced, because renal impairment will raise bisphosphonate concentrations, with the potential for further renal toxicity.

By the time treatment has restored a safe, stable level of hypercalcaemia the diagnosis of primary hyperparathyroidism should have been confirmed, and urgent parathyroidectomy can then be performed.

Parathyroid bone disease
A reduced bone mineral density is a common feature of all grades of primary hyperparathyroidism.[7] However, it is also important to identify those patients with a high pre-operative rate of bone turnover who are particularly at risk of post-operative hypocalcaemia (the hungry bone syndrome).

Bone turnover markers are commonly elevated in primary hyperparathyroidism but in terms of predicting those at risk of the hungry bone syndrome the total or bone-specific alkaline phosphatase has sufficient specificity and sensitivity. In those identified as being at risk, there is a choice between treating pre-operatively or immediately post-operatively. Treatment with hydroxylated metabolites of vitamin D pre-operatively runs the risk of worsening hypercalcaemia, thus delaying surgery, and does not always prevent post-operative hypocalcaemia. Awareness of the potential problem of the hungry bone syndrome means that appropriate treatment can be introduced early in the post-operative phase.

Patients with tertiary hyperparathyroidism due to active osteomalacia rarely present with hypercalcaemia of sufficient severity to warrant immediate surgery because it is offset by the vitamin D deficiency. Such patients should receive cautious vitamin D therapy but the serum calcium will rise as the osteomalacia heals, at which point parathyroidectomy should proceed according to the criteria already described.

Pre-operative localization of parathyroid tissue
A number of non-invasive techniques have been introduced for the pre-operative localization of parathyroid tissue. All have to be judged against the ability of the experienced surgeon, who will be able to localize the abnormal gland(s) in >90% of patients who have not previously had surgery.[17] Pre-operative localization with currently available techniques is effective in 60–75% of patients, but does not reduce failure rate or operating time. Since these techniques are expensive there is little to justify their use in first-time parathyroidectomy. Ultrasound might be an exception, because it is relatively inexpensive, but its success rate is very operator-dependent. It is not suitable for localizing retrosternal adenomas, nor does it perform well with multiple adenomas or hyperplasia. It does, however, identify thyroid pathology, which might cause confusion at operation or require treatment in its own right.

The situation is different in second neck explorations where ultrasound, thallium-technetium or [99mTc]-sestamibi scanning, CT and MRI have been employed. Overall there is probably little to choose between any of these methods and usage depends on local availability and expertise. In our centre the sequence of investigation of in-patients with persistent or recurrent primary hyperparathyroidism is to use imaging followed, if necessary, by PTH sampling from venous catheterization. The first stage is to perform CT or MRI of the thyroid/parathyroid area, including the anterior and posterior mediastinum. These techniques are particularly useful at identifying parathyroid tissue in ectopic localizations, which is one of the commonest causes of failed parathyroidectomy. MRI has a similar overall sensitivity of about 60%, but has the advantages that it has better tissue contrast than CT and is more helpful in separating adenomas from lymph nodes or blood vessels.

Radionucleotide scanning with thallium-technetium is tending to be replaced by [99mTc]-sestamibi as an alternative.[18] Sestamibi is taken up by both thyroid and parathyroid glands, but persists for longer in the latter site. Separation can be achieved using either single isotope kinetics or with dual isotope ([123I]–[99mTc]) subtraction scanning and this latter technique may be capable of detecting hyperplasia.[19] A recent review of radionucleotide scanning found that the technique detected 87% of solitary adenomas but only 55% of surgically proven multigland disease.[20] However, of much greater clinical significance was the ability to detect 75% of persistent or recurrent lesions in patients who had had a previous neck exploration.

Where the technology is available, intact PTH assays from 15–20 venous samples from the thyroid/parathyroid area, approached from iliac vein catheterization, are very sensitive at identifying small tumours not visible on CT or MRI. The recent demonstration that rapid intra-operative PTH measurements allow localization and confirmation of excision of hyperfunctioning parathyroid tissue awaits confirmation and general availability of the assay methodology.[21]

Surgical treatment

It is essential that parathyroidectomy is performed by an experienced endocrine surgeon.[22,23] A recent survey showed that specialist surgeons compared to non-specialists had significantly lower complication rates after primary surgery (1.0 vs 1.9%), with lower re-operation rates (1.5 vs 3.8) and lower in-hospital mortality (0.04 vs 1.0%). Overall the cure rate for first-time operations was 95.2% and for re-exploration was 82.7%. Even amongst specialist surgeons the outcome related to experience.[24]

The usual procedure is to explore the site identified by any pre-operative localization technique and then examine the site of the other three glands. If an adenoma is identified there is an 80% probability that it is single, and extensive exploration is unnecessary if one or two normal glands are identified. Around 5% of parathyroid glands may be ectopic and, apart from investigating the presence of abnormal vessels, usually from the inferior thyroid artery, that might supply a retrosternal adenoma, extensive exploration for ectopic tissue is unnecessary.

A modification of this approach is to identify an adenoma, and then to explore only that side of the neck for the second gland. If it is normal the other side is not examined[25] but most experienced surgeons will feel that the benefits of bilateral exploration outweigh the negligible risk. Unilateral neck exploration may be a viable option where there is the availability of a radiologist experienced in parathyroid ultrasound. Removal of an ultrasound identified adenoma in the presence of an ipsilateral normal gland had a lower complication rate, mainly as a result of decreased operation time and avoided post-operative hypocalcaemia and contralateral neck scarring.[26] In this particular study 93% of the adenomas were unilateral, but 40% of the patients had a bilateral exploration, either because an ipsilateral normal gland was not identified or because there was a question of hyperplasia.

If two or more adenomas are identified there should be extensive neck exploration on the presumption of a fourth abnormal gland. There may be considerable difficulty in distinguishing between multiple adenomata and hyperplasia, and this may not always be resolved by the subsequent histopathology.[27] It is for these reasons that parathyroidectomy should only be performed by specialist centres with access to skilled radiology, surgeons and pathologists.

In cases of primary four-gland disease, which is often found in familial primary hyperparathyroidism or in the multiple endocrine neoplasia syndrome, there are two management options. One is a $\frac{7}{8}$ resection, which means that three glands are removed in their entirety and a small portion of the remaining gland is left *in situ*. This can be marked with a clip or suture for later identification in case of recurrence. The other option is the removal of all enlarged glands, the smallest of which is cut into 1 mm cubes, which are then implanted in the muscles of the forearm or thigh. This technique of auto-transplantation is particularly useful in secondary or tertiary hyperparathyroidism due to chronic renal insufficiency. Part of the tissue may be deep-frozen and conserved in case the auto-transplantation is unsuccessful, so that reimplantation can then be performed.[28] There needs to be some reservation about auto-transplantation because the tissue may resume autonomous growth, leading to recurrent hyperparathyroidism, although re-exploration of the transplant site is easier than a second neck exploration.

It has been suggested that the percutaneous installation of alcohol under local anaesthetic into parathyroid adenomas under ultrasound control may be an alternative to removal in patients who are frail and a poor operative risk.[29] The problems with this approach are that parathyroid histology is unavailable, the procedure needs to be repeated several times until all the abnormal tissue is destroyed and the installation may be painful. The long-term results of this technique, particularly with respect to the recurrent laryngeal nerves, are unknown, and it cannot be recommended at the present time.

Another innovation is minimally invasive surgery for primary hyperparathyroidism. This is performed through a 1–2 cm transverse incision after localization of a single adenoma by ultrasound combined with CT imaging.[30] This procedure was successful in 60 out of 66 cases but it is too early to know whether this should be added to current surgical practice.

Post-operative management

Removal of a single adenoma in a specialist centre has a low morbidity and mortality.[24] The main problems are treatment failure, hypoparathyroidism and recurrent laryngeal nerve damage, with the last having an incidence of <1% in experienced hands.

Treatment failure is very dependent on surgical experience, but is also influenced by the type of hyperparathyroidism. Patients with multiple adenomata or hyperplasia have an overall relapse rate of about 10%, while the familial syndromes may have an immediate failure rate of 13% and a late relapse rate of 29%. However, after the removal of a single adenoma only 3% of patients can be expected to relapse over the next 9 years;[31] but this does emphasize the importance of an annual check of serum calcium after parathyroidectomy.

Immediately post-operatively there may be a transient phase of mild hypocalcaemia, which does not require treatment, as the normal, but suppressed, glands regain their calcium sensitivity. Permanent hypoparathyroidism is unusual,[32] but extensive neck exploration for an elusive adenoma may disturb the function of the remaining parathyroid glands for a short period of days or weeks, and this will require calcium and vitamin D therapy as detailed below. Permanent hypoparathyroidism is a rare event (<2% of cases), but this will require long-term supplementation (Chapter 2).

If overt hyperparathyroid bone disease was present pre-operatively or bone turnover markers such as alkaline phosphatase were elevated, there may be a prolonged, but ultimately reversible, phase of hypocalcaemia (hungry bone syndrome). This is partially due to the immediate decline in bone resorption due to correction of PTH excess, coupled with persis-

tence of bone formation due to the longer life-span (approximately 12 weeks) of the pre-operative osteoblast population. Bone gain after parathyroid surgery may continue over a period of 2–4 years,[33] with improvements of around 12% in trabecular bone at the lumbar spine as well as gains at the femoral neck. Symptomatic hypocalcaemia, particularly tetanic contractions of the hands and feet with circumoral paraesthesiae, may develop within days of parathyroidectomy and may last for weeks or even for 2–3 months. All patients should have a daily serum calcium estimation after parathyroidectomy but it is those high-risk patients with parathyroid bone disease that require calcium and vitamin D supplementation as soon as the serum calcium reaches the lower part of the normal range.

Very few of these patients will be adequately controlled by calcium supplements alone, and they should be given calcitriol 1–2 mcg daily to maintain gastrointestinal calcium absorption. Calcitriol is the preparation of choice because it acts directly, without the need for further metabolism within the body. It also has a rapid onset of action and a short half life, giving a good margin of safety from toxicity. Tetanic symptoms will require bolus injections of calcium gluconate (10 ml of a 10% solution) or, if severe, a continuous infusion of 100 ml of 10% calcium gluconate (22 mmol) over 24 hours. All calcium solutions are thrombophlebitic and must be infused into large veins. Once the initial tetanic spasms are controlled, calcium supplementation can be switched to the oral route (calcium lactate gluconate/calcium carbonate: Sandocal 400 mg (10 mmol) three times daily).

In patients with a low bone mass corresponding to the WHO criteria of osteoporosis (T score at either lumbar spine or hip below -2.5 SD) there is the option of waiting and measuring post-operative skeletal recovery or intervening early with antiresorptive therapy. In post-menopausal women there is the relatively easy option of hormone replacement therapy, which has been shown to improve BMD in untreated primary hyperparathyroidism.[34] Where there is uncertainty or resistance to early post-operative intervention, an

---

Table 3.5 Monitoring programme for patients with asymptomatic primary hyperparathyroidism (modified according to Consensus Development Conference Panel, 1991).[37]

Control measures (for all cases, with and without new symptoms)

- blood pressure (monthly)
- ECG (annually), echocardiography, ETT if indicated
- serum calcium (six-monthly)
- serum creatinine, creatinine-clearance
- abdominal radiograph or ultrasound
- 24-hour urinary calcium (selected cases)
- bone mass measurement (every 1 to 2 years)
- assessment of neuromuscular weakness, depression, symptoms related to skeletal, gastrointestinal, and renal systems (6 months)

Reasons for switching from observation to surgery

- development of typical parathyroid-related symptoms (skeletal, renal, gastrointestinal, neuromuscular, psychological)
- poor control of hypertension or cardiac disease
- sustained increase in serum calcium greater than 0.25 mmol/l
- substantial decline in renal function; nephrolithiasis; increase in hypercalciuria
- substantial decline in bone mass
- inability or unwillingness to continue under medical supervision

---

alternative is to measure the gain in BMD at 12 months and advise treatment based on the response and other risk factors for osteoporotic fracture. These patients should be treated in the conventional manner as described in Chapter 9.

Providing there is no urinary obstruction the treatment of renal caculi complicating primary hyperparathyroidism can be left until after parathyroidectomy. Treatment is along conventional lines, and the risk of recurrence after successful parathyroidectomy is low. However, idiopathic renal stone disease is a more common condition than primary hyperparathyroidism, and these conditions may co-exist in the same patient, so that the stone disease will have to be treated independently.[35] Nephrocalcinosis complicating primary hyperparathyroidism has a poorer prognosis, and kidney dysfunction often continues to deteriorate despite successful parathyroidectomy.

Only a minority of patients will experience stable renal function.[36]

MEDICAL MANAGEMENT

For the patient in whom a thorough evaluation has clearly defined 'mild asymptomatic' primary hyperparathyroidism (serum calcium <3 mmol/l) conservative management may be appropriate.[37] This should follow well-defined guidelines, with particular emphasis on a number of specific issues (Table 3.5). A prerequisite for this approach is that the patient should be prepared to accept regular monitoring at approximately six-monthly intervals. It is also appropriate to discuss at the outset the circumstances under which this approach would be abandoned in favour of parathyroidectomy.

General measures

It seems reasonable to avoid a very high dietary calcium intake, although the evidence that this has long-term clinical benefit is unavailable. Similarly, a low-calcium diet should be avoided, because the parathyroids continue to regulate secretion around the new (higher) set point and will increase secretion in the face of calcium deficiency. Although feedback inhibition of calcitriol on PTH secretion has been utilized in the secondary hyperparathyroidism of chronic renal failure (Chapter 6), there is little evidence for its use in primary hyperparathyroidism.

The recent reports that, despite parathyroidectomy, there is an increase in late cardiovascular deaths[2] have emphasized the need to identify and treat cardiovascular risk factors. Routine investigations should include electrocardiography and echocardiography. Hypertension and ischaemic heart disease should be adequately treated, but thiazide diuretics should be avoided because of their potential for exacerbating hypercalcaemia.[4]

Patients should be warned of the risks of dehydration and advised to increase their fluid intake in the appropriate circumstances. They should also be advised to seek prompt medical help for illnesses that carry a risk of diarrhoea or vomiting.

Regular assessment of renal function is important both for the maintenance of stable calcium and also because deterioration is a reason for abandoning conservative treatment in favour of surgery. Abdominal ultrasound is more sensitive than plain radiography for detecting and monitoring the presence of nephrocalcinosis. The frequency of repeat examinations would depend on the results of the initial evaluation. In the absence of any initial abnormality our practice would be to repeat this at intervals of 2–3 years.

Skeletal monitoring

An important requirement for conservative management is the absence of significant parathyroid bone disease, and this assessment must include measurement of BMD by DXA. In mild primary hyperparathyroidism the rate of bone loss at the spine, hip and distal radius appears to be appropriate for age, without evidence of any increase.[9] Since most of these patients will be in the osteopenic range of BMD (T scores between -1 and -2.5 SD) they require monitoring at about two yearly intervals to exclude more rapid rates of loss. If this is detected it should not be assumed to be due to hyperparathyroidism, but carefully investigated to exclude other conditions that might require treatment in their own right.

Hormone replacement therapy should be given serious consideration in postmenopausal women with primary hyperparathyroidism, because of its effect of reducing PTH-mediated bone resorption. Serum calcium may show a modest fall, and although PTH and serum phosphate are usually unchanged bone mineral density may increase slightly.[34,38] These patients should be monitored within a specialist clinic.

The place of currently available bisphosphonates in the maintenance of BMD is under investigation. They do not seem to have a role in the long-term reduction in the degree of hypercalcaemia. Oral or intravenous phosphate will reduce the serum calcium, and was used for the treatment of severe hypercalcaemia before the advent of the bisphosphonates. It does not have a place in the conservative management of hyperparathyroidism because of the risk of soft tissue (particularly renal) calcification due to an increase in the calcium-phosphate product.

More specific therapy to lower the serum calcium may be available in the future by targeting the extracellular calcium receptor of the parathyroid cell. Clinical trials are in progress with calcimimetic agents that act as agonists at the PTH calcium receptor to suppress PTH secretion.[39,40]

Although current evidence supports the view that patients with mild primary hyperparathyroidism do well with conservative management, it has to be recognized that they are a highly selected group.[22] The length of follow-up is also relatively short, and there is the concern that, even after parathyroidectomy, there may be an increase in cardiovascular mortality.[2]

Special conditions

Pregnancy

Untreated primary hyperparathyroidism is an unusual problem in pregnancy, but carries an increased risk to both the mother and child. A young woman with asymptomatic primary hyperparathyroidism who plans to become pregnant should be treated surgically prior to conception. Hyperparathyroidism diagnosed during the first two trimesters should be managed conservatively, with particular attention to the maintenance of hydration, the avoidance of a high-calcium diet and withdrawal of drugs such as thiazides. If severe hypercalcaemia is present then parathyroidectomy should be planned for the end of the second trimester.[41] If the diagnosis is made in late pregnancy and the condition is not too severe then operation should be postponed until after delivery. At birth the baby may develop tetany as a result of parathyroid suppression caused by the maternal hypercalcaemia. Calcium supplementation, either intravenous or oral, may be needed to control symptomatic hypocalcaemia. The problem can be expected to resolve spontaneously over a 2–3 week period.

Familial hypocalciuric hypercalcaemia (FHH)

This condition is caused by an inherited defect in the calcium receptor of the parathyroid cell that raises the set point about which the serum calcium is regulated. Most patients with this condition experience a benign course, and parathyroidectomy neither reduces the serum calcium nor brings clinical benefit.[42] It is important to make the diagnosis and screen family members in order to avoid unnecessary parathyroid surgery. In rare situations there is an indication for total parathyroidectomy:

1. The double dose of FHH gene may lead to severe neonatal hyperparathyroidism.
2. An adult with relapsing pancreatitis.
3. An adult or child with severe hypercalcaemia (>3.5 mmol/l).

Multiple endocrine neoplasia (MEN)

In MEN Type I (parathyroid, anterior pituitary and pancreatic tumours) primary hyperparathyroidism is the commonest clinical manifestation, often presenting at an earlier age than sporadic primary hyperparathyroidism.[43] Parathyroidectomy is the only definitive form of treatment, and the indications are the same as those for spontaneous primary hyperparathyroidism. MEN I is usually a multigland disorder, and resection of <3½ glands is likely to be followed by relapse of the hyperparathyroidism.[44] All these patients should be managed in a specialist centre.

In MEN Type II (medullary carcinoma of the thyroid, bilateral phaeochromocytoma, and parathyroid hyperplasia) primary hyperparathyroidism is seen histologically in 50% of cases, but owing to its milder course is only clinically relevant in 10% of patients. Although the basic lesion is hyperplasia the glands may vary in size, giving a misleading impression of an adenoma. Treatment should be in a specialist centre, and is the same as that for MEN Type I.[44]

Parathyroid carcinoma

This condition will often be diagnosed either at or following parathyroidectomy, where local invasion will be seen at operation and confirmed histologically. Treatment is by wide local excision (hemithyroidectomy), which may need to be repeated for local recurrence.[45] Metastases may be slow-growing and may be worth resecting, depending on their site. Bisphosphonates may be useful to reduce hypercalcaemia in the early stages, but advanced disease is usually refractory. Radiotherapy is useful palliation of painful metastases. Calcimimetic drugs may reduce the hypercalcaemia[40] and there is an isolated case report of a beneficial response to calcitriol,[46] which would however require close biochemical monitoring to avoid worsening hypercalcaemia.

REFERENCES

1. Posen S, Clifton-Bligh P, Reeves TS et al (1985). Is parathyroidectomy of benefit in primary hyperparathyroidism? *Q J Med 54*: 241–246.

2. Hedbäck G, Odén A (1998). Increased risk of death from primary hyperparathyroidism – an update. *Eur J Clin Invest 28*: 271–276.

3. Wermers RA, Sundeep K, Atkinson EJ et al. (1998). Survival after the diagnosis of hyperparathyroidism: a population-based study. *Am J Med 104*: 115–122.

4. Christenson T, Hellstrom K, Wengle B et al. (1976). Prevalence of hypercalcemia in a health screening in Stockholm. *Acta Med Scand 200*: 131–137.

5. Mundy GR, Cove DH, Fisken R (1980). Primary hyperparathyroidism: changes in the pattern of clinical presentation. *Lancet 1*: 1317–1320.

6. Kleerekoper M, Bilezikian JP (1994). Parathyroidectomy for non traditional features of primary hyperparathyroidism. *Am J Med 96*: 99–100.

7. Abdelhadi M, Nordenstrom J (1998). Bone mineral recovery after parathyroidectomy in patients with primary and renal hyperparathyroidism. *J Clin Endocrinol Metab 83*: 3845–3851.

8. Sancho JJ, Rouco J, Riera-Vidal R, Sitges-Serra A (1992). Long-term effects of parathyroidectomy for primary hyperparathyroidism on arterial hypertension. *World J Surg 16*: 732–736.

9. Parfitt AM, Rao DS, Kleerekoper M (1991). Asymptomatic primary hyperparathyroidism discovered by multi-channel biochemical screening: clinical course and considerations bearing on the need for surgical intervention. *J Bone Miner Res 6*(suppl 2): S97–S101.

10. Parfitt AM (1979). Equilibrium and disequilibrium hypercalcaemia: new light on an old concept. *Metab Bone Dis Rel Res 1*: 279–293.

11. Bilezikian JP (1992). Management of acute hypercalcaemia. *New Engl J Med 326*: 1196–1203.

12. Hosking DJ, Cowley A, Bucknall CA (1981). Rehydration in the treatment of severe hypercalcaemia. *Q J Med 50*: 473–481.

13. Suki WN, Yium JJ, von Minden M et al. (1970). Acute treatment of hypercalcemia with furosemide. *New Engl J Med 382*: 836–842.

14. Fleisch H (1997). *Bisphosphonates in bone disease*, 3rd edn, pp. 86–111, The Parthenon Publ. Group, New York and London.

15. Ralston SH, Gardner MD, Dryburgh FJ, Jenkins AS, Cowan RA, Boyle IT (1985). Comparison of aminohydroxypropylidene diphosphate, mithramycin, and corticosteroids/calcitonin in treatment of cancer-associated hypercalcaemia. *Lancet 2*: 907–910.

16. Hosking DJ, Gilson D (1984). Comparison of the renal and skeletal action of calcitonin in the treatment of severe hypercalcaemia of malignancy. *Q J Med 53*: 359–368.

17. Doppman JL, Miller DL (1991). Localisation of parathyroid tumours in patients with asymptomatic hyperparathyroidism and no previous surgery. *J Bone Miner Res 6*(suppl 2): S153–S158.

18. Ishibashi M, Nishida H, Okuda S et al. (1998). Localization of parathyroid glands in hemodialysis patients using Tc-99m sestamibi imaging. *Nephron 78*: 48–53.

19. Neumann DR, Esselstyn CBJR, Madera A, Wong CO, Lieber M (1998). Parathyroid detection in secondary hyperparathyroidism with $^{123}I/^{99m}Tc$-sestamibi subtraction single photon emission computed tomography. *J Clin Endocrinol Metab 83*: 3867–3871.

20. Pattou F, Hugo D, Proye C (1998). Radionucleide scanning in parathyroid diseases. *Br J Surg 85*: 1605–1616.

21. Patel PC, Pellitteri PK, Patel NM, Fleetwood MK (1998). Use of rapid intra-operative parathyroid hormone assay in the surgical management of parathyroid disease. *Arch Otolaryngol Head Neck Surg 124*: 559–562.

22. Bilezikian JP (1996). Primary hyperparathyroidism. In: *Primer on the metabolic bone diseases and disorders of mineral metabolism*, ed. MJ Favus, 3rd edn, pp. 181–186. Lippincott-Raven, Philadelphia and New York.

23. Grey AB (1997). The skeletal effects of primary hyperparathyroidism. *Baillière's Clin Endocrin Metab 11*: 101–116.

24. Sosa JA, Powe NR, Levine MA, Udelsman R, Zeigler MA (1998). Profile of clinical practice: threshold for surgery and surgical outcomes for patients with primary hyperparathyroidism: a national survey of endocrine surgeons. *J Clin Endocrinol Metab 83*: 2658–2665.

25. Russell CFJ (1992). Unilateral parathyroid exploration. *Br J Surg 79*: 861–862.

26. Vogel LM, Lucas R, Czako P (1998). Unilateral parathyroid exploration. *Am Surg 64*: 693–696.

27. Dietel M (1982). *Functional morphology and pathology of parathyroid glands*. Fischer, Stuttgart, 1982.

28. Rothmund M (1991). Chirurgische Therapie des primären Hyperparathyreoidismus. In: *Hyperparathyreoidismus*, ed. M Rothmund, pp. 101–119. Thieme, Stuttgart and New York.

29. Bennedbaek FN, Karstrup S, Hegedüs L (1997). Percutaneous ethanol injection therapy in the treatment of thyroid and parathyroid diseases. *Eur J Endocrin 136*: 240–250.

30. van Vroonhoven RJMV, van Dalen A (1998). Successful minimally invasive surgery in primary hyperparathyroidism after combined preoperative ultrasound and computed tomography imaging. *J Int Med 243*: 581–587.

31. Rudberg C, Akerström G, Palmer M et al. (1986). Late results of operation for primary hyperparathyroidism in 441 patients. *Surgery 99*: 643–651.

32. Brasier AR, Wang C, Nussbaum SR (1988). Recovery of parathyroid hormone secretion after parathyroid adenomectomy. *J Clin Endocrinol Metab 61*: 495–500.

33. Silverberg SJ, Gartenberg F, Jacobs TP et al. (1995). Increased bone mineral density after parathyroidectomy in primary hyperparathyroidism. *J Clin Endocrin Metab 80*: 729–734.

34. Grey AB, Stapleton JP, Evans MC, Reid IR (1995). Accelerated bone loss in postmenopausal women with primary hyperparathyroidism. *J Clin Endocrin Metab 44*: 697–702.

35. Niederle B, Roka R, Fritsch A (1986). Long-term results after surgical treatment of primary hyperparathyroidism. In: Parathyroid Surgery, *Progr Surg* eds M Rothmund, SA Wells, *18*: 146–164.

36. Dixon J, Smith JF (1981). Progressive renal failure in surgically treated hyperparathyroidism. *J Clin Pathol 34*: 730–737.

37. Consensus Development Conference Panel (1991). Diagnosis and management of asymptomatic primary hyperparathyroidism: Consensus Development Conference Statement. *Ann Int Med 114*: 593–597.

38. Selby PL, Peacock M (1986). Ethinyl estradiol and norethindrone in the treatment of primary hyperparathyroidism in postmenopausal women. *New Engl J Med 314*: 1481–1485.

39. Ott SM (1998). Calcimimetics – new drugs with the potential to control hyperparathyroidism. *J Clin Endocrinol Metab 83*: 1080–1082.

40. Collins MR, Skarulis MC, Bilezikian JP et al. (1998). Treatment of hypercalcaemia secondary to parathyroid carcinoma with a novel calcimimetic agent. *J Clin Endocrinol Metab 83*: 1083–1088.

41. Ziegler R (1987). Erkrankungen der Nebenschilddrüsen. In: *Internistische Erkrankungen und Schwangerschaft*, ed. H Huchzermeyer, Vol. 2, pp. 52–70. Kohlhammer, Stuttgart, Berlin, Köln and Mainz.

42. Marx SJ (1996). Familial hypocalciuric hypercalcemia. In: *Primer on the metabolic bone diseases and disorders of mineral metabolism*, ed. MJ Favus, 3rd edn, pp. 190–192, Lippincott-Raven, Philadelphia and New York.

43. Burgess JR, Greenaway TM, Shepherd JJ (1998). Expression of the MEN-1 gene in a large kindred with multiple endocrine neoplasia type 1. *J Int Med 243*: 465–470.

44. Heath H, Hobbs MR (1996). Familial hyperparathyroid syndromes. In: *Primer on the metabolic bone diseases and disorders of mineral metabolism*, ed. MJ Favus, 3rd edn, pp. 187–189, Lippincott-Raven, Philadelphia and New York.

45. Vetto JT, Brennan MF, Woodruf J, Burt M (1993). Parathyroid carcinoma: diagnosis and clinical history. *Surgery 114*: 882–892.

46. Palmieri-Sevier A, Palmieri GMA, Baumgartner CJ, Britt LG (1993). Case report: long-term remission of parathyroid cancer: possible relation to vitamin D and calcitriol therapy. *Am J Med Sci 306*: 309–312.

4

Bone Disease and Malignancy

Henry Bone

Overview • Hypercalcaemia of malignancy • Skeletal metastases • Multiple myeloma
• Osteoporosis secondary to the treatment of malignancy • Summary

OVERVIEW

Malignant disease can affect the skeleton systemically or locally. Hypercalcaemia of malignancy generally causes multi-systemic effects, such as depression of consciousness, nausea and extracellular volume depletion. Metastases to the skeleton may result in local pain, fracture or other complications. Patients with myeloma may suffer from either lytic lesions or generalized osteoporosis as well as from hypercalcaemia. Furthermore, patients with malignant diseases may suffer from osteoporosis as a consequence of their treatment. In rare cases, malignancy may cause renal phosphate wasting and oncogenic osteomalacia.

Biology of tumour–osteoclast interactions

The skeletal complications of malignancy are principally mediated by the interaction of tumour cells with osteoclasts through either local or systemic biochemical signals. The osteoclast is a giant cell that is differentiated to resorb bone and is characterized by its 'ruffled border' and the presence of calcitonin receptors.

In the space under the ruffled border, between the cell body and the bone mineral surface, the osteoclast secretes acid in order to dissolve bone mineral; proteolytic enzymes then digest the matrix that remains. Osteoclasts are either directly responsive to cytokines and growth factors or indirectly regulated by cells of the osteoblast lineage. These cells respond to modulators such as parathyroid hormone through the activation of cell surface receptors. Osteoclasts, even when highly stimulated in primary or secondary hyperparathyroidism, do not respond to direct application of PTH.[1] However, when osteoblasts are also present, the indirect stimulatory effects of parathyroid hormone on osteoclast activity are quite apparent.[2] This indirect regulatory process is important in normal physiology, and is commonly involved in the pathogenesis of bone disease in malignancy. Of the systemically acting factors that are important in cancer patients, the most commonly found, and best characterized, is parathyroid hormone-related peptide (PTHrP), which acts through the PTH receptor on osteoblasts and is frequently elevated in patients with humoral hypercalcaemia of malignancy.[3] Osteoclasts can also be indirectly stimulated to resorb bone by the effects of 1,25-dihydroxyvitamin D,[4] again acting through an effect on osteoblasts. Cytokines are locally acting factors, which appear to be responsible for osteolysis at the margins of bone tumours. A number of cytokines have been identified that can, in the presence of osteoblasts, stimulate osteoclastic osteolysis. These include the interleukins, tumour necrosis factors alpha and beta and the prostaglandins.[5–7] Any or several of these may play a role in the development of metastases, and there may be as yet other undiscovered substances responsible for this activity. The exact nature and roles of the biochemical messengers secreted by the osteoblasts to stimulate osteoclasts are not fully characterized.

Drugs that suppress tumour-induced osteoclastic activity

Calcitonin, a naturally occurring peptide hormone for which osteoclasts have specific receptors, acts by suppressing resorbing activity, but also increases renal calcium excretion. Due to these effects it has a role in the treatment of hypercalcaemia,[8] but it has not been useful in controlling the spread of metastases.

Bisphosponates are pyrophosphate analogues that suppress osteoclast activity[9] and have proved to be very effective in controlling hypercalcaemia. Bisphosphonates adhere to the exposed bone mineral, particularly at sites of bone resorption such as the perimeter of lytic lesions. Although tightly adherent to exposed mineral, the bisphosphonate may be released at the low pH encountered under the ruffled border of the osteoclast and then ingested by the cell. This results in a shift towards apoptosis, and in the case of many nitrogen-containing bisphosphonates also inhibits the normal prenylation of structural proteins[10,11] interfering with the ability of osteoclasts to form the ruffled border and secrete acid. Thus bisphosphonates reliably inhibit the resorption of bone by osteoclasts but they may have additional benefits. A number of bisphosphonates have been successfully employed in the treatment and prevention of osteolytic metastases through their ability to inhibit further invasion of adjacent normal bone. Clodronate and pamidronate have found the greatest use in this application, which has been particularly well demonstrated in cases of breast cancer and multiple myeloma.

HYPERCALCAEMIA OF MALIGNANCY

Mechanisms (Table 4.1)

Hypercalcaemia of malignancy is characterized by elevation of the serum calcium concentration with suppression of normal parathyroid hormone secretion. Carcinomas of the lung or breast and multiple myeloma commonly involve bone, but many other tumours can also produce such effects. Although extremely destructive osteolytic metastases may cause hypercalcaemia of malignancy, this probably only occurs in the absence of a humoral mechanism when there is also impairment of renal calcium excretion (Figure 4.1). Elevation of the serum calcium concentration due to direct tumour-mediated osteolysis suppresses PTH, thereby reducing distal calcium reabsorption and increasing calciuria, thus tending to offset the hypercalcaemia. Thus even very aggressive local bone destruction alone is not usually sufficient to produce hypercalcaemia unless renal calcium excretion is impaired by structural or functional changes.

In contrast to metastatic hypercalcaemia, the humoral hypercalcaemia of malignancy is usually due to a generalized stimulation of osteoclast-mediated bone resorption throughout the skeleton together with decreased renal calcium clearance. For many years, it was thought that parathyroid hormone (PTH) was secreted ectopically by certain solid malignancies. However, it is now clear that a peptide with the ability to bind to the parathyroid hormone receptor is responsible for virtually all the cases once attributed to PTH.[3,12,13] This peptide, because of its homology to the N-terminal active region of PTH and its action on the PTH receptor, is known as parathyroid hormone-related peptide (PTHrP). PTHrP has only limited

---

Table 4.1   Pathophysiology of hypercalcaemia of malignancy.

Bone
Increased osteolysis
  a.   Local mediators: interleukins, TNF, prostaglandins
  b.   Systemic hormones: PTHrP, calcitriol
Impaired osteoblastic function: multiple myeloma

Kidney
Increased filtered load of calcium: bone resorption
Increased proximal calcium (and sodium) reabsorption: ECF volume contraction
Increased distal tubular calcium reabsorption: PTHrP

Intestine (minimal contribution)
Reduced calcium intake: nausea, vomiting
Increased active calcium transport: calcitriol

---

homology to PTH; but the homologous sites in the first 13 amino acids of the N-terminal region are crucial. Although PTHrP is widely present in normal humans and animals, its physiological role is poorly understood. PTHrP indirectly activates osteoclasts in much the same manner as human parathyroid hormone, resulting in accelerated osteolysis. Renal calcium excretion is also decreased, owing to an effect on the distal tubule. The combination of increased osteolysis and decreased calcium clearance results in hypercalcaemia. This is an important defence against the development of hypercalcaemia, and invariably occurs when the increased filtered load of calcium overwhelms the effect of PTHrP on the distal nephron.

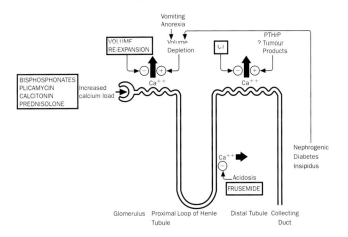

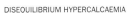

Figure 4.1   Renal mechanisms for the development of severe (disequilibrium) hypercalcaemia. Treatment modalities shown in boxes.

PTHrP is not the only humoral mediator of hypercalcaemia in malignancy. A small number of cases have been reported where calcitriol is produced in excessive quantities, causing pathological acceleration of bone resorption, as is commonly seen in granulomatous disorders. This has been described with lymphomas, in which elevation of 1,25-dihydroxyvitamin D and suppression of PTHrP and PTH are associated with hypercalcaemia.[14,15] In this situation, as in most patients with malignancy-induced hypercalcaemia, calcium absorption from the intestine plays little part, because it is limited by nausea and vomiting, which occur early in the course of the development of hypercalcaemia. Cases have also been described in which prostaglandin-mediated hypercalcaemia has been implicated.[16,17] The problem of hypercalcaemia in myeloma is discussed below.

Clinical presentation (Table 4.2)

Patients with hypercalcaemia of malignancy often present *in extremis*. The elevated serum calcium clouds consciousness, and often causes nausea and vomiting. In addition, hypercalcaemia impairs renal concentrating ability, resulting in progressive dehydration, thereby further impairing the ability to excrete the increased calcium load causing a spiralling cycle of increasing hypercalcaemia. By the time patients reach medical attention they may have an extracellular fluid deficit of several litres and may have experienced profound losses of magnesium, phosphate, and potassium. However, owing to decreased renal clearance, serum levels of these principally intracellular electrolytes may be normal on initial presentation so that their loss may only be appreciated after fluid repletion.

Therapy (Table 4.3)

General principles
Primary therapy consists of expansion of the extracellular fluid space with isotonic saline (at least 3 litres in the first 24 hours) and appropriate electrolyte supplementation to restore renal function and thereby promote renal excretion of calcium. If renal function is adequate, a tolerable serum calcium concentration can be achieved in most patients simply with ample fluid replacement and extracellular fluid volume expansion, producing a saline and calcium diuresis. Owing to an unfortunate, but widespread, misunderstanding of an early

---

Table 4.2 Hypercalcaemic symptoms.	
Non-specific:	Weakness, tiredness, anorexia, vomiting, constipation
	Thirst. Polyuria
Renal impairment:	Nephrocalcinosis
	Calculi
	Myeloma of the kidney
Hypercalcaemic crisis:	Confusion, coma
	Hypotension
	Fits
	Anuric renal failure

Table 4.3 Treatment of hypercalcaemia of malignancy.

Increase renal excretion of calcium

    Rehydration: Correct ECF volume depletion

                                       Restore GFR

    Saline diuresis: Reduce proximal tubular sodium (and calcium) reabsorption

    Furosemide (frusemide):   Reduce calcium reabsorption in loop of Henle,
    (not recommended):   *but* benefits offset by volume depletion

    Calcitonin: Inhibit distal tubular calcium reabsorption
                                       (requires prior saline volume expansion to deliver calcium
                                       to distal tubule)

Decrease bone resorption

    Primary treatment of tumour

    Bisphosphonate-induced decrease in osteolysis

    Corticosteroids (restrict to haematological malignancies)

Limit calcium absorption

    Usually limited by nausea and vomiting

Removal of calcium

    Dialysis

---

report of the use of furosemide (frusemide) in the treatment of hypercalcaemia,[18] loop diuretics are often given as the primary treatment of hypercalcaemia. This practice is to be discouraged since a saline diuresis, with its associated loss of calcium, can be produced in most patients simply by saline infusion. The use of furosemide or other loop diuretics should be restricted to relieving volume overload in patients whose cardiac or renal function is insufficient to tolerate the rate of infusion that is required. The use of furosemide as a primary therapy may be self-defeating since the diuresis so caused will partially offset the benefits of fluid administration and volume re-expansion, reducing rather than increasing renal calcium clearance. As the patient's fluid and electrolyte status is restored, antiresorptive therapy should be introduced for medium-term control of the

hypercalcaemia. Effective treatment of the cancer itself is always the best approach; if this is not possible then control of the mechanism of hypercalcaemia is the next best option.

Drug therapy

Calcitonin

Calcitonin is a 32-amino acid peptide. The most widely used preparation is synthetic salmon calcitonin. It is more potent than mammalian calcitonins. It rarely produces the type of immune reactions that one might anticipate with a foreign peptide. The major effects of calcitonin on bone and calcium homeostasis are mediated via receptors on osteoclasts and distal renal tubular cells. The effects of calcitonin on the osteoclast are to suppress motility, ruffled border formation, acid secretion and resorptive activity. The main renal effects of calcitonin (given in doses usually ranging from 100–400 μ subcutaneously or intramuscularly at 8–12 hour intervals) are to decrease distal renal tubular reabsorption and increase phosphaturia. Although it is a moderately powerful antiresorptive agent, it is much less effective than the bisphosphonates and is generally inadequate to overcome the stimulatory effects of tumour-secreted osteolytic messengers. Perhaps its most important mode of action in the treatment of hypercalcaemia is its direct calciuric effect on the kidneys. This is particuarly effective where prior saline volume re-expansion delivers more calcium to the distal nephron[19] (Figure 4.2). For this reason it still has

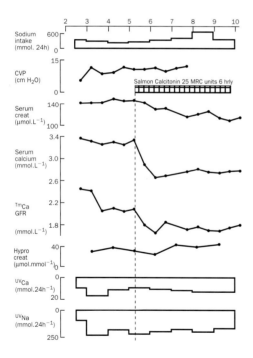

Figure 4.2 Effect of saline rehydration and calcitonin in the treatment of hypercalcaemia (Creat: serum creatinine. TmCa/GFR: notional setting of calcium reabsorption. Hypro/Creat: hydroxyproline excretion in μmol/mmol creatinine. UVCa, UVNa: excretion of calcium and sodium).

a place in the early treatment of hypercalcaemia, and has been used in combination with bisphosphonates. The effect of calcitonin may become blunted with continued use, perhaps as a result of down-regulation of its receptors, although this may be prevented by corticosteroid therapy.[19,20]

Bisphosphonates

It has been well established that potent bisphosphonates, usually administered intravenously, provide effective control of hypercalcaemia over a period of days to weeks. The most extensively characterized, and widely used of these drugs, are clodronate[21–24] and pamidronate;[25–27] but similar effects have been seen with etidronate, alendronate and ibandronate. Etidronate has largely been abandoned owing to its relatively low potency, its renal toxicity and its tendency to cause phosphate retention and inhibit mineralization. An infusion of an adequate (60–90 mg) dose of pamidronate in conjunction with the supportive therapy described above, will usually inhibit bone resorption sufficiently to reduce the serum calcium to within the normal range over three to five days. This inhibition of bone resorption will typically last for a period of several days to a few weeks, and retreatment is generally effective. About 50% of the dose of pamidronate is retained in the skeleton after intravenous adminstration, while the remaining 50% is excreted in the urine over 24–48 hours. No dosage reduction is required unless the serum creatinine level exceeds 440 μmol/l[27], in which case a reduction of 30–50% and slow administration (0.5 mg/min) seem to be reasonable. It must be borne in mind that the extraskeletal effects of PTHrP are not in any way inhibited by bisphosphonate treatment. Thus the phosphate and magnesium wasting associated with PTHrP continue and require constant attention, even when a normal serum calcium has been achieved. Intravenous clodronate 300 mg/d for 5 days or a single dose of 1500 mg[24,28,29] has a similar but perhaps less prolonged effect compared to pamidronate. Results similar to those described for pamidronate have been obtained with alendronate,[30,31] ibandronate[32,33] and other new bisphosphonates.

Combined therapy with a bisphosphonate and calcitonin

The independent actions of calcitonin and bisphosphonates on osteoclasts, together with the renal effect of calcitonin, suggest that combined therapy might have an additive effect. This is in fact the case, since combination therapy results in a more rapid reduction of the serum calcium than bisphosphonate monotherapy, and a much more complete and durable reduction of the serum calcium than does calcitonin alone.[26,34,35] In fact, care must be taken with combined treatment because hypocalcaemia may occur rapidly in the absence of adequate monitoring.

Definitive management

It is crucial for the clinician to bear in mind that the period of normocalcaemia achieved by antiresorptive treatment is by no means a victory over the underlying disease process. It is merely a window of opportunity for the establishment of a definitive diagnosis, when this is not known, and initiation of treatment to the underlying tumour. All too often, when the focus of attention is on control of hypercalcaemia, efforts to establish a precise diagnosis and introduce specific therapy for the underlying tumour are instituted too slowly to prevent recurrence of hypercalcaemia. It is therefore essential that diagnostic studies and therapeutic decisions are initiated promptly so that the inevitable recurrence of hypercalcaemia is prevented.

SKELETAL METASTASES

Mechanism

The frequency of skeletal metastases varies with different malignancies. Breast cancer is particularly noted for remote skeletal spread, while prostate cancer may affect both local and remote skeletal sites. Other frequent causes of skeletal metastases include bronchial, renal and thyroid malignancies. The most fundamental characteristic of a tumour is growth. Key requirements for 'successful' metastatic spread include adequate blood supply, tissue adhesion and a favourable environment for growth. Adhesion to matrix proteins and responsiveness to growth factors in bone matrix appear to be important determinants of metastatic potential. Once a tumour cell has lodged in bone as a result of haematogenous or lymphatic spread, its ability to proliferate beyond a very limited number of cell divisions will depend on removal of the normal bone, which constrains further expansion. A key mechanism of metastasis to bone is induction by the tumour cells of bone resorption by normal osteoclasts, which are the only cells equipped to dissolve bone mineral and remove the matrix (Figure 4.3). They are responsive to the effects of a variety of chemotactic and growth factors, some of which may be produced by the tumours themselves.

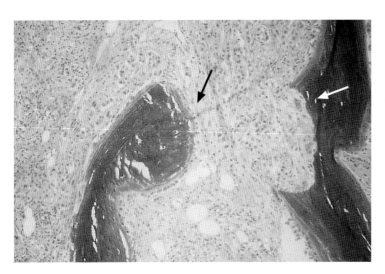

Figure 4.3 Effect of breast cancer metastases in bone marrow in relation to osteoclastic bone resorption. The bone marrow contains extensive infiltration with breast cancer cells. Active osteoclastic resorption is seen (white arrow). Extensive osteoblastic repair/formation is also seen (black arrow)

Alternatively it may be that tumours induce local marrow stromal cells or osteoblastic cells at the metastatic site to produce secondary stimulatory substances. Induction of adjacent osteoclastic bone resorption appears to be a general mechanism by which metastases expand, and PTHrP is probably important in this process, as well as being a systemic humoral factor.[36]

Presentation

For the most part, the significance of skeletal metastases is related to their destructive effect on bone. However, spinal metastases may result in compression of the cord or nerve roots, producing pain or a functional deficit. As a lesion enlarges and destroys the immediately adjacent normal tissue, it will eventually weaken the bone sufficiently to produce pain and structural instability. The clinical significance of the lesion is related to these two effects, and treatment is directed at their mitigation. For the most part, bone pain and structural damage go hand in hand, and in many cases those interventions that are required to stabilize bone are also effective in reducing or eliminating pain.

Surveillance

Regular clinic visits for a review of history and physical examination with careful attention to patients' symptoms are of paramount importance. Beyond these very basic principles, the approach to surveillance is dependent upon the specific type of tumour. When the presence of skeletal metastases is suspected, a radionucleotide bone scan using radio-labelled bisphosphonate tracers may be very helpful (Figure 4.4). The exposed mineral surface at sites of tumour invasion avidly binds radio-labelled bisphosphonate tracer, which is then detected by scintigraphy. This is most effective when there is osteoblastic repair, and the lack of this response is a particular problem with multiple myeloma. Areas that demonstrate uptake on scintigraphy or that can be localized by clinical symptoms or physical examination are then further evaluated by plain radiography, CT, or MRI. This last is currently regarded as the most definitive imaging technique for tumour, especially in bone marrow and the axial skeleton. Bone expansion and thinning or disruption of the cortex are particularly important signs to seek on plain radiography (Figure 4.5).

Breast cancer presents a particular problem, because it is common, and although bone scans are frequently employed for post-treatment

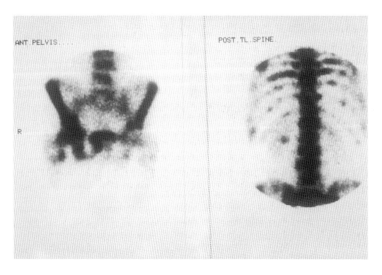

Figure 4.4 Isotope bone scan showing multiple metastases in ribs and pelvis.

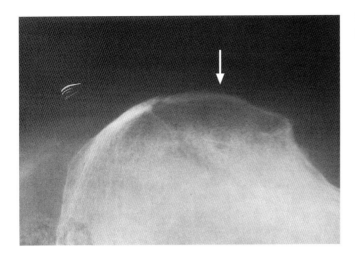

Figure 4.5 Cortical thinning of metastases from breast cancer.

follow-up, a recent consensus-guideline panel found that a positive scan is rarely the first sign of metastasis. The panel did not recommend routine scintigraphy in asymptomatic patients[37,38] because false positive scans are fairly common. If isotope scans are to be used for surveillance, a baseline scan obtained at the time of the initial evaluation is an important reference point for future management. Current technology does not provide a fully satisfactory means of detecting the presymptomatic patient with metastases.

The most useful approach includes regular physician-obtained medical history and physical examination, mammography and patient education regarding self-examination as well as awareness of signs and symptoms. Limited evidence exists concerning the use of biochemical markers of bone resorption to monitor for the development of bone metastases, or for monitoring the response to bisphosphonate therapy, although the latter use seems far more promising.[29]

The unresolved question is how best to approach the management of women with soft tissue, but not bone, metastases. The dilemma is whether all such patients should be treated empirically with bisphosphonates, or whether they should be followed, with institution of treatment only when skeletal metastases are identified. Once skeletal metastases are apparent, the effectiveness and safety of bisphosphonate therapy argue strongly for treatment of asymptomatic patients. The long-term results of such a strategy have not been formally compared with the results of very early treatment prior to the development of bone metastases.

In patients with prostatic carcinoma, skeletal metastases are relatively common and scintigraphy is the preferred method for their detection, although MRI may be helpful for further evaluation. Occasionally biopsy is required for final diagnosis but in most cases evaluation with MRI and CT will reliably distinguish this malignancy from such lesions as Paget's disease of bone. This may occasionally have a similar appearance on an isotopic bone scan or plain radiography.

Management

Radiation therapy

When osteolytic lesions are detected, intervention should be prompt and relatively aggressive unless the patient is in a terminal stage. In most cases, radiation therapy to the local lesion is effective in controlling pain and local tumour growth. Some radiographic evidence of remineralization may occur, but the bone is likely to be somewhat devitalized and locally weakened. Radiation therapy must be planned in conjunction with surgical management to minimize structural damage and interference with bone healing.

Surgical intervention

Surgical intervention is required when a fracture has occurred or is thought to be imminent.[39] Healing of pathologic fractures is often poor, in part because of the local effects of the tumour and in part because of the effects of radiation, so that surgical fixation is usually required. When long bones are involved, intramedullary fixation with local curettage of tumour and insertion of cement is greatly preferred, since the adjacent bone is often of insufficient strength for effective extramedullary fixation. Weight-bearing is obviously a special consideration when the femur is involved. Femoral neck fractures are usually treated with an endoprosthesis or total hip arthroplasty, depending upon the condition of the acetabulum. When the acetabulum is involved then special techniques are necessary to support the arthroplasty cup. Polymethylmethacrylate is often used, as well as bone grafts as reinforcement. Vertebral compression fractures that do not affect the neural structures usually do well with local radiation but surgical intervention by an anterior approach should be considered when there is cord involvement or instability. The new technique of percutaneous vertebroplasty may prove to be useful.[40]

Chemotherapy

The approach to chemotherapy is highly specific to the particular malignancy and its clinical presentation. Skeletal metastases are often a late occurrence after initial treatment, including primary or secondary chemotherapy, so that therapeutic options may be limited. However, many patients with skeletal metastases are clearly capable of responding to chemotherapy and such treatment can be regarded as being complementary to radiotherapy, surgery, and systemic treatment with antiresorptive agents.

Antiresorptive drug therapy

It is highly desirable to prevent the development of bone metastases, or at least to delay their growth. Primary treatment of the tumour by preventing haematogenous spread is the optimal approach for control of metastases, but inhibition of the proliferation of lesions once they have seeded is also of great importance. It is in this respect that modern bisphosphonates have proved to be of enormous importance. In addition to their antiresorptive effect, recent studies have also suggested that bisphosphonates may reduce metastatic spread by blocking adhesion of tumour cells to bone surfaces.[41,42]

Bisphosphonates have long half lives in bone, and therefore may be given intermittently by the intravenous route. The bisphosphonates with the most extensively demonstrated effect in the control of skeletal metastases are pamidronate and clodronate with some evidence for a more durable effect of pamidronate.[43] Since they are poorly absorbed, oral treatment usually requires daily administration, as well as much larger doses than are given intravenously.

Pamidronate can be given as a daily oral preparation,[44,45] but it is not well tolerated in an oral formulation and is more commonly used as an intermittent intravenous infusion.[46–48] It has been shown to inhibit the growth of skeletal metastases of breast cancer, and thereby to reduce the number of serious events such as fracture and the need for radiation therapy or orthopaedic surgery. The usual dosage is a dose of 90 mg, given intravenously every 3 to 4 weeks.

Clodronate is widely used in its oral form, although an intravenous preparation has also been used for the same indication.[49–52] Typical doses of clodronate are 1600 mg daily by mouth or 600 mg IV. This medication is not available in the United States, but is extensively used in Europe. Once absorbed or infused, clodronate has a similar fate to that of pamidronate, with about 50% excreted unchanged in the urine and the remainder retained within the skeleton. As with all other bisphosphonates, the oral absorption of clodronate is limited to less than 2% of the administered dose.[53]

It is important that patients maintain a good calcium and vitamin D intake while being treated with potent bisphosphonates. Their antiresorptive effect typically results in secondary hyperparathyroidism due to continued deposition of mineral in bone, while calcium efflux is decreased. This effect will be amplified if vitamin D and calcium status is poor. There do not appear to be any important long-term adverse effects of the chronic administration of pamidronate or clodronate. These drugs do not generally induce the mineralization defect associated with etidronate. Ocular symptoms have been reported in a small number of patients who were treated with pamidronate, but no causative mechanism has been demonstrated.[54]

Clodronate, pamidronate, alendronate and olpadronate have all been shown to have beneficial effects in metastatic prostate carcinoma.[55–68] However, as might be expected in a disease less likely to cause fracture than breast cancer, these benefits have been mainly symptomatic, in terms of decreased bone pain.

MULTIPLE MYELOMA

Myeloma is a monoclonal malignancy of plasma cells which may produce hypercalcaemia, diffuse osteopenia, osteoporosis, or discrete osteolytic lesions, causing localized pain and/or fracture. The condition is typically widespread in the marrow space by the time of diagnosis, although it occasionally presents as an isolated lytic lesion. Myeloma is almost always associated with secretion of a monoclonal globulin and clues to its presence include elevation of the erythrocyte sedimentation rate, anaemia and rouleaux formation. It is not unusual to detect a monoclonal gammopathy by serum protein electrophoresis in the course of evaluating patients with osteoporosis. The nature of this monoclonal protein may be confirmed by immunoelectrophoresis or immunofixation. Myeloma may occasionally present as 'light-chain' disease, with kappa or lambda light chains in the urine, but little or no paraprotein in serum. When a monoclonal protein is detected, a bone marrow biopsy is usually performed to determine whether myeloma is present. Marrow biopsy may disclose frank myeloma (>10% plasmacytosis) or the presence of plasma cells in numbers too small to make the diagnosis. In the latter case, the diagnosis is 'monoclonal gammopathy of uncertain significance', and while many such cases progress to frank myeloma, this is not inevitable. The effect of such a gammopathy on bone mass has not been fully characterized.

Myeloma can produce either or both of two well-recognized patterns of bone damage. There may be a diffuse loss of bone mass similar in appearance to osteoporosis, or there may be typical 'punched-out' lytic areas where the myeloma cells are clustered into plasmacytomas (Figure 4.6). These changes together with hypercalcaemia constitute the major effects of myeloma on bone and mineral homeostasis. Owing to its origin within the bone marrow, this plasma cell malignancy is strategically situated to cause considerable skeletal damage. Since the disease is generally widespread when first detected, chemotherapy is not usually curative, and disease management is one of containment on a chronic basis. Where discrete plasma cell lesions (plasmacytomas) are present, they may lead to focal bone destruction in much the same way as solid tumour metastases. In general myeloma appears to cause generalized bone destruction as a result of direct diffusion of osteoclast-stimulating agents within the bone marrow, rather than requiring their general circulation. The lack of an osteoblastic response suggests that these cells may be suppressed by the myeloma,[59] and this may contribute to the lack of tracer uptake by affected bones on scintigraphy.

Pathogenesis

While cytokines appear to be the major factor in the pathogenesis of myeloma-induced osteolysis, several cases have been described in which secretion of parathyroid hormone-related peptide (PTHrP) has resulted in hypercalcaemia.[60,61] Myeloma may influence the serum calcium concentration by two mechanisms.

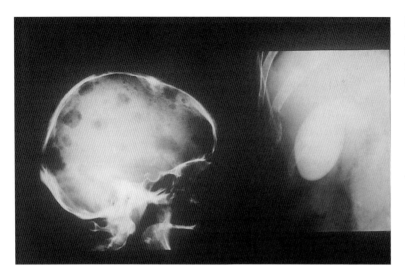

Figure 4.6 Typical lytic lesions in a rib and the skull in multiple myeloma. The rib lesion was detected during a cholecystogram (opacified gall bladder)

Osteolysis may lead to hypercalcaemia by virtue of massive release of calcium into the circulation, overwhelming the ability of the kidney to maintain homeostasis. Typically, PTH will be suppressed under these circumstances, and the absence of a parathyroid hormone-like effect on renal tubular calcium reabsorption will lead to hypercalciuria. This is a particular feature of myeloma even with minimal hypercalcaemia, and measurement of urinary calcium excretion may be useful in monitoring such patients. Secondly, the presence of very high levels of myeloma protein may artefactually elevate the total serum calcium concentration without a proportionate increase in the ionized or filterable fraction. It must be borne in mind, however, that since the myeloma proteins are globulins with lower binding affinities for calcium than albumin, the elevation of the total protein must be substantial in order to account fully for the hypercalcaemia. Calculation of the corrected serum calcium concentration or careful measurement of the serum-ionized calcium together with measurement of intact PTH is useful in making this distinction.

Treatment of the skeletal effects of myeloma depends very much on that of the underlying disease, as with other malignancies. The usual treatment consists of cycles of an alkylating agent with high-dose glucocorticoids. If the patient responds to a course of chemotherapy, stimulation of osteoclastic bone resorption will be reduced, as will calcium release from the skeleton with preservation of bone mass. Unfortunately, it is not always possible to adequately control the skeletal effects of myeloma by chemotherapy, and other antiresorptive agents such as the bisphosphonates are then required.

Treatment of hypercalcaemia in myeloma
The treatment of hypercalcaemia in myeloma is similar to that employed for other tumours. Fluid and electrolyte replacement is of primary importance, but bisphosphonate therapy is usually required in addition. A convenient approach is to use an infusion of 90 mg of pamidronate[62,63] given at 3–5-day intervals until hypercalcaemia is controlled, and then followed with 4-weekly infusions to maintain normocal-

caemia. Although 'myeloma kidney' is a concern in this disease, the dosage of pamidronate need not be reduced unless renal function is significantly impaired (serum creatinine >440 µmol/l).[27] Even in patients with end-stage renal failure, the dose need not be reduced by more than 50%, and in patients on dialysis a similar 50% dose reduction seems reasonable (given just after a dialysis treatment). In patients with renal insufficiency, it seems prudent to infuse pamidronate somewhat more slowly than usual (over 6–12 hours) in order to reduce the peak serum concentration, thereby minimizing any possible toxic effect on remaining kidney function. Clodronate is also effective in myeloma-related hypercalcaemia, and has been used extensively for this purpose.[64]

It is now generally accepted that bisphosphonate treatment is an important part of the overall approach to myeloma.[65–67] Evidence is emerging from preclinical studies to suggest that potent bisphosphonates may not only reduce the risk of skeletal events, but may also appear to induce apoptosis of the myeloma cells.[68,69] Myeloma is the only currently known example where the bisphosphonate may not only affect the osteoclast, but also the malignant cell itself. It may be that the development of future bisphosphonates will involve some selection for anti-myeloma-cell effects.

Lytic lesions in myeloma
Management of focal lytic lesions in myeloma is similar to that of metastatic solid tumours. Primary attention is given to the prevention of complications and the relief of symptoms. Radiation therapy can be helpful in both respects but when there is a structural defect, orthopaedic intervention can be critical to efforts to preserve function. Nailing, with local removal of tumour and insertion of cement is of particular importance, since weakening of structures adjacent to a fracture may render extramedullary fixation unreliable. Efforts to introduce structural materials such as plastic cements in order to reinforce threatened bone are at an early but promising stage.

Bisphosphonates have been shown to be highly effective in reducing the progression and morbidity of myeloma lesions,[62,63,65] and should be routinely employed in management.

Monitoring in myeloma

Monitoring of the patient with myeloma is somewhat different from that of patients with solid tumours. Scintigraphy is less sensitive for myeloma deposits than it is for other tumours, and cases in which abnormal radiographs have coincided with normal scintigraphy are well described. Thus a skeletal survey with plain radiographs remains the mainstay for myeloma evaluation and follow-up. Scintigraphy nevertheless has a role in detecting new lesions in the vertebrae, ribs and sternum.

It may be useful to use biochemical markers of bone resorption, such as the pyridinoline cross-links, for monitoring the response of patients to bisphosphonate treatment. Markers of bone formation, such as the serum alkaline phosphatase, will of course be inappropriate for this purpose.

Because of the generalized loss of bone mass often seen in myeloma, dual-energy X-ray absorptiometry can also be used in the evaluation and monitoring of affected patients.

OSTEOPOROSIS SECONDARY TO THE TREATMENT OF MALIGNANCY

Gonadal steroid deficiency

Androgen deficiency
Treatment for cancer is associated with an increased risk of osteoporosis for a variety of reasons. Orchiectomy or medical suppression of gonadal steroid secretion is a critical element of the treatment of prostatic cancer and this has a similar effect to that of testosterone deficiency encountered for any other reason. Since men with prostate cancer may survive for many years, particularly when such treatment is used as adjuvant therapy, the opportunity for the development of osteoporosis is certainly present and well described. Although men tend to be somewhat less susceptible to the conse-

quences of hypogonadism than women under similar circumstances, because of their greater peak bone mass, it is reasonable to monitor axial bone density. In other situations with declining bone mass as a consequence of hypogonadism the patient would be treated with testosterone. This option is of course precluded in the management of prostate cancer. In such circumstances, intervention takes two forms. Firstly, contributory causes of osteoporosis, such as poor dietary calcium or vitamin D intake and disorders of mineral metabolism such as renal calcium wasting or calcium malabsorption, must be excluded or corrected. Secondly, effective antiresorptive treatment must be instituted. While in most countries there is no drug currently registered for this specific indication, the experience with potent bisphosphonates, particularly alendronate (10 mg daily), suggests that they provide effective and well-tolerated treatment.[70] In general, it appears prudent to evaluate bone mineral density at the time of institution of anti-androgen treatment for prostate carcinoma. Thus treatment can be started early if the bone mass is low, or perhaps delayed when there is evidence of a relatively normal baseline bone mass. This implies that bone densitometry will be performed at baseline and at intervals (of approximately 2 years). Obviously, it is important that bone densitometry is performed at sites unaffected by osteoblastic metastases.

Oestrogen deficiency
As in the case of men with prostate cancer, women with breast cancer often undergo gonadal ablation, either as a result of oophorectomy or as a consequence of chemotherapy.[71] Because many breast cancers are oestrogen-dependent, few women with this tumour are ever subsequently treated with oestrogens. The same principles of ensuring adequate vitamin D and calcium intake apply equally well to women as in men, and one must also be aware of the risks of calcium wasting or malabsorption, as in other women with osteoporosis. Tamoxifen has been shown in large long-term studies to reduce the risk of recurrent breast cancer, and is widely used for this purpose. It is

of some comfort that tamoxifen has a mitigating effect on the bone loss associated with oestrogen deficiency,[72] although the effect is less than that of conventional replacement doses of oestrogen. The newer agent, raloxifene, has a better-documented effect on bone mass,[73] and may also be capable of reducing the recurrence rate of breast cancer.[74] Raloxifene (60 mg daily) may have an advantage in that, unlike tamoxifen, it does not stimulate uterine endometrial tissue.

Bisphosphonates do not have any known antiproliferative effect on breast tissue. However, they appear to be more potent than raloxifene or tamoxifen in protecting or even enhancing bone mass. As a consequence, they may play a role in treatment of osteoporosis associated with gonadal steroid deficiency in women who have been treated for breast cancer. Alendronate (10 mg daily) appears to be substantially more effective from a purely skeletal standpoint, while intravenous pamidronate (60 mg every 3 months) has also been shown to be effective in the treatment of this type of osteoporosis.[75] Recent studies in women without breast cancer have indicated an additive effect of the combination of oestrogen (0.625 mg conjugated equine oestrogen) and alendronate (10 mg daily).[76] It is conceivable, although unproven, that there may be a similar additive effect of alendronate and a selective oestrogen receptor modulator that could be used in breast cancer.[77]

Awareness of the likely development of osteoporosis in women who have been treated for breast cancer is important, and surveillance with a baseline bone densitometry is advisable, with further measurement at approximately 2-yearly intervals, if no intervention is initially required.

Other skeletal consequences of cancer therapy

Treatment of certain malignancies, such as lymphomas, involves administration of high doses of glucocorticosteroids. Management is broadly similar to that of patients being treated with high-dose steroids for a benign disease.

It is also important to note that children and adolescents treated for malignancies often have reduced bone mass, which will be carried forward into adult life.[78,79]

Less common complications of the treatment of cancer, which may have a major effect on the skeleton, include radiation enteritis. This can result in malabsorption and the same type of metabolic problems that are encountered in patients with inflammatory bowel disease.

Osteonecrosis

The direct effects of radiation therapy on bone, producing radiation osteonecrosis, must also be considered, and may require surgical intervention.

Osteonecrosis is also a well-described complication of cancer therapy with glucocorticosteroids, and cytotoxic agents. It is an important diagnostic consideration when pathological fractures occur, since treatment may be constrained by the need to avoid what would, under different circumstances, be useful therapeutic strategies.

Oncogenic osteomalacia

One special case, which should be considered as both an initial manifestation and as a complication of certain tumours, is oncogenic osteomalacia. Typically the rare tumours that cause this syndrome are of mesenchymal origin. In this syndrome characteristic features of osteomalacia are associated with hypophosphataemia, increased phosphate clearance and a relatively low serum 1,25 dihydroxyvitamin D level. There appears to be a humoral mechanism that stimulates renal phosphate excretion, but the exact pathogenesis of this syndrome remains obscure.[80,81] Treatment with calcitriol and phosphate may control the symptoms, but treatment of the underlying malignancy is the only truly effective approach.

SUMMARY

Management of the skeletal complications of malignant diseases depends heavily on a careful consideration of the underlying pathophysiological mechanisms and precise application of therapeutic principles to their correction.

Advances in pharmacological control of pathological bone resorption have greatly facilitated medical intervention.

REFERENCES

1. Chambers TJ, McSheehy PM, Thomson BM, Fuller K (1985). The effect of calcium-regulating hormones and prostaglandins on bone resorption by osteoclasts disaggregated from neonatal rabbit bones. *Endocrinology 116*: 234–239.
2. McSheehy PM, Chambers TJ (1986). Osteoblastic cells mediate osteoclastic responsiveness to parathyroid hormone. *Endocrinology 118*: 824–828.
3. Broadus AE, Mangin M, Ikeda K et al. (1988). Humoral hypercalcemia of cancer. Identification of a novel parathyroid hormone-like peptide. *New Engl J Med 319*: 556–563.
4. McSheehy PM, Chambers TJ (1987). 1,25-dihydroxyvitamin D3 stimulates rat osteoblastic cells to release a soluble factor that increases osteoclastic bone resorption. *J Clin Invest 80*: 425–429.
5. Chambers TJ, Fuller K, McSheehy PM, Pringle JA (1985). The effects of calcium regulating hormones on bone resorption by isolated human osteoclastoma cells. *J Pathol 145*: 297–305.
6. Thomson BM, Saklatvala J, Chambers TJ (1986). Osteoblasts mediate interleukin 1 stimulation of bone resorption by rat osteoclasts. *J Exp Med 164*: 104–112.
7. Thomson BM, Mundy GR, Chambers TJ (1987). Tumor necrosis factors alpha and beta induce osteoblastic cells to stimulate osteoclastic bone resorption. *J Immunol 138*: 775–779.
8. Hosking DJ, Gilson D (1984). Comparison of the renal and skeletal actions of calcitonin in the treatment of severe hypercalcemia of malignancy. *Q J Med 53*: 359–368.
9. Fleisch H (1997). *Bisphosphonates in bone disease: from the laboratory to the patient*, 3rd edn.
10. Luckman SP, Coxon FP, Ebetino FH, Russell RG, Rogers MJ (1998). Heterocycle-containing bisphosphonates cause apoptosis and inhibit bone resorption by preventing protein prenylation: evidence from structure–activity relationships in J774 macrophages. *J Bone Miner Res 13*: 1668–1678.
11. Fisher JE, Rogers MJ, Halasy JM et al. (1999). Alendronate mechanism of action: geranylgeraniol, an intermediate in the mevalonate pathway, prevents inhibition of osteoclast formation, bone

resorption, and kinase activation in vitro. *Proc Nat Acad Sci USA* 96: 133–138.

12. Stewart AF, Burtis WJ, Wu T, Goumas D, Broadus AE (1987). Two forms of parathyroid hormone-like adenylate cyclase-stimulating protein derived from tumors associated with humoral hypercalcemia of malignancy. *J Bone Miner Res* 2: 587–593.

13. Strewler GJ, Stern PH, Jacobs JW et al. (1987). Parathyroid hormone like protein from human renal carcinoma cells. Structural and functional homology with parathyroid hormone. *J Clin Invest* 80: 1803–1807.

14. Johnston SR, Hammond PJ (1992). Elevated serum parathyroid hormone related protein and 1,25-dihydroxycholecalciferol in hypercalcaemia associated with adult T-cell leukemia-lymphoma. *Postgrad Med J* 68: 753–755.

15. Seymour JF, Gagel RF, Hagemeister FB, Dimopoulos MA, Cabanillas F (1994). Calcitriol production in hypercalcemic and normocalcemic patients with non-hodgkin lymphoma. *Ann Intern Med* 121: 633–640.

16. Mundy GR (1989). Hypercalcemic factors other than parathyroid hormone-related protein. *Endocrinol Metab Clin North Am* 18: 795–806.

17. LaForga JB, Vierna J, Aranda FI (1994). Hypercalcemia in Hodgkin's disease related to prostaglandin synthesis. *J Clin Pathol* 47: 567–568.

18. Suki WN, Yium JJ, VonMinden M, Saller-Hebert C, Eknoyan G, Martinez-Maldonado M (1970). Acute treatment of hypercalcemia with furosemide. *New Engl J Med* 283: 836–840.

19. Hosking DJ, Stone MD, Foote JW (1990). Potentiation of calcitonin by corticosteroids during the treatment of the hypercalcemia of malignancy. *Eur J Clin Pharmacol* 38: 37–41.

20. Binstock ML, Mundy GR (1980). Effect of calcitonin and glutocorticoids in combination on the hypercalcemia of malignancy. *Ann Intern Med* 93: 269–272.

21. Siris ES, Sherman WH, Baquiran DC, Schlatterer JP, Osserman EF, Canfield RE (1980). Effects of dichloromethylene diphosphonate on skeletal mobilization of calcium in multiple myeloma. *New Engl J Med* 302: 310–315.

22. Chapuy MC, Meunier PJ, Alexandre CM, Vignon EP (1980). Effects of disodium dichloromethylene diphosphonate on hypercalcemia produced by bone metastases. *J Clin Invest* 65: 1243–1247.

23. Jung A, Chantraine A, Donath A et al. (1983). Use of dichloromethylene diphosphonate in metastatic bone disease. *New Engl J Med* 308: 1499–1501.

24. Kanis JA, McCloskey EV (1997). Clodronate (review). *Cancer* 80 (8 Suppl): 1691–1695.

25. Body JJ, Pot M, Borkowski A, Sculier JP, Klastersky J (1987). Dose/response study of aminohydroxypropylidene bisphosphonate in tumor-associated hypercalcemia. *Am J Med* 82: 957–963.

26. Thiébaud D, Jaeger P, Jacquet AF, Burckhardt P (1988). Dose-response in the treatment of hypercalcemia of malignancy by a single infusion of the bisphosphonate AHPrBP. *J Clin Oncol* 6: 762–768.

27. Nussbaum SR, Younger J, Vandepol CJ et al. (1993). Single-dose intravenous therapy with pamidronate for the treatment of hypercalcemia of malignancy: comparison of 30-, 60-, 90-mg dosages. *Am J Med* 95: 297–304.

28. O'Rourke NP, McCloskey EV, Vasikaran S et al. (1993). Effective treatment of malignant hypercalcemia with a single intravenous infusion of clodronate. *Br J Cancer* 67: 560–563.

29. Kanis JA, McCloskey EV (1997). Bone turnover and biochemical markers in malignancy. *Cancer* 80 (8 Suppl): 1538–1545.

30. Zysset E, Ammann P, Jenzer A et al. (1992). Comparison of a rapid (2-h) versus a slow (24-h) infusion of alendronate in the treatment of hypercalcemia of malignancy. *Bone Miner* 18: 237–249.

31. Nussbaum SR, Warrell RP Jr, Rude R et al. (1993). Dose-response study of alendronate sodium for the treatment of cancer-associated hypercalcemia. *J Clin Oncol* 11: 1618–1623.

32. Pecherstorfer M, Herrmann Z, Body JJ et al. (1996). Randomized phase II trial comparing different doses of the bisphosphonate ibandronate in the treatment of hypercalcemia of malignancy. *J Clin Oncol* 14: 268–276.

33. Ralston SH, Thiébaud D, Herrmann Z et al. (1997). Dose-response study of ibandronate in the treatment of cancer-associated hypercalcemia. *Br J Cancer* 75: 295–300.

34. Ralston SH, Gardner MD, Dryburgh FJ, Jenkins AS, Cowan RA, Boyle IT (1985). Comparison of aminohydroxypropylidene diphosphonate, mithramycin, and corticosteroids/calcitonin in treatment of cancer-associated hypercalcemia. *Lancet* ii: 907–910.

35. Thiébaud D, Jacquet AF, Burckhardt P (1990). Fast and effective treatment of malignant hypercalcemia. Combination of suppositories of calci-

tonin and a single infusion of 3-amino 1-hydroxypropylidine-1-bisphosphonate. *Arch Intern Med 150*: 2125–2128.

36. Guise TA (1997). Parathyroid hormone-related protein and bone metastases. *Cancer 80* (8 Suppl): 1572–1580.

37. ASCO (1997). Recommended Breast Cancer Surveillance Guidelines. *J Clin Oncol 15*: 2149–2156.

38. Smith TJ, Davidson NE, Schapira DV et al. (1999). American Society of Clinical Oncology 1998 Update of Recommended Breast Cancer Surveillance Guidelines. *J Clin Oncol 17*: 1080–1082.

39. Harrington KD (1997). Orthopedic surgical management of skeletal complications of malignancy. *Cancer 80* (8 suppl): 1614–1627.

40. Weill A, Chiras J, Simon JM et al. (1996). Spinal metastases: indications for and results of percutaneous injection of acrylic surgical cement. *Radiology 199*: 241–247.

41. Van der Pluijm G, Vloedgraven H, van Beek E, van der Wee-Pals L, Lowik C, Papapoulos S (1996). Bisphosphonates inhibit the adhesion of breast cancer cells to bone matrices in vitro. *J Clin Invest 98*: 698–705.

42. Boissier S, Magnetto S, Frappart L et al. (1997). Bisphosphonates inhibit prostate and breast cell adhesion to unmineralized and mineralized bone extracellular matrices. *Cancer Res 57*: 3890–3894.

43. Purohit OP, Radstone CR, Anthony C, Kanis JA, Coleman RE (1995). A randomized double-blind comparison of intravenous pamidronate and clodronate in the hypercalcemia of malignancy. *Br J Cancer 72*: 1289–1293.

44. van Holten-Verzantvoort AT, Bijvoet OL, Cleton FJ et al. (1987). Reduced morbidity from skeletal metastases in breast cancer patients during long-term bisphosphonate (APD) treatment. *Lancet ii*: 983–985.

45. Cleton FJ, van Holten-Verzantvoort AT, Bijvoet OL (1989). Effect of long-term bisphosphonate treatment on morbidity due to bone metastases in breast cancer patients. *Recent Result Cancer Res 116*: 73–78.

46. Conte PF, Latreille J, Mauriac L et al. (1996). Delay in progression of bone metastases in breast cancer patients treated with intravenous pamidronate: results from a multinational randomized controlled trial. The Aredia Multinational Cooperative Group. *J Clin Oncol 14*: 2552–2559.

47. Hortobagyi GN, Theriault RL, Lipton A et al. (1998). Long-term prevention of skeletal complications of metastatic breast cancer with pamidronate. Protocol 19 Aredia Breast Cancer Study Group. *J Clin Oncol 16*: 2038–2044.

48. Theriault RL, Lipton A, Hortobagyi GN et al. (1999). Pamidronate reduces skeletal morbidity in women with advanced breast cancer and lytic bone lesions: a randomized, placebo-controlled trial. *J Clin Oncol 17*: 846–854.

49. Elomaa I, Blomqvist C, Porkka L et al. (1988). Clodronate for osteolytic metastases due to breast cancer. *Biomed Pharmacother 42*: 111–116.

50. Paterson AH, Ernst DS, Powles TJ, Ashley S, McCloskey EV, Kanis JA (1991). Treatment of skeletal disease in breast cancer with clodronate. *Bone 12* (Suppl 1): S25–S30.

51. Paterson AH, Powles TJ, Kanis JA, McCloskey E, Hanson J, Ashley S (1993). Double-blind controlled trial of oral clodronate in patients with bone metastases from breast cancer. *J Clin Oncol 11*: 59–65.

52. Kanis JA, Powles T, Paterson AH, McCloskey EV, Ashley S (1996). Clodronate decreases the frequency of skeletal metastases in women with breast cancer. *Bone 19*: 663–667.

53. Yakatan GJ, Poyner WJ, Talbert RL et al. (1982). Clodronate kinetics and bioavailability. *Clin Pharmacol Therap 31*: 402–410.

54. Macarol V, Fraunfelder FT (1994). Pamidronate disodium and possible ocular adverse drug reactions. *Am J Ophthalmol 118*: 220–224.

55. Adami S, Salvagno G, Guarrera G et al. (1985). Dichloromethylene-diphosphonate in patients with prostatic carcinoma metastatic to the skeleton. *J Urol 134*: 1152–1154.

56. Masud T, Slevin ML (1989). Pamidronate to reduce bone pain in normocalcaemic patient with disseminated prostatic carcinoma. *Lancet i*: 1021–1022.

57. Adami S (1997). Bisphosphonates in prostate carcinoma. *Cancer 80* (8 Suppl): 1674–1679.

58. Pelger RC, Hamdy NA, Zwinderman AH, Lycklama A, Nijeholt AA, Papapoulos SE (1998). Effects of the bisphosphonate olpadronate in patients with carcinoma of the prostate metastatic to the skeleton. *Bone 22*: 403–408.

59. Roodman GD (1997). Mechanisms of bone lesions in multiple myeloma and lymphoma. *Cancer 80* (8 Suppl): 1557–1563.

60. Beaudreuil J, Cohen-Solal M, Dore MX et al. (1996). Secretion of parathyroid hormone-related peptide in patients with multiple myeloma. *Rev Rhum*, English Ed. *63*: 502–503.

61. Horiuchi T, Miyachi T, Arai T, Nakamura T, Mori M, Ito H (1997). Raised plasma concentrations of parathyroid hormone related peptide in hypercalcemic multiple myeloma. *Horm Metab Res 29*: 469–471.

62. Berenson JR, Lichtenstein A, Porter L et al. (1996). Efficacy of pamidronate in reducing skeletal events in patients with advanced multiple myeloma. *New Engl J Med 334*: 488–493.

63. Berenson JR, Lichtenstein A, Porter L et al. (1998). Long-term pamidronate treatment of advanced multiple myeloma patients reduces skeletal events. *J Clin Oncol 16*: 593–602.

64. Paterson AD, Kanis JA, Cameron EC et al. (1983). The use of dichloromethylene diphosphonate for the management of hypercalcaemia in multiple myeloma. *Br J Haematol 54*: 121–132.

65. Bloomfield DJ (1998). Should bisphosphonates be part of the standard therapy of patients with multiple myeloma or bone metastases from cancers? An evidence-based review. *J Clin Oncol 16*: 1218–1225.

66. Bataille R (1996). Management of myeloma with bisphosphonates. *New Engl J Med 334*: 529–530.

67. Bataille R, Harousseau JL (1997). Multiple myeloma. *New Engl J Med 336*: 1657–1664.

68. Aparicio A, Gardner A, Tu Y, Savage A, Berenson J, Lichtenstein A (1998). In vitro cytoreductive effects on multiple myeloma cells induced by bisphosphonates. *Leukemia 12*: 220–229.

69. Shipman CM, Rogers MJ, Apperley JF, Russell RG, Croucher PI (1997). Bisphosphonates induce apoptosis in human myeloma cell lines: a novel anti-tumour activity. *Br J Haematol 98*: 665–672.

70. Orwoll E, Ettinger M, Weiss S et al. (1999). Alendronate treatment of osteoporosis in men. *J Bone Miner Res 14* (Suppl. 1): S184.

71. Saarto T, Blomqvist C, Valimaki M, Makela P, Sarna S, Elomaa I (1997). Chemical castration induced by adjuvant cyclophosphamide, methotrexate, and fluorouracil chemotherapy causes rapid bone loss that is reduced by clodronate: a randomized study in premenopausal breast cancer patients. *J Clin Oncol 15*: 1341–1347.

72. Turken S, Siris E, Seldin D, Flaster E, Hyman G, Lindsay R (1989). Effects of tamoxifen on spinal bone density in women with breast cancer. *J Nat Cancer Inst 81*: 1086–1088.

73. Balfour JA, Goa KL (1998). Raloxifene [review]. *Drugs Aging 12*: 335–341.

74. Powles TJ (1998). Status of antiestrogen breast cancer prevention trials [review]. *Oncology 12* (3 suppl 5): 28–31.

75. Thiébaud D, Burckhardt P, Melchior J et al. (1994). Two years' effectiveness of intravenous pamidronate (APD) versus oral fluoride for osteoporosis occurring in the postmenopause. *Osteoporosis Int 4*: 76–83.

76. Bone HB, Lombardi A, Greenspan SL et al. Alendronate and estrogen effects in postmenopausal women with low bone mineral density. *J Clin Endocrinol Metab* (in press).

77. Johnell O, Scheel W, Lu Y, Lakshmanan M (1999). Effects of raloxifene (RLX) and alendronate (ALN) and RLX+ALN on bone mineral density (BMD) and biochemical markers of bone turnover in postmenopausal women with osteoporosis. *J Bone Miner Res 14* (Suppl. 1): S85.

78. Aisenberg J, Hsieh K, Kalaitzoglou G et al. (1998). Bone mineral density in young adult survivors of childhood cancer. *J Pediatr Hematol Oncol 20*: 241–245.

79. Henderson RC, Madsen CD, Davis C, Gold SH (1998). Longitudinal evaluation of bone mineral density in children receiving chemotherapy. *J Pediatr Hematol Oncol 20*: 322–326.

80. Schapiro D, Ben Izhak O, Nachtigal A et al. (1995). Tumor-induced osteomalacia. *Semin Arthritis Rheum 25*: 35–46.

81. Nelson AE, Robinson BG, Mason RS (1997). Oncogenic osteomalacia: is there a new phosphate regulating hormone? *Clin Endocrinol 47*: 635–642.

5

Paget's Disease

David Hosking

Clinical features • Investigations • Aims of treatment • Treatment strategies

Paget's disease is a focal disorder of bone remodelling where the primary abnormality is a greatly accelerated rate of osteoclastic resorption with a secondary increase in bone formation. Although the osteoclasts show a variety of ultrastructural changes,[1] the normal osteoblast morphology confirms that their increased activity is a coupled response to the accelerated resorption. As a consequence of these changes the normal lamellar bone becomes progressively replaced by mechanically compromised woven bone, leading to pain, deformity and fracture.

Paget's osteoclasts are commonly seen to contain nuclear inclusions which resemble paramyxovirus nucleocapsids. Immunocytochemical and *in situ* hybridization studies suggest that these might be measles, respiratory syncytial virus or canine distemper virus.[2,3] Although intact virus has not been isolated from any of these cells, nor infection transmitted by co-culture, the virus could still spread by infected osteoclast precursors fusing with mature cells. The demonstration of virus mRNA in osteoclast precursors, marrow and peripheral blood mononuclear cells in patients with Paget's disease is consistent with such a hypothesis.[3]

An unresolved problem is how these changes might interrelate with a genetic predisposition to the disease as shown by the observation that about 15% of patients have an affected first-degree relative. A potential link might be through the chromosome 18q, which carries the locus for familial expansile osteolysis (which in some respects resembles Paget's disease) and also that for the proto-oncogene Bcl-2. Upregulation of the expression of this proto-oncogene, which is suppressor of apoptosis, by a viral infection could lead to enhanced osteoclast lifespan and increased bone resorption.[4]

The extent of skeletal involvement varies greatly between individuals, ranging from limited monostotic disease to extensive polyostotic abnormality. The explanation for this variability is uncertain, as is the reason why the disease may spread within a bone but never extends to involve previously unaffected bones. The initial distribution may be determined by a particularly appropriate marrow environment, for example one secreting interleukin 6, which provides a seeding site for abnormal circulating osteoclast precursors.[3]

The prevalence of Paget's disease seems to be declining, as is the proportion of new patients with very active disease, either assessed bio-chemically or in terms of the volume of affected bone.[5] Since initial disease activity and extent are important determinants of response these changes have important implications for the development of current therapeutic strategies.

CLINICAL FEATURES

The symptoms of Paget's disease, while having a substantial effect on the quality of life,[6] also determine the mode of presentation and con-tribute to the diagnosis of the condition. They are also important in terms of the extent that they influence, and themselves can be modified by, the choice of treatment.

Bone pain

This is the commonest presenting symptom,[7] but is both non-specific and multifactorial, in that it may be due to direct bone involvement, fractures or neurological compression syn-dromes (Table 5.1). Pain probably arises from distortion of the periosteum, and potential mechanisms include traction due to deformity or expansion of the bone, or the consequences of increased vascularity.

Pretreatment assessment
The first step is to make sure that the site of pain coincides with clear radiographic and scinti-graphic evidence of disease; and local tenderness to deep pressure may also be helpful. The skin over a pagetic bone may be warmer than its sur-roundings, owing to the increased vascularity and this presentation is more commonly associated with painful disease.[8] The next step is to charac-terize the pain, which is often described as boring or nagging. It is often present at rest, and may dis-turb sleep, although mechanical pain from degen-erative disease of the spine and hip may also become worse in the recumbent position. Pain relief with simple analgesics is not a reliable guide to the origin of pain, and symptoms correlate poorly with the absolute level of bone turnover. However, within an individual, bone pain may increase in parallel with disease activity.

Degenerative joint disease

Involvement of periarticular bone leads to dis-tortion of the adjacent joint surface and acceler-ation of degenerative changes, particularly at major weight-bearing sites, such as spine, hip or knee. These changes may be made worse by the effects of local deformity, particularly of long bones, which leads to limb shortening and abnormal stresses on adjacent joints.

Pretreatment assessment
The major distinguishing feature of pain from degenerative joint disease is that it is usually made worse by movement or weight-bearing. Radiographic evidence of joint changes (or their absence) is also helpful, but the usual problem is mixed bone and joint involvement.[9] The par-tition of pain between these two components is often very difficult. Pain in these circumstances may often respond, totally or in part, to a thera-peutic trial. The presence of severe degenera-tive joint disease in a symptomatic patient should not preclude a trial of medical therapy before referral for joint replacement, as responses to medical treatment do occur.

Fractures

The abnormal bone architecture of Paget's dis-ease often results in a bowing deformity of long bones that develops slowly over many years. It is most common in the femur or tibia, although the upper limbs may also be involved, particu-larly if they are regularly stressed. As the bone bends it tends to develop stress fractures on the convex margin of the deformity. These stress fractures have well-defined margins, so that both their position and their appearance distin-guish them from the Looser's zones of osteoma-lacia (Figure 5.1). The stress fracture is a site of very active bone remodelling, similar to that of fracture callus, which, together with increased vascularity, makes these lesions appear 'hot' on an isotope bone scan. This type of fracture is relatively common, and most are probably asymptomatic. However, they represent an area of weakness in a weight-bearing bone, and may

Table 5.1 Clinical features of Paget's disease.

Symptom	Mechanism	Assessment
Bone pain	Abnormal bone structure. Stress fractures. Compression of nervous tissue. Periosteal traction, deformity	Relation of symptoms to radiographic evidence of disease. Pain at rest, disturbance of sleep
Degenerative joint disease	Periarticular disease. Abnormal stress on joint	Pain on weight-bearing or exercise. Radiographic appearance
Fractures	Abnormal bone texture. Fissure fractures, deformity	Sudden increase in pain. Radiographic evidence of fissure fractures, lytic defect
Deformity	Abnormal bone architecture. Mechanical stress	Standardized radiographs. Stereophotography
Neurological syndromes	Vascular steal. Direct compression by bone	Myelography. Therapeutic trial of antiresorptive therapy
Immobilization hypercalcaemia	Short-term reduction in bone turnover. Increased bone resorption	Active Paget's disease. Exclusion of other causes of hypercalcaemia

extend to completion with minimal or absent trauma. Sudden onset of pain, or exacerbation of existing pain, over a fissure fracture may indicate that it is extending to produce the typical transverse type of fracture (Figure 5.2). This process may occur rapidly over a few days, and any patient with a significantly bowed limb who develops rapidly progressive pain should not weight-bear until the diagnosis is established. Fractures may also occur through lytic intracortical defects (Figure 5.3), as well as through pagetic bone in the absence of fissure

fractures; but these two scenarios are relatively uncommon.

Pretreatment assessment
Stress fractures commonly present as a complete fracture in patients with previously asymptomatic or unrecognized Paget's disease. In patients where the presence of fissure fractures has been recognized, the sudden development of severe and fairly localized pain may give a clue to impending extension. This localization contrasts with the diffuse pain of other-

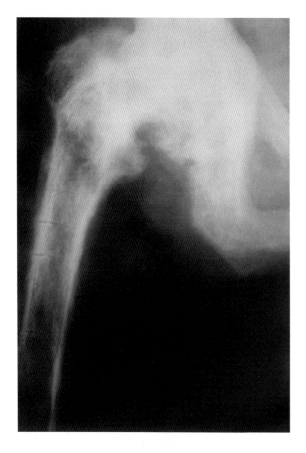

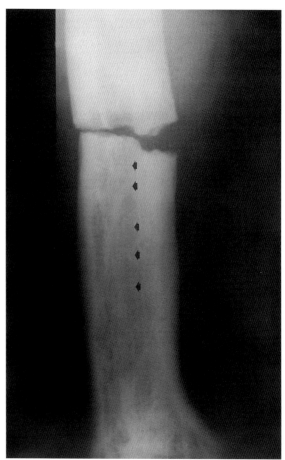

Figure 5.2 Complete transverse fracture. Arrows indicate fissure fractures.

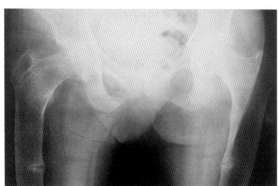

Figure 5.1 Fissure fractures in Paget's disease (top) and Looser's zones in osteomalacia (bottom).

wise uncomplicated Paget's disease.[10]

Fissure fractures are often multiple, and localization of the one which is extending can be difficult. Bone turnover markers are not of value in this regard, since they may be normal

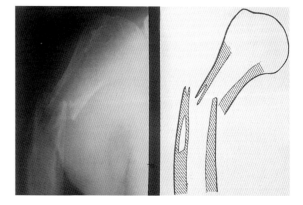

Figure 5.3 Intracortical lytic defect and fracture.

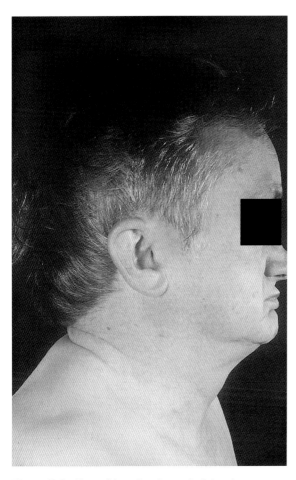

Figure 5.4 Frontal bossing from skull involvement.

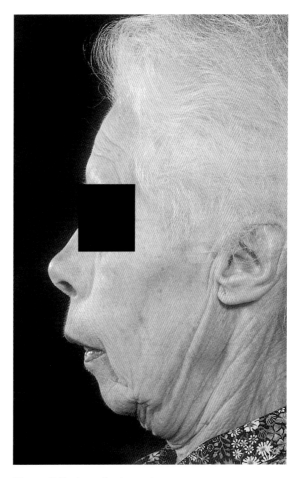

Figure 5.5 Leontiasis ossium.

or raised.[11] Identification of the site of maximum tenderness on deep palpation allows placement of a radio-opaque marker on the skin. This can be followed by a good-quality radiograph to show whether the site of pain corresponds to an underlying fissure.

Since fissure fractures have high rates of bone turnover and increased vascularity they will tend to preferentially accumulate antiresorptive drugs such as the bisphosphonates. These may disrupt the steady state and precipitate extension. It is therefore important to obtain good-quality radiographs of all affected weight-bearing bones before starting antiresorptive treatment. This is important so

that all fissure fractures or other foci of potential weakness can be identified, in order that the patient and physician can be alerted to the significance of sudden exacerbations of pain at these sites.

Deformity

In addition to long bone deformity and involvement of the neural envelope (which will be considered in the next section), Paget's disease of the skull and face may rarely give rise to distressing symptoms. Skull involvement may lead to frontal bossing (Figure 5.4), headaches, and more rarely to cognitive impairment due to the diversion of blood from the internal to the external carotid system. Paget's disease of the maxilla leads to leontiasis ossium (Figure 5.5), which, apart from its physical appearance, leads to anterior displacement of the upper teeth. Expansion of the mandible results in a similar anterior displacement of the lower jaw, and both syndromes may lead to atypical facial pain, particularly over the temporomandibular joint on chewing, as well as poor dental health.[12]

Pretreatment assessment
The extent of malocclusion is best assessed radiographically, but good-quality clinical photographs may also help. Progression is fortunately slow, but makes it difficult to assess natural history or the response to treatment.

Neurological syndromes

The main neurological syndromes in Paget's disease arise from the consequences of basilar invagination or the encroachment on cranial nerve exit foraminae. Distortion of the fourth ventricle and brain stem by basilar invagination may result in internal hydrocephalus, brainstem or cerebellar syndromes, or vertebrobasilar insufficiency.[13] Encroachment on cranial nerve exit foraminae leads to lower motor neurone lesions. The foraminae of the auditory and ocular nerves are the most commonly affected. However, such changes are relatively uncommon given the predilection of Paget's disease for the skull. Deafness is always difficult to evaluate because hearing declines with age; both ossicular involvement and auditory nerve compression can be caused by Paget's disease.

Paget's disease of the spine leads to compressive symptoms due to vertebral collapse or bony expansion encroaching into the spinal canal or intervetebral foraminae. Since the cervical spine is uncommonly involved in Paget's disease, most spinal syndromes are due to involvement of the thoracic and lumbar segments, giving rise to paraparesis or radicular symptoms. Cauda equina lesions occur with Paget's disease below L2.

Pretreatment assessment
The main issue here is to separate symptoms due to direct compression of nervous tissue from those due to vascular steal syndromes. The latter are probably more common than is usually recognized and arise because of diversion of arterial blood away from nervous tissue to the vascular bone. Direct encroachment can usually be identified by MRI or CT myelography, but vascular steal syndromes may only be identified by a therapeutic trial of a potent antiresorptive agent, which may rapidly relieve symptoms.[14]

Miscellaneous symptoms

A variety of other symptoms have been attributed to Paget's disease, such as high-output cardiac failure and dementia. All of these are multifactorial in aetiology and more common in the elderly. Specific syndromes, such as immobilization hypercalcaemia and sarcomatous change, are exceedingly rare.

INVESTIGATIONS

The next step in management is to assess the activity and extent of the disease, because this will influence the dose and duration of antiresorptive therapy.

Biochemistry

Biochemical markers of bone turnover provide an easy method of assessing disease activity and its response to treatment (Figure 5.6). The most widely available measurements are those of total alkaline phosphatase (AP), reflecting bone formation, and fasting urinary hydroxyproline excretion (HYPRO), reflecting resorption. However neither is entirely specific for bone turnover because they also receive significant contributions from non-skeletal sources. This is not a major problem when bone turnover is high, but becomes progressively more important as activity falls with treatment, particularly when monitoring changes within the reference range. Several newer alternatives have recently been introduced with the aim of improving sensitivity and specificity. Their advantages, however, are relatively small, being 73% and 64% for the respective sensitivities of pyridinoline and hydroxyproline and 84% and 78% for both bone-specific (BAP) and total alkaline phosphatase.[15] Other markers, such as osteocalcin, deoxypyridinoline, tartrate-resistant acid phosphatase and the telopeptide of type I collagen, seem much less sensitive and have little to offer compared with the relatively inexpensive traditional markers.

A pragmatic approach is to use total AP and HYPRO to monitor the early phase of treatment and to add measurements of BAP and the best currently available cross-link marker as activity approaches and falls within the reference range. Currently, there are no available data to show whether these aspirations can be realized and which of the resorption assays is best for this purpose.

After a single intravenous infusion of a bis-phosphonate, resorption markers fall to a nadir value within about a week, while AP declines over about six weeks. Measurement of resorption and formation markers at approximately 4–6-weekly intervals therefore provides adequate information with which to assess the response to treatment. This approach is also suitable for the monitoring of oral treatment, particularly since antiresorptive drugs are often licensed for use in three-monthly courses. Measurements at weeks 0, 6, 12 and 18 therefore provide good data upon which to assess response and the need for retreatment. The current aim of treatment is to reduce bone turnover to near the middle of the normal range, since this is associated with an extended duration of control once therapy is withdrawn (Figure 5.7).[6,17]

Radiology and scintigraphy

Skeletal imaging is an essential stage in the evaluation of the new patient with Paget's disease, and selective examination may be needed

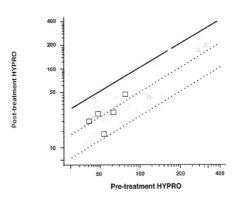

Figure 5.6 Pretreatment bone turnover predicts post-treatment nadir.

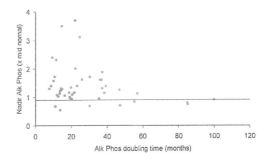

Figure 5.7 Post-treatment nadir and duration of remission.

to reassess established cases. An isotope bone scan is the best first step, because although increased uptake is non-specific it is the most sensitive way of assessing the distribution and extent of the disease. With modern software particular areas of interest can be identified and their activity quantitated in relation to an unaffected reference site (commonly a contralateral limb). This may be particularly useful with limited or monostotic disease where the affected bone is too small to raise 'whole body' biochemical markers of bone turnover.[18]

Radiographs of all affected sites should be obtained for all new patients, both to confirm the diagnosis and to evaluate the potential for

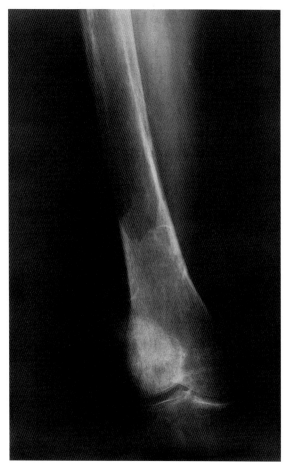

Figure 5.8 Extensive lytic resorption front in shaft of femur.

Finally, radiology is also useful to assess bowing deformity of long bones[11] and the contribution this may make to the development of degenerative joint disease adjacent to the pagetic areas. It is also highly relevant to the clinical assessment of the probability of symptomatic relief with medical treatment.

The diagnosis of Paget's disease is generally straightforward, and relies on the combination of typical clinical symptoms, bone turnover markers, and the characteristic changes on bone radiology and scintigraphy. Occasionally there may be diagnostic problems, and these are summarized in Table 5.2. Bone biopsy is rarely indicated in the routine management of Paget's disease, but is occasionally required where investigations of a particular lesion are equivocal.

current or future complications. Although some sites may be asymptomatic, they should be examined because they may lead to future problems and therefore may have a bearing on the choice of treatment.

All affected weight-bearing bones should be examined radiographically to identify areas of mechanical weakness such as fissure fractures, intracortical lytic defects or extensive resorption fronts (Figure 5.8), because over-enthusiastic antiresorptive treatment may increase the risk of a complete fracture. The skull (particularly the base) and the spine also require evaluation in terms of the current or future potential to cause neurological 'compression' syndromes.

Table 5.2 Diagnostic sequences in Paget's disease.

Identification of symptoms and their relationship to skeletal involvement

Assessment of pretreatment disease activity:
   Total alkaline phosphatase, fasting urine hydroxyproline
   Newer markers: bone-specific alkaline phosphatase, urinary cross-links

Skeletal scintigraphy:
   Identification of distribution of disease
   Quantification of areas of focal activity

Radiology:
   Confirmation of diagnosis of Paget's disease
   Exclusion of other metabolic bone disease
   Identification of areas of skeletal weakness
      Fissure fractures
      Intracortical lytic defects
      Extensive resorption fronts

AIMS OF TREATMENT

Pain relief

Assessment of pain relief is complicated, because its aetiology is multifactorial and there is little correlation between its severity and either the extent or the activity of the disease.

Pain localized to the middle of the diaphysis responds better than that near the epiphysis because of the complicating influence of degenerative joint disease. However, osteoarthritis should not be a bar to medical treatment, because this may improve symptoms sufficiently to make them tolerable, or may even give sufficient relief to avoid joint replacement.

Treatment with etidronate, one of the earliest bisphosphonates, has been shown to reduce bone pain in a dose-dependent manner[19–21] and in a recent study with risedronate the time course of pain relief mirrored changes in bone turnover.[22] Few of the bisphosphonates have been compared in terms of their effects on pain, but two recent controlled studies showed no difference between etidronate and tiludronate[23] and etidronate and alendronate.[24] Anecdotally, some patients show recurrence of symptoms at a particular level of bone turnover (sometimes within the reference range), and this remains reproducible in each relapse over a period of years.

Neurological symptoms

Acute onset of paraparesis or quadriparesis in the presence of MRI evidence of cord compression is an indication for urgent neurosurgical decompression. This is not without technical difficulties, because of the vascularity of the abnormal bone and the increased risk of compression at more than one site.[25] Although benefit has been reported in up to 85% of patients,[26] there may be a 10% mortality.[27] Where symptoms are less acute, particularly where direct compression of the cord is minimal or absent, medical treatment has been shown to be of benefit. The rapid response to calcitonin[28] or bisphosphonates[14,27] is consistent

with the vascular steal aetiology. Since in this situation the degree of clinical improvement correlates well with the magnitude of the biochemical response,[13,27] treatment should be maintained as long as bone turnover is decreasing, with the aim of achieving values within the reference range. Even where there is some evidence of cord compression, antiresorptive therapy may still produce clinical benefit but responses are generally slower, and myelographic evidence of improvement has been variable.[28]

Headaches due to skull vault involvement often respond well to medical treatment, but the response of deafness has been inconsistent.[29] This almost certainly reflects the multifactorial and non-pagetic component of this symptom.

Pre-operative reduction in bone vascularity

The increased vascularity of pagetic bone has been reported to double blood loss during total hip replacement,[30] although another study showed no effect on operative variables such as blood loss, operation time or post-operative complications.[31] Since bone blood flow can be rapidly reduced by antiresorptive therapy there seems no reason why patients should not be pretreated before elective surgery. There is, of course, much less potential in the case of emergency surgery. The rapid vascular response to calcitonin[32] may be of value, but in general the disadvantages of delaying surgery usually outweigh possible advantages.

Reduction in deformity

The current ability to restore and maintain normal bone turnover over a period of years has stimulated interest in the prevention or correction of deformity. There are interesting studies using specialized techniques such as stereophotography of superficial skeletal sites that show small reductions in deformity with long-term control of bone turnover.[33] These findings support the reasonable (but as yet unproven) expectation that prolonged control of bone turnover may prevent the emergence of clinical deformity or degenerative joint disease. Since the typical skeletal deformities of Paget's disease develop slowly over a period of years and their distorting force increases as the deformity progresses, it is unlikely that medical treatment will have noticeable effects. If deformity, and therefore the orientation of the distorting forces, is corrected surgically, as may happen after a complete long-bone fracture, then modelling over a period of years may restore a relatively normal appearance.

Fissure fractures present a particular management problem, in that they reflect a dynamic equilibrium between deformity-mediated distraction forces and healing through fracture callus. The blood flow to the affected site is also increased, so that over-enthusiastic therapy with bisphosphonates, the deposition of which is partly blood flow-dependent, may suppress the reparative process, so that the fissure fracture extends to completion. The need to have good-quality radiographs of fissure fractures has already been emphasized. Low-dose bisphosphonate therapy should also be employed and, if there is an option, oral treatment is probably safer than the intravenous route.

Immobilization hypercalcaemia

This is an uncommon problem even in patients with extensive and very active Paget's disease who are immobilized, either as a consequence of a fracture or systemic illness. The hypercalcaemia responds rapidly to intravenous bisphosphonate, and a recurrence can be prevented by maintenance oral therapy.

High-output cardiac failure

Paget's disease is rarely the main contributory factor in elderly cardiovascular patients, but where the disease is very active it is reasonable to add antiresorptive therapy to the conventional treatment with diuretics and angiotensin-converting enzyme inhibitors.

Sarcoma

There is no evidence that the emergence of this very rare complication is reduced by control of bone turnover, nor is the outcome of the tumour influenced by antiresorptive therapy.

Restoration of normal bone turnover

Biochemical markers of bone turnover are the most practical and objective method of evaluating the response to treatment and comparing different therapies or schedules. For the reasons already discussed, monitoring centres around the regular measurement of serum alkaline phosphatase and urinary hydroxyproline excretion.

Normal bone turnover

Several studies have shown that the achievement of normal bone turnover is associated with a prolonged duration of remission once treatment is discontinued.[16,34] The real issue is what is meant by 'normal' bone turnover.

For any individual their normal alkaline phosphatase lies (with a 95% probability) somewhere within the reference range; but if they develop Paget's disease, then this value will rise, although the original will be unknown at the time of clinical presentation. However, the lower the post-treatment alkaline phosphatase then the greater the probability that it lies below the pre-pagetic normal value for that individual. Experience suggests, therefore, that the duration of biochemical remission once treatment is withdrawn will vary directly with the post-treatment bone turnover. This has led to the current practice of aiming to reduce bone turnover to below the mid-point of the reference range as a compromise aimed at maximizing the duration of remission while avoiding over-suppression of bone turnover.

Biochemical relapse

The concept of relapse is somewhat arbitrary, and there are a number of options. Relapse can be equated with a bone turnover above a particular value, such as the upper limit of the reference range or a multiple of this value. Clearly, in view of what has been discussed above, the magnitude of this change will depend on the individual's true normal bone turnover. While this is an entirely arbitrary cut-off, it has the advantage of simplicity and pragmatism.

A more logical approach is to consider relapse as being that change in bone turnover of which there is a low probability ($P < 0.01$) that it is due to the chance factors such as random biological or assay variability. For serum alkaline phosphatase this equates with a change of +25%.[34]

A refinement is to calculate the rate of increase in bone turnover to predict the point in time when this 25% threshold is likely to be exceeded. Since relapse shows a log-linear increase with time, the increase can be expressed as the time that it takes for the alkaline phosphatase to double.[35] With the newer bisphosphonates this doubling time will be about 12–24 months, so that regular measurements at 3–4-monthly intervals will give some indication as to when retreatment will be required.

Monitoring frequency

Bone resorption falls rapidly over 5–10 days after an intravenous infusion of a potent bisphosphonate followed by a slower decline in formation markers over about six weeks.[35] In practical terms measurement of serum total alkaline phosphatase and fasting urine HYPRO/creatinine at 4–6-weekly intervals gives a good indication of the effects of repeated bisphosphonate infusions. The same monitoring frequency is also appropriate for oral bisphosphonate therapy. A measurement 4–6 weeks after completion of either treatment schedule gives an indication of the final response.

For monostotic or limited disease more frequent measurements at 3–4 weekly intervals during treatment may allow the identification of a trend within the reference range that can be used to judge dose and duration of treatment. Newer and more specific markers are theoretically attractive, but their practical utility has yet to be demonstrated.

Monitoring the maintenance of remission or relapse requires bone turnover measurements at about 3–4-monthly intervals.

TREATMENT STRATEGIES

Treatment strategy falls into two broad categories, namely, regular intravenous infusions and oral therapy. Each has its advantages and disadvantages, which are summarized in Table 5.3. However, with currently available bisphosphonates, optimal control of disease activity can be achieved with either route of administration. The choice therefore depends on the facilities available in the treatment centre and patient preference.

Intravenous administration equates with a known compliance and avoids uncertainties about the efficacy of gastrointestinal bisphosphonate absorption. While it is convenient for patients living near the treatment centre, it may not be for those who live at a distance. Specimens for monitoring response are much easier to collect in those who attend regularly for intravenous infusions, and, apart from the occasional acute phase response with aminobisphosphonates,[36] this route is generally trouble-free.

Bisphosphonates need to be taken fasting, because of their poor gastrointestinal absorption. This is sometimes difficult to assess, as is overall compliance with treatment when patients on oral therapy are only seen for monitoring visits. For patients living some distance from the treatment centre, oral therapy, which can be supervised in primary care, is the only realistic option. Side-effects such as upper gastrointestinal irritation or diarrhoea may be a problem with oral therapy, and may lead to discontinuation of treatment if this is supervised in a non-specialist centre.

Table 5.3	Treatment options in Paget's disease.	
	Intravenous	Oral
Compliance	Known with certainty	Less certain
Administered dose	50% to bone, rest excreted by kidney	Must be taken fasting to optimize absorption (1–10% administered dose)
Patient convenience	Good if near treatment centre. Avoids regular tablet ingestion	Convenient for treatment managed in primary care
Monitoring	Easy to perform before each infusion	Generally restricted to monitoring visits
Side-effects	Acute phase response with aminobisphosphonate	Upper gastrointestinal dyspepsia or diarrhoea

Intravenous therapy

Pamidronate is currently the only bisphosphonate licensed for treatment of Paget's disease by the intravenous route in the UK. The situation may change as newer bisphosphonates are introduced.

Pamidronate

Pamidronate is irritant to the mucous membranes of the mouth and the upper gastrointestinal tract,[36] and as a consequence it is usually given intravenously. It has been used extensively, and is currently the best option for this route of administration. Most published studies[36–42] have given about 200 mg over a period of about 10 days (Table 5.4). For a pretreatment bone turnover of approximately 3 times the upper limit of normal this regimen will decrease the excess bone turnover (above the mid-point of the reference range) by 65–95% and restore normal values in 60–95% of

patients. Shorter courses or single infusions[39–42] tend to be less effective and predictable, but some are impressive.[41] None of these regimens has been associated with significant side-effects except for the acute phase reaction,[36–40] transient exacerbations of bone pain after the first infusion,[38,42] and transient hypocalcaemia.[38] Although pamidronate is generally free from the problem of defective mineralization, occasional complications of this nature have been reported with high-dose pamidronate therapy.

Since the pretreatment bone turnover is the most readily identifiable indicator of the probability of achieving normal bone turnover, it seems reasonable to stratify dose accordingly. Our practice is summarized below:

1. Mildly active disease (pre-treatment alkaline phosphatase $< \times 3$ upper limit of normal) should be treated with 30–60 mg of pamidronate at 4–6-weekly intervals to achieve full assessment of the response after each dose. This regimen is not suitable

for more active disease because only about 30% of patients will achieve normal turnover by 6 months and treatment is too protracted.[43]

2. Moderately active disease (pre-treatment alkaline phosphatase < × 10 the upper limit of normal) should be treated with 60 mg of pamidronate at 2-weekly intervals to a total dose of about 300 mg (Figure 5.6).

3. For very active disease (pre-treatment alkaline phosphatase > × 10 the upper limit of normal) the above regimen should be extended in duration (6 months) and dose (up to 1000 mg). New cases with this degree of activity are uncommon,[5] and if available the use of one of the more potent bisphosphonates would be an advantage.[44]

Once bone turnover has reached a stable minimum value, pamidronate should be withdrawn and the subsequent changes in disease activity monitored. This is best achieved with sequential measurements of alkaline phosphatase, which has greater precision and reproducibility compared to hydroxyproline.[34] One of the characteristic features of bisphosphonate treatment is that remissions may be prolonged (3–25 months),[16,38,42] though the disease will eventually relapse. This is conventionally taken as an increase in alkaline phosphatase of 25% above the minimum post-treatment value. The main determinants of relapse after the withdrawal of pamidronate therapy are the pre-treatment and minimum alkaline phosphatase concentrations and the rate of response to the first dose of pamidronate.[16] Of these it is the initial response to treatment that is most predictive. If patients achieve a normal post-treatment alkaline phosphatase then 41% can be expected to be in remission at one year, in contrast to 4% of those who do not achieve normal turnover. Even so, there is tremendous variability of remission, even in those who achieve normal bone turnover,[16] and in one study remission extended to 2.7 years.[36] The most probable explanation for this variability is the uncertainty of what a normal alkaline phosphatase actually means for an individual.

Clodronate

This bisphosphonate is of intermediate potency between etidronate and pamidronate, but does not impair mineralization even at high therapeutic doses. The intravenous route avoids the problem of gastrointestinal side-effects, and a number of regimes have been compared and found to be similar.[45]

1. Five daily infusions of 300 mg over 4 hours reduced bone turnover by almost 60% within 1–3 months, and this response was sustained in the majority of patients six months later, but only in 22% by a year later.

2. A single infusion of 1500 mg produced a similar response (Table 5.4), but with a slightly higher proportion (40%) of patients still in remission at a year. However, this difference in this small study was not statistically significant.

3. Five monthly infusions of 300 mg clearly reduced bone turnover more slowly, but the effect, by comparison with the other options, was similar.

This study seemed to suggest that it is the total dose of clodronate rather than the duration of treatment that is the main determinant of response. Clodronate is less effective than pamidronate for a comparable level of disease activity, but is suitable for patients with only modest bone turnover. As with all bisphosphonates, the duration of remission is heavily influenced by the degree to which bone turnover is suppressed by treatment.[34,35]

Oral therapy

As bisphosphonate potency is increased this has enabled the dose needed to control Paget's disease to be decreased, thereby reducing local irritation and opening the way for effective, well-tolerated oral therapy.

Etidronate

Etidronate was the first bisphosphonate introduced for the treatment of Paget's disease over 25 years ago. It transformed management,

Table 5.4 Response to intravenous bisphosphonates in the treatment of Paget's disease.

Bisphosphonate	Ref.	Total dose (mg)	Duration (days)	n	Alk. phos. (×ULN)	3 months		6 months	
						% decrease*	Normal %	% decrease*	Normal %
Pamidronate	37	120	2–8	31	1.57	93.3	90	97.8	94
		180	2–8	18	3.71	84.4	50	88.4	67
		240	2–8	13	9.20	82.3	0	89.3	15
Pamidronate	36	200	10	32	2.43	—	—	87.9	81
Pamidronate	38	180	42	30	4.80	—	—	87.0	53
Pamidronate	39	200	10	14	3.29	76.6	55	82.0	60
		200	5	16	2.55	64.2	54	58.1	66
		40	4	15	2.18	59.9	9	48.4	36
		10	1	13	2.22	3.7	0	1.8	0
Pamidronate	40	105	1	14	3.04	75.6	71	82.3	71
	41	60	1	26	7.44	94.8	85	99.3	78
Pamidronate	42	75	5	11	6.90	—	—	56.7	50
		180	84	9	4.35	—	—	94.4	78
Clodronate	45	1500	5	20	2.94	—	—	59.8**	32**
		1500	1	20	1.99	—	—	51.1**	16**
		1500	150	20	2.74	—	—	62.8**	15**

* Decrease of excess above mid-point of reference range.
** Time of minimum not stated.

because its potency and persistence of action greatly exceeded that of currently available drugs. However, use of the most effective dose was limited by the development of defective mineralization, and it has largely been superseded by more potent bisphosphonates.

Over the range 2.5 to 20 mg/kg/day (200–1600 mg/day) etidronate decreased bone turnover in a dose-dependent fashion (40–60% decrease in alkaline phosphatase) and also relieved pain.[46–48] The major limiting factor was the development of defective mineralization in 10–20% of patients given more than 800 mg/day for 6 months. Clinically this presented with severe bone pain or fractures (not necessarily in pagetic bone); and although the defect regressed when the drug was withdrawn, it does limit treatment to suboptimal doses.

Since pretreatment disease activity is the major determinant of whether treatment will induce a remission, there is still a place for etidronate in the treatment of modest disease. In patients with an alkaline phosphatase approximately twice the upper limit of normal, about 75% of patients will achieve a remission with 400 mg daily for 6 months. An alternative is to give 1600 mg daily for one month, which may be more convenient for the patient, although this may be accompanied by a transient mineralization defect. As the pretreatment disease activity increases, the proportion of patients achieving remission with these doses will diminish and more potent bisphosphonates should be used if they are available.

All bisphosphonates are badly absorbed from the upper gastrointestinal tract and they must be given on an empty stomach, with food being delayed for at least one hour. They should be taken with large volumes of water (and not with other liquids) in the upright position.

Clodronate

Oral therapy with clodronate has been investigated over a wide dose range of 400–2400 mg per day, but the optimum dose, balancing effectiveness against side-effects, seems to be 800 mg daily. This dose given for 6 months can be expected to reduce bone turnover by 70–80% by the end of treatment.[49,50] This response seems largely independent of pre-treatment activity, and about 50% of patients will achieve stable, normal levels of bone turnover. More active disease (pre-treatment bone turnover $> \times 10$ the upper limit of normal) may respond better to 1600 mg per day; and in one study 73% of patients achieved normal bone turnover by 6 months.[49]

The transient uncoupling of bone resorption and formation that occurs with the early phase of bisphosphonate treatment[35] leads to a transient (3–4 month) 2–4-fold increase in parathyroid hormone. This can be prevented by calcium and vitamin D supplements, and although this results in lower levels of alkaline phosphatase it does not influence the degree of control of bone resorption.[50] Serum calcium is maintained within the normal range by this secondary hyperparathyroidism, and there is no evidence that supplementation is a clinically useful adjunct to bisphosphonate therapy.

Tiludronate

In vitro studies with tiludronate, a bisphosphonate with a thiomethylene side chain, show it to be ten times more active than etidronate; comparative studies in Paget's disease confirm its greater activity, although not with such a wide margin.

Over a range of 100–800 mg/day, tiludronate produced a dose-dependent decrease in bone turnover that only reaches significance compared to placebo at 400 mg/day or more.[51] In patients with a 4–5-fold increase in bone turnover 400–800 mg/day reduces bone turnover by 45–50% at 3 months, with 15–18% achieving normal values. In this particular study there was a marginal benefit in terms of efficacy of the 800 mg dose without a significant increase in side-effects. However, subsequent studies, using a formulation (200 mg tablet) that was better absorbed, have centred on the 400 mg dose, which represents the best balance between efficacy and side-effects.

This formulation (400 mg per day) was used in a large open labelled 6-month treatment study[52] where the pretreatment alkaline phosphatase was 3.44 times the upper limit of normal. Bone turnover was reduced by 47.2% at 3 months and by 58.3% at the end of the 6-month treatment period, with 28% of patients achieving values in the normal range.

In another study,[23] tiludronate (400 mg/day) given for either 3 or 6 months was considerably more effective than etidronate given in a dose of 400 mg daily for 6 months (Table 5.5). In the tiludronate group the responses at 3 and 6 months were similar, and this has led to the recommendation that the initial course of treatment should be for 3 months, which can be repeated in 3 months in those patients who have not achieved normal turnover. Another important observation in this study was the influence of previous bisphosphonate therapy. The response to etidronate was diminished by prior etidronate therapy, whereas this had no effect on the response to tiludronate. Subsequent studies with other bisphosphonates suggest that responses may be improved by changing the class of bisphosphonate from one treatment course to another. Recent studies of the mechanism of action of bisphosphonates at a cellular level provide a possible explanation for these differing clinical responses.[53]

Tiludronate is clearly more effective than etidronate, which is the only bisphosphonate to which it has been compared in a randomized study. As with all bisphosphonates, gastrointestinal side-effects such as dyspepsia and nausea are the main problem. Early, but usually mild, diarrhoea seems a particular effect of tiludronate. Patients with very active disease will generally require a second 3-month course of treatment in order to achieve normal bone turnover. However, it is clear that response is maintained once treatment is withdrawn and the 3-month interval between treatment courses is not usually attended by a significant relapse. This pattern of treatment also allows the full effects of the first course of tiludronate to be evaluated before embarking on a more extended therapy.

Alendronate
Extension of the amino side chain of pamidronate by another carbon atom produces alendronate, with an approximate 10-fold increase in potency compared with pamidronate. Osteoporosis is the main licensed indication for alendronate (in a dose of 10 mg daily), but several studies of a larger dose (40 mg/day) in Paget's disease have confirmed its efficacy.

In an early study of mild Paget's disease,[54] 40 mg/day of alendronate was shown to be more effective than 20 mg/day in terms both of the reduction in disease activity (50% compared to 24%) and the proportion of patients who achieved a normal level of bone turnover. However, in three of the ten patients given the 40 mg dose, treatment had to be withdrawn because of gastric or oesophageal irritation. This seemed to be a particular problem, because the beneficial effects of the higher dose could not be reproduced by giving the lower dose for longer.

In a larger double-blind randomized placebo-controlled trial over 6 months the efficacy of the 40 mg dose was confirmed (Table 5.5).[55] Compared to the other reported studies, the response to alendronate for the level of pre-treatment bone turnover seems superior to other oral therapies and comparable to that achieved with intravenous pamidronate (Table 5.4). This study also showed improvement in osteolytic lesions seen radiographically in just under half the patients, while only 4% of those receiving placebo improved. Bone histology in a subset of patients confirmed the absence of defective mineralization with this regimen, and also showed the deposition of lamellar rather than woven bone during treatment. The 40 mg dose was well tolerated, and in this double-blind study there was a low incidence of treatment-related gastrointestinal side-effects. Treatment was subsequently extended beyond 6 months in some patients, who showed a continuing response, with 74% ultimately achieving normal bone turnover.

Alendronate (40 mg daily) has also been compared to etidronate (400 mg daily) in a randomized double-blind study extending over 6 months.[24] Both groups included very active disease, and the superiority of alendronate was demonstrated in terms both of the reduction in

Table 5.5 Comparison of oral bisphosphonates in the treatment of Paget's disease.

Bisphosphonate	Ref.	Daily dose (mg)	Duration (months)	n	Alk. phos. (×ULN)	3 months		6 months	
						% decrease*	Normal %	% decrease*	Normal %
Etidronate	23	400	6	79	4.30	44.3	5	54.2	11
	24	400	6	47	5.33	39.8	11	50.1	17
Tiludronate	23	400	3	78	4.80			81.5	24
		400	6	77	4.52	75.2	14	83.5	27
Alendronate	54	40	6	10	2.03	74.2	—	82.2	60
	55	40	6	55	4.70	69.1	12	85.4	48
	24	40	6	42	6.50	71.7	27	88.1	63
Risedronate	22	30	3	20	6.10	63.0	5	79.5	40
	57	30	3	160	6.95	66.3	12	75.1	33
	58	30	1	21	7.00	72.2	14	—	—

* Percentage decrease of excess alkaline phosphatase above mid-point of reference range.

disease activity and of the achievement of normal bone turnover (Table 5.5). The study also confirmed the earlier work, showing an absence of defective mineralization and improvement in radiographic osteolysis. The safety profile of alendronate was similar to that of etidronate, even in terms of upper gastrointestinal adverse experiences.

The duration of alendronate treatment required to achieve normal bone turnover depends on the pre-treatment activity. In patients with a pre-treatment bone turnover of 2–3 times the upper limit of normal, 6 months' treatment with 40 mg or 80 mg daily will achieve normal bone turnover in all patients.[56] More active disease will require a longer treatment period but this aim seems to be achieved with a 40 mg dose.[55]

The rapid inhibition of bone resorption relative to formation leads to secondary hyperparathyroidism which may persist to some degree for up to a year,[56] but does not seem to be clinically significant. Alendronate, like other aminobisphosphonates, may be accompanied by an acute phase response with a transient fall (over about 3 days) in total white cell count, neutrophils, lymphocytes, and platelets, which, on recovery, may stabilize above normal.[56]

Risedronate
Risedronate is a pyridinyl bisphosphonate, which in animal studies has been shown to be 1000 times more potent, as an antiresorptive agent, than etidronate. It does not impair mineralization even at 3000 times the minimum effective antiresorptive dose.

Clinical studies have utilized a 30 mg dose given for 3 months, with retreatment after a 3-month interval if bone turnover remains elevated.[22,57,58] In disease of moderate to severe activity it reduces turnover by 75–80% after a single course (Table 5.5), and with retreatment restores normal activity in just over half the patients.[22,57]

In these open label studies there was a significant reduction in pain due to pagetic bone involvement and the drug seemed to have a good safety profile. Upper gastrointestinal side-effects, mainly dyspepsia and nausea, occurred in 20% of patients, but were generally mild and did not lead to withdrawal of treatment.

As with tiludronate, the three-monthly on–off–on treatment schedule allows a complete evaluation of the first course of treatment before the next is commenced. Bone turnover remains stable during the period off treatment and there is no evidence that cyclical therapy leads to loss of disease control.

None of the newer bisphosphonates (tiludronate, alendronate and risedronate) have been compared directly in the same clinical trial. As a consequence, their relative merits can only be assessed from the type of criteria set out in Table 5.5. This is a significant handicap, since it is well recognized that there is substantial individual variation in the response to treatment. All these agents seem potent and will control even very active disease if given in optimal doses for a sufficient period of time. None of them seems to cause defective mineralization and there do not seem to be major differences in their side-effect profile. The choice therefore seems to be determined by experience with a particular drug, its availability (licensed for the indication of Paget's disease), and its cost.

Calcitonin
Calcitonin has been superseded as an antiresorptive agent by the bisphosphonates because of their greater potency, acceptability and better safety profile. The role of calcitonin in the current management of Paget's disease is limited. There is some evidence that its effects on bone blood flow[32] are more rapid than those of the bisphosphonates. As a consequence it may have a role in the emergency treatment of severe neurological compression syndromes such as paraparesis, or in the short-term preparation for joint replacement. However, calcitonin and bisphosphonates have not been directly compared; but in these desperate circumstances there is no reason why these two agents should not be administered concurrently. A suitable regimen would be 100 IU daily of salmon calcitonin given intramuscularly or subcutaneously.[28] Although calcitonin can be given intranasally, the bioavailability is less certain than the parenteral route.

REFERENCES

1. Rebel A, Malkani K, Basle M, Bregeon C (1976). Osteoclast ultrastructure in Paget's disease. *Calcif Tissue Res 20:* 187–199.
2. Reddy SV, Singer FR, Mallette L, Roodman GD (1996). Detection of measles virus nucleocapsid transcripts in circulating blood cells from patients with Paget's disease. *J Bone Miner Res 11:* 1602–1607.
3. Roodman GD (1996). Paget's disease and osteoclast biology. *Bone 19:* 209–212.
4. Mee AP, Hillarby C, Selby PL, Mawer EB, Hoyland JA (1997). Up-regulation of Bcl-2 mRNA in Paget's disease: the link between viral infection and genetic susceptibility. *Bone 20* (suppl 4): 10S.
5. Cundy T, McAnulty K, Wattie D, Gamble G, Rutland M, Ibbertson HK (1997). Evidence for secular change in Paget's disease. *Bone 20*: 69–71.
6. Gold DT, Boisture J, Shipp KM, Pieper CF, Lyles KW (1996). Paget's disease of the bone and quality of life. *J Bone Miner Res 11:* 1897–1904.
7. Nagant de Deuxchaisnes C, Krane SM (1964). Paget's disease of bone: clinical and metabolic observations. *Medicine 43:* 233–266.
8. Ring EFJ, Davies J, Barker JR (1977). Thermographic assessment of calcitonin therapy in Paget's disease. In: *Bone disease and calcitonin,* ed. JA Kanis, pp. 39–48. Armour Pharmaceuticals, Eastbourne.
9. Franck WA, Bress NM, Singer FR, Krane SM (1974). Rheumatic manifestations of Paget's disease of bone. *Am J Med 56:* 592–603.
10. Khairi MRA, Wellman HN, Robb JA, Johnston CC (1973). Paget's disease of bone (osteitis deformans): symptomatic lesion and bone scan. *Ann Intern Med 79:* 348–351.
11. Redden JF, Dixon J, Vennart W, Hosking DJ (1981). Management of fissure fractures in Paget's disease. *Int Orthop 5:* 103–106.
12. Wheeler TT, Alberts MA, Dolan TA, McGorray SP (1995). Dental, visual, auditory and olfactory complications in Paget's disease of bone. *J Am Geriatr Soc 43:* 1384–1391.
13. Kanis JA (1991). *Pathophysiology and treatment of Paget's disease of bone.* Martin Dunitz, London.
14. Wallace E, Wong J, Reid IR (1995). Pamidronate treatment of the neurologic sequelae of pagetic spinal stenosis. *Arch Int Med 155:* 1813–1815.
15. Alvarez L, Guanabens N, Peris P et al. (1995). Discriminative value of biochemical markers of bone turnover in assessing the activity of Paget's disease. *J Bone Miner Res 10:* 458–465.
16. Patel S, Stone MD, Coupland C, Hosking DJ (1993). Determinants of remission of Paget's disease of bone. *J Bone Miner Res 8:* 1467–1473.
17. Hosking DJ, Meunier PJ, Ringe JD, Reginster J-Y, Gennari C (1996). Paget's disease of bone: diagnosis and management. *BMJ 312*: 491–494.
18. Patel S, Pearson D, Hosking DJ (1995). Quantitative bone scintigraphy in the management of monostotic Paget's disease of bone. *Arthritis Rheum 38:* 1506–1512.
19. Altman RD, Johnston CC, Khairi MRA et al. (1973). Influence of disodium etidronate on clinical and laboratory manifestations of Paget's disease of bone (osteitis deformans). *N Engl J Med 289:* 1379–1384.
20. Canfield R, Rosner W, Skinner J (1977). Diphosphonate therapy of Paget's disease of bone. *J Clin Endocrinol Metab 44:* 96–106.
21. Ibbertson HK, Henley JW, Frazer TR et al. (1979). Paget's disease of bone – clinical evaluation and treatment with diphosphonate. *Aust NZ J Med 9:* 31–35.
22. Hosking DJ, Eusebio RA, Chines AA (1998). Paget's disease of bone: reduction of disease activity with oral risedronate. *Bone 22:* 51–55.
23. Roux C, Gennari C, Farrerons J et al. (1995). Comparative prospective, double-blind, multicenter study of the efficacy of tiludronate and etidronate in the treatment of Paget's disease of bone. *Arthritis Rheum 38:* 851–858.
24. Siris E, Weinstein RS, Altman R et al. (1996). Comparative study of alendronate versus etidronate for the treatment of Paget's disease of bone. *J Clin Endocrinol Metab 81:* 961–967.
25. Schmidek HM (1977). Neurologic and neurosurgical sequelae of Paget's disease of bone. *Clin Orthop 127:* 70–77.
26. Sadar ES, Walton RJ, Grossman HM (1972). Neurological dysfunction in Paget's disease of the vertebral column. *J Neurosurg 37:* 661–665.
27. Douglas DL, Kanis JA, Duckworth T et al. (1981). Paget's disease: improvement of spinal cord dysfunction with diphosphonate and calcitonin. *Metab Bone Dis Rel Res 3:* 327–336.
28. De Rose J, Singer FR, Avramides A et al. (1974). Response of Paget's disease to porcine and salmon calcitonins. Effects of long term treatment. *Am J Med 56:* 858–866.
29. Lando M, Hoover LA, Finerman G (1988). Stabilisation of hearing loss in Paget's disease with calcitonin and etidronate. *Arch Otolaryngol Head Neck Surg 114:* 891–894.

30. Goutallier D, Sterkers Y, Cadeau F (1984). Expérience de la prosthèse totale au cours de la coxopathie pagetique. *Rheumatologie 36:* 81–82.

31. Stauffer RN, Sim FH (1976). Total hip arthroplasty in Paget's disease of the hip. *J Bone Joint Surg 58A:* 76–78.

32. Wooton R, Reeve J, Spellacy R et al. (1978). Skeletal blood flow in Paget's disease of bone and its response to calcitonin therapy. *Clin Sci Mol Med 54:* 69–74.

33. Kanis JA, Gray RES (1987). Long term follow up observations on treatment in Paget's disease of bone. *Clin Orthop 217:* 99–125.

34. Gray RES, Yate AJP, Preston CJ et al. (1987). Duration of effect of oral diphosphonate therapy in Paget's disease of bone. *Q J Med 64:* 755–767.

35. Frijlink WB, Te Velde J, Bijvoet OLM, Heynen G (1979). Treatment of Paget's disease with (3-amino-1-hydroxypropylidene)-1,1 bisphosphonate (APD). *Lancet I:* 799–803.

36. Harinck HIJ, Papapoulos SE, Blanksma HJ, Mookenaar AJ, Vermeij P, Bijvoet OLM (1987). Paget's disease of bone: early and late responses to three different modes of treatment with aminohydroxypropylidene bisphosphonate (APD). *BMJ 295:* 1301–1305.

37. Gutteridge DH, Retallack RW, Ward LC et al. (1996). Clinical, biochemical, haematological and radiographic responses in Paget's disease following intravenous pamidronate disodium: a 2 year study. *Bone 19:* 387–394.

38. Ryan PJ, Sherry M, Gibson T et al. (1992). Treatment of Paget's disease by weekly infusions of 3 aminohydroxypropylidene-1,1-bisphosphonate (APD). *Br J Rheum 31:* 97–101.

39. Pepersack T, Karmali R, Gillet C et al. (1994). Paget's disease of bone: five regimens of pamidronate treatment. *Clin Rheum 13:* 39–44.

40. Watts RA, Skingle SJ, Bhambhani MM et al. (1993). Treatment of Paget's disease of bone with single dose intravenous pamidronate. *Ann Rheum Dis 52:* 616–618.

41. Chakravarty K, Merry P, Scott DGI (1994). A single infusion of bisphosphonate AHPrBP in the treatment of Paget's disease of bone. *J Rheumatol 21:* 2118–2121.

42. Cantrill JA, Buckler HM, Anderson DC (1986). Low dose intravenous 3-amino-1-hydroxypropylidene-1,1-bisphosphonate (APD) for the treatment of Paget's disease of bone. *Ann Rheum Dis 45:* 1012–1018.

43. Stone MD, Hawthorne AB, Kerr D et al. (1990). Treatment of Paget's disease with intermittent low-dose infusions of disodium pamidronate (APD). *J Bone Miner Res 5:* 1231–1235.

44. Schweitzer DH, Zwinderman AH, Vermeij P et al. (1993). Improved treatment of Paget's disease with dimethylaminohydroxypropylidene bisphosphonate. *J Bone Miner Res 8:* 175–182.

45. Khan SA, McCloskey EV, Eyres KS et al. (1996). Comparison of three intravenous regimens of clodronate in Paget's disease of bone. *J Bone Miner Res 11:* 178–182.

46. Russell RGG, Smith R, Preston C et al. (1974). Diphosphonates in Paget's disease. *Lancet I:* 894–898.

47. Canfield R, Rosner W, Skinner J et al. (1977). Diphosphonate therapy of Paget's disease of bone. *J Clin Endocrinol Metab 44:* 96–106.

48. Khairi MRA, Altman RD, DeRosa GP et al. (1977). Sodium etidronate in the treatment of Paget's disease of bone. *Ann Intern Med 87:* 656–663.

49. Douglas DL, Duckworth TL, Kanis JA et al. (1990). Biochemical and clinical responses to dichloromethylene diphosphonate (Cl_2 MDP) in Paget's disease of bone. *Arthritis Rheum 23:* 1185–1192.

50. Delmas PD, Chapuy MC, Vignon E et al. (1982). Long-term effects of dichloromethylene diphosphonate in Paget's disease of bone. *J Clin Endocrinol Metab 54:* 837–844.

51. Reginster JY, Colson F, Morlock G et al. (1992). Evaluation of the efficacy and safety of oral tiludronate in Paget's disease of bone. *Arthritis Rheum 35:* 967–974.

52. Reginster JY, Treves R, Renier JC et al. (1994). Efficacy and tolerability of a new formulation of oral tiludronate (tablet) in the treatment of Paget's disease of bone. *J Bone Miner Res 9:* 615–619.

53. Luckman SP, Hughes DE, Coxon FB et al. (1998). Bisphosphonates act by inhibiting protein prenylation. *J Bone Miner Res 13:* 581–589.

54. Adami S, Mian M, Gatti P, Rossini M et al. (1994). Effects of two oral doses of alendronate in the treatment of Paget's disease of bone. *Bone 15:* 415–417.

55. Reid IR, Nicholson MD, Weinstein RS et al. (1996). Biochemical and radiologic improvement in Paget's disease of bone treated with alendronate: a randomised, placebo-controlled trial. *Am J Med 101:* 341–348.

56. Khan SA, Vasikaran S, McCloskey EV et al. (1997). Alendronate in the treatment of Paget's disease of bone. *Bone 20:* 263–271.

57. Siris ES, Chines AA, Altman RD et al. (1998). Risedronate in the treatment of Paget's disease: an open label, multicenter study. *J Bone Miner Res 13:* 1032–1038.

58. Brown JP, Kylstra JW, Bekker PJ et al. (1994). Risedronate in Pagets disease: preliminary results of a multicentre study. *Sem Arthrit Rheum 23:* 272.

6

Renal Bone Disease

Michael Schömig, Badri Lamichhane and Eberhard Ritz

OVERVIEW

Maintenance of an appropriate concentration of ionized calcium within the extracellular fluid (ECF Ca^{2+}) is critical to the normal functioning of a wide range of tissues. It depends on the integrated effects of the parathyroid hormone (PTH)–vitamin D endocrine system, acting predominantly through the kidney, bone and intestine. The kidney plays a pivotal role in the system not only through the excretion of waste products and the reabsorption of nutrients but as the site of production of 1.25 dihydroxyvitamin D ($1.25(OH)_2D$), a hormone with a wide range of physiological actions. It is therefore to be expected that when renal function becomes impaired there will be widespread consequences for mineral homeostasis in general and the skeleton in particular.

Renal bone disease is a major clinical problem in patients with terminal renal failure[1] and contributes significantly to their poor quality of life. It is mainly, but not exclusively, due to the consequences of secondary hyperparathyroidism and accelerated bone turnover. However, with the more efficient prevention and treatment of parathyroid hyperplasia, a significant number of patients are encountered with low bone turnover (adynamic bone disease). In the past this latter problem was usually due to aluminium toxicity, either derived from the dialysate or ingested as aluminium containing phosphate binders. Although this iatrogenic complication has virtually disappeared, the problem of adynamic bone disease remains. The cause of this condition is uncertain, and whether it has any clinical consequences, other than the propensity to hypercalcaemia, remains an unresolved question.

The pathogenesis of renal bone disease is at the same time complex, multifactorial and incompletely understood. Rather than comprising well-defined histopathological subtypes, it represents a spectrum of histological change ranging from a high turnover state driven by hyperparathyroidism through osteomalacia to a low turnover (adynamic) bone disease. While some of the cases of adynamic bone disease are due to vitamin D deficiency, and in the past some were due to aluminium toxicity, the removal of aluminium as a problem has left many cases unexplained. The two main subtypes will be briefly described, although it must be recognized that mixed changes where secondary hyperparathyroidism is combined with osteomalacia are common, and probably reflect the multifactorial nature of the condition.

HIGH TURNOVER (HYPERPARATHYROID) BONE DISEASE (TABLE 6.1)

Hyperphosphataemia: Phosphate retention is a well-recognized factor, which leads to secondary hyperparathyroidism through a number of different processes. A rise in serum phosphate has a direct effect to reduce serum calcium and also inhibits the renal 1α hydroxylase, which reduces the synthesis of 1,25(OH)$_2$D. It may also have a direct effect on the parathyroid cell to increase PTH synthesis.[2] Many of these changes are synergistic, in that, for example, a fall in 1,25(OH)$_2$D concentration reduces the direct inhibitory effect on PTH secretion as well as leading to impaired calcium absorption, thereby reinforcing the tendency to hypocalcaemia and secondary hyperparathyroidism.

Calcitriol deficiency: The hepatic metabolite (25(OH)D) is converted in the proximal tubular epithelial cells to the active vitamin D metabolite 1,25(OH)$_2$D. Synthesis is stimulated by PTH and inhibited by hyperphosphataemia. Even in early renal failure, there is a tendency for 1,25(OH)$_2$D concentration to decrease, although this is often offset by increased PTH secretion. As renal failure progresses, the prevalence of 1,25(OH)$_2$D deficiency increases. One specific problem is that vitamin D metabolites, bound to plasma-binding protein (DBP), may be lost in the urine in patients with heavy proteinuria, so that vitamin D deficiency may ensue. The renal 1αhydroxylase is normally substrate-independent, but becomes dependent on the availability of 25(OH)D substrate in renal patients, so that vitamin D deficiency aggravates the defect in the synthesis of 1,25(OH)$_2$D.

Diminished feedback inhibition of PTH: A number of factors have been proposed as having pathogenetic importance. A decrease in vitamin D receptor expression by parathyroid cells[3] will reduce the inhibitory effect of 1,25(OH)$_2$D on PTH secretion. The basis of this effect is unclear, but it could be that low levels of 1,25(OH)$_2$D lead to a failure of receptor upregulation, or the phenomenon might be due to the effects of uraemia itself.

Parathyroid hyperplasia, once established, may also initiate a self-perpetuating cycle. In patients whose estimated parathyroid mass exceeds 1–1.5 g, nodular hyperplasia is usually found, and these nodules frequently exhibit

---

Table 6.1   Pathogenesis of high turnover (hyperparathyroid) bone disease.

Hyperphosphataemia
  Hypocalcaemia leading to secondary hyperparathyroidism
  Reduced 1α hydroxylase and renal 1,25(OH)$_2$D synthesis
  Direct stimulatory effect on PTH secretion

Impaired feedback inhibition of PTH
  Decrease in vitamin D receptor expression in parathyroid gland
  Increased setpoint at which calcium inhibits PTH secretion
  Increase in parathyroid cell number/basal PTH secretion

Skeletal resistance to PTH
  Impaired calcaemic response to PTH (abnormal vitamin D metabolism)

monoclonal growth.[4] Furthermore, microsatellite analysis shows loss of heterozygosity for many alleles, including putative tumour suppressor genes.[5] It appears that continuous stimulation of the parathyroid gland selectively favours cells with higher proliferative potential, so that the gland progressively escapes from growth inhibitory control mechanisms.

Finally, there is debate as to whether the set point at which ionized calcium inhibits PTH secretion becomes increased in renal failure.[6] *In vitro* studies suggest that there may be cellular abnormalities, including lower expression of the calcium sensing molecule, implying a higher set point. On the other hand *in vivo* studies do not support this view and an alternative is that this effect is a reflection of the increased parathyroid cell number. Since there is an intrinsic non-suppressible basal secretion of PTH,[7] an increase in parathyroid cell number would lead to an increased non-suppressible level of PTH and an apparent elevation of the set point.

Skeletal resistance to PTH: Infusions of PTH are less effective in correcting hypocalcaemia in patients with moderate renal failure compared to normal subjects. This apparent skeletal resistance to PTH[8] will tend to drive up serum concentrations until the tendency to hypocalcaemia is corrected. At these very high levels of PTH the skeletal response may be different, in that the normal role of the osteocyte lining cell system may be replaced by osteoclastic bone reabsorption with the development of parathyroid bone disease.

LOW TURNOVER (ADYNAMIC) BONE DISEASE AND OSTEOMALACIA (TABLE 6.2)

Parathyroid function: Circulating levels of parathyroid hormone are relatively normal in most patients with adynamic bone disease, in marked contrast to the situation in hyperparathyroid bone disease.[9] This may be an important causative factor, and a number of interrelated mechanisms may be involved.

a. Aluminium toxicity was a problem but recognition of its role and reduction in the intake from phosphate binders or dialysate have greatly reduced or eliminated this factor. Aluminium inhibits PTH release at the cellular level, and this may be of particular significance, since hyperparathyroidism seems protective, and parathyroidectomy deleterious, to the deposition of aluminium in bone.

b. Vitamin D therapy may have a direct suppressant effect on PTH secretion, and it is used clinically for this purpose in the prophylaxis of renal bone disease.[10] A similar mechanism of

---

Table 6.2 Pathogenesis of low turnover (adynamic) bone disease.

Relative hypoparathyroidism
> Direct suppressant effect of aluminium on PTH secretion
> Over-suppression of PTH secretion by calcitriol therapy
> Hypercalcaemia (high dialysate calcium, poor skeletal uptake of calcium)

Decreased bone formation
> Inhibition of osteoblast proliferation and differentiation (aluminium)
> Relative hypoparathyroidism
> Miscellaneous factors (diabetes mellitus, glucocorticoids, age)

Defective mineralization
> Aluminium deposition at calcification front with inhibition of hydroxyapatite crystal formation

suppression may follow the use of a high dialysate calcium. Once adynamic bone disease has developed there is a tendency towards hypercalcaemia, probably due to poor exchange with the adynamic bone, and this will also contribute to PTH suppression.

Decreased bone formation: Aluminium toxicity reduces bone formation through inhibition of the proliferation and differentiation of osteoblasts. Since PTH is a major regulator of bone turnover any resistance to its skeletal action or inappropriately low levels will also decrease bone formation. Other factors may also play a role, such as the presence of diabetes mellitus, the effects of glucocorticoids or ageing, all of which tend to be associated with adynamic bone disease.

Defective mineralization: Deposition of aluminium at the calcification front inhibits the growth of hydroxyapatite crystals and may impair mineralization. However, in most cases the reduction in bone formation rate is comparable and there is little increase in osteoid. By contrast, in the presence of vitamin D deficiency a significant mineralization defect will occur with the typical appearance of osteomalacia.

CLINICAL FEATURES

The clinical features of renal bone disease are often non-specific (Table 6.3), but predomi-

---

Table 6.3   Clinical features of renal bone disease.

Bone pain		
Muscle weakness:	Vitamin D deficiency	
	Aluminium toxicity	
	Severe secondary hyperparathyroidism	
Skeletal deformity:	Children:	Rickets
		Slipped epiphyses
		Abnormal dentition
	Adults:	Scoliosis/kyphosis
		Pseudoclubbing of fingers
		Brown tumours/fractures
Growth retardation (children)		
Soft tissue calcification:	Periarticular	
	Vascular	
	Ischaemic tissue necrosis (calciphylaxis)	
	Visceral calcification	
Amyloid depositions:	Bones:	Cysts (multiple > single) at end of long bones
		Fractures through cystic areas
	Joints:	Generalized/focal
		Spondyloarthropathy (scapulo-humeral)
		Erosive arthropathy
	Tendons:	Carpal tunnel syndrome
	Soft tissues:	Rare

nantly comprise bone pain and deformity, muscle weakness, extraskeletal calcification and growth retardation in children. The clinical picture needs to be complemented by biochemical and radiographic measurements (Table 6.4), which also form an important basis for the monitoring of treatment.

Bone pain is often diffuse, but tends to be worse on weight-bearing. It tends to be more severe with aluminium toxicity or osteomalacia as against parathyroid bone disease. Muscle weakness apears to be a specific feature, but may be difficult to assess in patients with bone pain. Muscle weakness is particularly pronounced in the musculature of the pelvis and shoulder girdles.

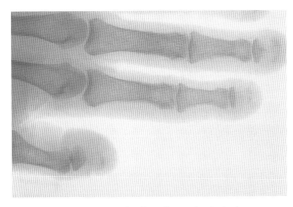

Figure 6.1 Erosion of tufts of terminal phalanges, which may give rise to pseudo-clubbing.

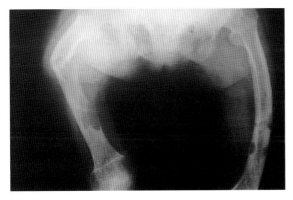

Figure 6.2 Fracture through 'brown tumours' of severe secondary hyperparathyroidism in chronic renal failure.

Skeletal deformities are common in children, and usually present with the features of rickets (epiphyseal swelling and pain, bowing of weight-bearing bones and rib cage or skull deformity). Other skeletal manifestations in childhood include slipped epiphyses (commonly femoral), abnormal dentition and growth retardation.

In adults the deformities usually reflect the presence of severe osteitis fibrosa, and include kyphosis/scoliosis, pseudoclubbing due to erosion of the terminal phalanx (Figure 6.1) and palpable 'brown tumours' through which fractures may occasionally occur (Figure 6.2).

Soft tissue calcification may be a particular problem, being most common around joints (Figure 6.3) and reflecting the presence of hyperphosphataemia and an increased calcium phosphate product. Other sites of pathological calcification include small limb arteries (Figure 6.4), a site that is particularly common amongst diabetics. Rare features include tissue necrosis (calciphylaxis) and visceral calcification, which is common at post-mortem but difficult to diagnose in life.

Amyloid deposits, derived from β2 microglobulin, mainly involve bone (bone cysts, fractures), joints (diffuse or focal arthropathy, spondyloarthropathy) or tendon sheaths (carpal tunnel syndrome), and only rarely other soft tissues. They tend to be more common in the older patient who starts dialysis in late middle life. The musculoskeletal symptoms may be diffuse and relatively non-specific, and may be difficult to distinguish from renal osteodystrophy or aluminium toxicity. A detailed clinical examination complemented by skeletal radiography and biochemical measurements will generally separate these conditions.

BIOCHEMICAL AND RADIOGRAPHIC EVALUATION (TABLE 6.4)

Serum calcium, phosphate and alkaline phosphatase are the standard measurements needed to assess the progress of mineral metabolism as renal function deteriorates, and are essential for monitoring the response to treatment. Serum alkaline phosphatase is a generally available

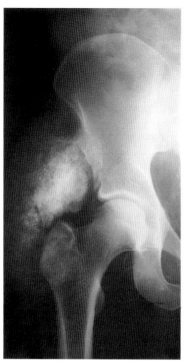

Figure 6.3 Subcutaneous calcification around the hip joint.

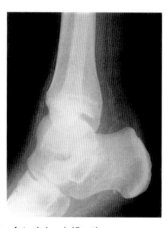

Figure 6.4 Arterial calcification.

Table 6.4 Laboratory and radiographic investigations.
Serum calcium, albumin, phosphate, alkaline phosphatase (measure monthly during treatment)
Intact PTH, 25 OHD (measure 6-monthly during treatment)
Aluminium and magnesium (only if patients are exposed to these ions)
Desferrioxamine infusion test (to assess aluminium load)
Skeletal radiograph ± bone scintigraphy
Measurement of bone mineral density (DXA)
Iliac crest bone biopsy (with double tetracycline label)

guide to the severity of hyperparathyroid bone disease, particularly if the bone-specific component is measured. The availability of measurements for intact PTH are an improvement on the older assays, which measured carboxy or amino terminal fragments. While levels are generally lower in adynamic bone disease compared to high turnover (hyperparathyroid) bone disease, there may be substantial overlap. The only certain way to distinguish the two is by iliac crest bone biopsy. In patients exposed to aluminium the serum concentration should be monitored but this reflects current exposure and not total body content, which is better assessed from the desferrioxamine test. Serum magnesium levels are generally within the upper part of the normal range even when renal failure is advanced. Levels should be measured if magnesium-containing medications are being used, since they carry a substantial risk of hypermagnesaemia. The newer bone turnover markers do not seem to have the sensitivity to provide additional information within the individual patient.

Radiographs may show the classical features of osteitis fibrosa (subperiosteal erosions, brown tumours or a 'rugger jersey' spine) (Figure 6.5) or osteomalacia (osteopenia, Looser's zones) (Figure 6.6), but may be normal despite moderately severe disease. These lesions may be detected by an isotope scan, which has greater sensitivity at detecting

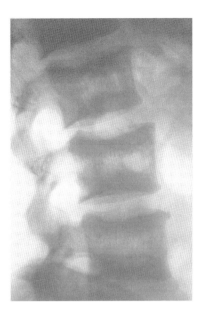

Figure 6.5 'Rugger jersey spine', showing sclerotic end plates.

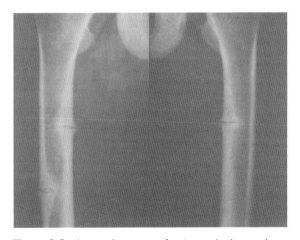

Figure 6.6 Looser's zones of osteomalacic renal osteodystrophy.

abnormality, although it is non-specific. Measurement of bone mineral density (BMD) by DXA is increasingly being included in the evaluation of renal bone disease. Osteoporosis, either linked directly or indirectly to renal failure, or as an indepenent process (due to post-menopausal osteoporosis or corticosteroid-induced bone loss) may often accompany renal bone disease, and its presence will influence management.

TREATMENT OF RENAL BONE DISEASE

Prophylaxis of secondary hyperparathyroidism (Table 6.5)

Secondary hyperparathyroidism is the combined result of failing exocrine function of the kidney (leading to phosphate excess) and failing endocrine function of the kidney (leading to calcitriol deficiency). Consequently, appropriate management of this condition requires that both these abnormalities are corrected as far as is possible.

It is important to recognize that abnormal calcium/phosphate metabolism impacts not only on the parathyroid glands and bone, but also on cardiovascular function, by increasing the risk of cardiac death, aortic stenosis and coronary plaque calcification. This adds a new dimension to the importance of normalizing calcium/phosphate metabolism in renal patients.

Table 6.5　Prophylaxis of secondary hyperparathyroidism.

Monitor serum calcium, phosphate, albumin, alkaline phosphatase at 2–6 month intervals.
Monitor serum 25(OH)D, intact 1-84 iPTH yearly and non frequent drug therapy

Low 25(OH)D (< 50 nmol/l)
Cholecalciferol 1000 IU/day

Low serum calcium and/or hyperphosphataemia
Calcium carbonate 0.5–1.5 g with each meal

Raised intact 1-84 iPTH above 18 pmol/l (×3 upper limit of normal) plus normal calcium and phosphate (spontaneously or with intervention)
Calcitriol or alfacalcidol 0.125–0.25 mcg g/day

Phosphate control

Hyperphosphataemia reduces the activity of the renal 1α-hydroxylase,[11] the rate-limiting enzyme in the synthesis of calcitriol $(1,25(OH)_2D)$, and also has a direct effect in stimulating parathyroid cells,[2] both processes contributing to the development of secondary hyperparathyroidism. Hyperphosphataemia is an important cause of soft tissue calcification, and since administration of active vitamin D also increases intestinal phosphate absorption and the plasma phosphate concentrations, it will also increase the propensity to develop soft tissue calcification. Normalization of plasma phosphate is therefore absolutely necessary before the administration of active vitamin D is considered.

Phosphate is present in virtually all foods, and reduction of dietary intake is therefore difficult without incurring the risk of malnutrition. Patients should, however, be advised to avoid foods in which the phosphate content is high. These include dairy products and foods to which phosphate is added (sausages, and phosphate-rich soft drinks). Dietary protein restriction is usually recommended to patients with renal insufficiency, and one desirable consequence is that this will also reduce the intake of phosphate.

Since severe dietary restriction is usually not feasible nor sufficient on its own, most uraemic patients remain in positive phosphate balance, unless oral phosphate binders are administered. The usual recommendation is to commence phosphate-lowering therapy once the plasma phosphate concentrations exceed the upper limit of the normal range (> 1.4 mmol/l).[1,9,11] This usually occurs when the creatinine clearance is approximately 30 ml/min. Plasma phosphate depends not only on renal clearance, but also on dietary phosphate intake, protein catabolism and other confounding factors. The aim is to trap phosphate in the intestinal lumen by forming insoluble calcium phosphate complexes.

Phosphate binders must be taken together with meals, because phosphate in the food can only be precipitated within the intestinal lumen when phosphate binders are present. Ingestion of calcium-containing phosphate binders without meals increases the risk of hypercalcaemia. The dose of phosphate binders should be divided between the meals according to the phosphate intake, with the highest dose at the main meal. The most commonly used phosphate binders are calcium carbonate or calcium acetate. Calcium citrate is not used, since this greatly increases aluminium absorption from the intestine. The most convenient preparations of calcium carbonate are Calcichew and Titralac, which should be given in a dose of 0.5–1.5 g with each meal. Aluminium-containing substances have been widely used in the past, but because of the risk of aluminium intoxication (encephalopathy, osteopathy, anaemia) they should be avoided. If hyperphosphataemia cannot be controlled without aluminium-containing binders (because of hypercalcaemia with calcium-containing binders) plasma aluminium concentrations must be monitored at regular intervals (relatively safe range: <60 mcg/l). Currently, phosphate binders without calcium or aluminium, such as sevelamer hydro-chloride, are under investigation and may offer the potential for safe control of plasma phosphate in the future.

The most important risk of calcium carbonate therapy is hypercalcaemia, particularly

1. if patients are also taking vitamin D
2. when patients are immobilized
3. when bone turnover is low (adynamic bone disease or aluminium intoxication).

If hyperphosphataemia does not respond to intervention, one should consider

1. non-compliance
2. increased phosphate release from the skeleton (e.g. marked osteitis fibrosa)
3. inadequate dialysis.

Pre-dialytic plasma phosphate concentration is markedly influenced by the efficiency of dialysis. The elimination kinetics of phosphate during dialysis are complex, since the major portion of the phosphate which is transferred into the dialysate must be mobilized from intracellular compartments. As a consequence, the amount of phosphate removed in the first two hours is relatively high, but after 1–2 hours, when plasma phosphate concentrations have been lowered, only small amounts of phosphate are subsequently eliminated. Prolongation of dialysis sessions therefore only modestly increases phosphate elimination, while more frequent dialysis results in a greater increase in phosphate removal. If hyperphosphataemia persists in a dialysis patient, then factors that could potentially reduce dialysis efficacy must be evaluated, such as dialyser surface, duration and frequency of dialysis sessions, or recirculation in the arterio venous (AV) fistula.

Correction of cholecalciferol deficiency

Deficiency of the parent compound vitamin D_3 (cholecalciferol) is common among renal patients as a result of altered lifestyle, with poor sunlight exposure, uraemic hyperpigmentation of the skin and loss of protein-bound vitamin D metabolites into proteinuric urine or peritoneal dialysis fluid. Vitamin D deficiency can be diagnosed when plasma 25(OH)D concentrations are low (< 50 nmol/l). In renal failure the synthesis of calcitriol $(1,25(OH)_2D)$ by the substrate-dependent, rate-limiting enzyme 1α-hydroxylase depends on the concentration of the precursor substance calcidiol, (25(OH)D). As a consequence, the administration of only 1000 IU vitamin D per day in vitamin D-deficient patients will restore normal levels of serum 25(OH)D and lead to an increase in calcitriol and a decrease in iPTH.

Administration of active vitamin D

Although not universally accepted,[1] one option is to administer prophylactic calcitriol or alfacalcidol $(1\alpha(OH)D)$ when 1-84 iPTH concentrations exceed 2–3 fold the upper limit of the normal range, despite measures to correct plasma phosphate and calcium concentrations.[10,12,13] Complete normalization of iPTH concentrations is undesirable, at least in end-stage renal failure. Normal bone turnover seems to require a slightly elevated PTH level[8] while suppression of PTH increases the risk of adynamic bone disease. It is currently unknown whether this high level reflects resistance of the skeleton to PTH or insufficient specificity of the PTH assay, which may also measure some inactive fragments.

It has emerged that relatively low doses of calcitriol (0.125 mcg g or 0.25 mcg g per day) or alternative active vitamin D preparations (1-alpha-calcidiol) are necessary to prevent the progres- sive increase of iPTH in patients with renal failure.[10,13] The rationale for the administration of calcitriol is not only to reverse over-secretion of PTH by the hypertrophic/hyperplastic parathyroid gland, but also to prevent parathyroid hyperplasia. This process, once established, is at least partially irreversible, and as a consequence every effort should be made to prevent its development. Administration of active vitamin D is fraught with risks of hypercalcaemia and accelerated loss of renal function. This can be prevented by the frequent (monthly) monitoring of plasma calcium, and with very low doses of calcitriol (0.125 µg/day) the risk is negligible.

Selection of dialysate calcium concentration

In renal failure, several factors tend to contribute to a negative calcium balance. On self-selected diets, the calcium intake of anorectic uraemic patients is usually suboptimal. Active vitamin D-dependent calcium absorption in the upper segments of the small intestine is markedly reduced because of the decreased calcitriol synthesis, while passive calcium absorption in lower intestinal segments is unaffected. As a consequence, adaptation of upper intestinal calcium absorption to a low dietary intake is impaired, but hypercalcaemia may develop if high doses of calcium carbonate are administered and absorbed in the distal bowel.

Once the patient is on dialysis, calcium may be lost into the dialysate. With ultrafiltration, convective calcium loss is obligatory, and this may amount to 200–400 mg/week. Diffusive loss of calcium into the dialysate occurs if the plasma concentration of diffusible calcium is higher than the dialysate calcium concentration. In the past, a dialysate calcium concentration of 7 mg/100 ml (1.75 mmol/l) was commonly used, which gives a concentration of ionized calcium that is higher than that of the blood. At this concentration, net uptake of calcium into the patient occurs during dialysis and compensates for convective loss of calcium via ultrafiltration and negative intestinal calcium balance between dialysis sessions. If calcium-containing phosphate binders or active vitamin D preparations are administered, intestinal uptake of calcium will be high, and the patients may develop hypercalcaemia under these circumstances. Lowering the dialysate calcium concentration to 6 mg/100 ml (1.5 mmol/l) or even temporarily to 5 mg/100 ml (1.25 mmol/l) will counteract this tendency to hypercalcaemia. It is important, however, to confirm that patients are taking their medication when low dialysis calcium concentrations are being used. If calcium carbonate and/or active vitamin D preparations are omitted, then there is a definite risk that calcium balance will become negative, with the result that secondary hyperparathyroidism will be exacerbated.[14,15]

TREATMENT OF ESTABLISHED HYPERPARATHYROIDISM (TABLE 6.6)

Administration of hydroxylated vitamin D metabolites

In the patient with advanced hyperparathyroidism, with serum levels of 1-84 iPTH above about 50 pmol/l (or 8-fold above the upper limit of normal) higher doses of active vitamin D are required. It is important to emphasize that active vitamin D must only be administered if hyperphosphataemia and hypercalcaemia are absent or have been reversed by appropriate treatment. We recommend starting with relatively modest doses of calcitriol (0.5 mcg g per day), and if this dose is tolerated without provoking hyperphosphataemia or hypercalcaemia, then the dose can be gradually increased until plasma 1-84 iPTH decreases.

Currently, several alternative schedules of active vitamin D administration are in use, but a consensus as to the optimum regimen has not yet emerged.

Continuous vs pulse administration
In experimental studies, continuous (daily) administration of calcitriol is less effective than

Table 6.6   Treatment of advanced hyperparathyroidism (PTH > 50 pmol/l).

Normalize plasma calcium and phosphate (active vitamin D metabolites are contraindicated in the presence of hypercalcaemia/hyperphosphataemia)

Hyperphosphataemia
→ Calcium carbonate or acetate with meals
→ Reduce excess dietary intake of phosphate
→ Increase efficiency of dialysis (higher blood flow, longer or more frequent dialysis sessions)

Hypercalcaemia
→ Reduce or withdraw calcium-containing phosphate binders
→ Reduce dialysate calcium to 1.5 mmol/l or (transiently) to 1.25 mmol/l

Normal serum calcium and phosphate
→ Increase calcitriol/alfacalcidol to 0.5–3.0 µg daily or 1–3 times/week
→ Adjust dose to maintain intact PTH at ×3 upper limit of normal
→ Long-term low-dose prophylaxis (calcitriol 0.25 µg weekly) if PTH tends to rise

Failure to obtain adequate control of intact PTH or therapy limited by hypercalcaemia/hyperphosphataemia
→ Consider parathyroidectomy

intermittent (pulse) administration in terms of lowering PTH concentrations and preventing parathyroid hyperplasia.[16] However, at the present time there is no good evidence that this effect is sufficiently marked to be of clinical importance.[17] At least in mild to moderate secondary hyperparathyroidism, direct comparisons showed similar efficacy of daily vs intermittent (once- or twice-weekly) calcitriol administration. In the dialysis patient, intermittent administration has the advantage that the drug can be taken under supervision, which is important given the poor compliance of these chronically ill patients.

Oral vs intravenous administration

It has been shown that intravenous administration causes a rapid lowering of 1-84 iPTH concentrations,[16] but direct comparisons of intravenous vs oral administration have failed to show any superiority of the intravenous route.[18]

Active vitamin D analogues

The major side effects of treatment with active vitamin D, such as calcitriol and 1-alpha calcidiol, are hypercalcaemia and hyperphosphataemia. There has, as a consequence, been an intense search for vitamin D analogues that suppress the parathyroid gland while having less hypercalcaemic and hyperphosphataemic potential. Several of these analogues are currently available and include 19-nor-1.25-dihydroxyvitamin D_2 (Paricalcitol) and 19-nor-22-oxa-1alpha,25-dihydroxyvitamin D_3 (22-oxacalcitriol), and these are currently in clinical trials. So far there is no evidence that they cause less hypercalcemia than equipotent doses of calcitriol or 1-alpha calcidiol.

Investigational drugs (calcimimetics)

The parathyroid cell expresses a membrane receptor that senses calcium and thus monitors extracellular calcium concentration. Substances have been developed (R-568) that mimic the effects of calcium on the calcium receptor, and as a consequence decrease PTH secretion. The hope is that they may impede the development of parathyroid hyperplasia; but they are currently in clinical trials, and not yet available for routine treatment.

Active vitamin D therapy

Under normal circumstances, the 1-84 iPTH concentration decreases relatively rapidly within 4–6 weeks if patients are going to respond to treatment with active vitamin

D. Many patients with advanced hyperparathyroidism are refractory to active vitamin D and this can be predicted by:

1. large parathyroid glands on imaging
2. hyperphosphataemia
3. hypercalcaemia.

It is arguable whether very high doses of calcitriol (in excess of 2 mcg g per single administration) should be tried in such patients because this may provoke hypercalcaemia/hyperphosphataemia and still fail to induce regression of parathyroid hyperplasia.

PARATHYROIDECTOMY

Recently, it has been recognized that severe parathyroid hyperplasia is a process similar to tumour growth. This is illustrated by the fact that after subtotal parathyroidectomy or autotransplantation of parathyroid tissue, regrowth, including local invasion, occurs in a high proportion (approximately one-third) of the patients. The relative resistance of patients with massive nodular hyperplasia to treatment with active vitamin D is explained by the fact that nodules fail to express the vitamin D receptor, so that the molecular machinery on which the response to vitamin D depends is absent.[3]

These and other arguments have led to a recommendation for parathyroidectomy in patients with a substantial elevation of 1-84 iPTH (above 50 pmol/l) who:

1. fail to respond within 4–8 weeks by decreasing their PTH concentration; and
2. have massive parathyroid enlargement on imaging (estimated mass greater than 1–1.5 g).[1,19]

An absolute indication for parathyroidectomy is calciphylaxis (ischaemic skin necrosis secondary to calcification of skin arteries). A relative indication is severe pruritus or biomechanical problems that require urgent stabilization (rupture of the patella or epiphyseolysis in uraemic children), all of which tend to be associated with a high PTH.

There is an ongoing discussion as to whether total parathyroidectomy or subtotal parathyroidectomy (with a remnant left *in situ* or autotransplanted into the subcutaneous abdominal fat or forearm musculature) is the best option. Subtotal parathyroidectomy is associated with a relatively high risk of recurrence, presumably because of the higher growth potential of the remaining parathyroid tissue. The risk can be reduced if the surgeon does not include large nodules in the autotransplant. As an alternative to surgery, alcohol injection into the enlarged parathyroid under ultrasonographic guidance has been tried successfully, but this procedure is not completely devoid of risk (damage to the recurrent laryngeal nerve).

Adynamic bone disease

There is no consensus at the present time as to the optimal treatment of adynamic bone disease. It is important to avoid over-suppression of PTH by calcitriol/alfacalcidol, and these metabolites are ineffective in the presence of established adynamic bone disease. Current treatment should include general measures such as HRT in postmenopausal women.

REFERENCES

1. Felensfeld AJ (1998). Considerations for the treatment of secondary hyperparathyroidism in renal failure. *J Am Soc Nephrol 20*: 993–1004.
2. Almaden Y, Canelejo A, Hernandez A et al. (1996). Direct effect of phosphorus on parathyroid hormone secretion from whole rat parathyroid glands in vitro. *J Bone Miner Res 11*: 970–976.
3. Fukuda AN, Tanaka H, Tominaga Y, Fakagawa M, Kurokawa K, Seino Y (1993). Decreased 1,25 dihydroxyvitamin D_3 receptor density is associated with a more severe form of parathryoid hyperplasia in chronic uremic patients. *J Clin Invest 92*: 1436–1443.
4. Arnold A, Brown MF, Urena P, Gaz RD, Sarfati E, Drueke TB (1995). Monoclonality of parathyroid tumours in chronic renal failure and in primary parathyroid hyperplasia. *J Clin Invest 95*: 2047–2053.
5. Chudek J, Ritz E, Kovacs G (1998). Genetic abnormalities in parathyroid nodules of uremic patients. *Clin Cancer Res 4*: 211–214.
6. Cardinal H, Brossard JH, Roy L, Lepage R, Rousseau L, D'Amour P (1998). The setpoint of parathyroid stimulation by calcium is normal in progressive renal failure. *J Clin Endocrinol Metab 83*: 3839–3844.
7. Brown E (1991). Extracellular Ca^{2+} sensing, regulation of parathyroid cell function and role of Ca^{2+} and other ions as extracellular (first messengers). *Physiol Rev 71*: 371–411.
8. Quarles LD, Lobaugh B, Murphy G (1992). Intact parathyroid hormone over estimates the presence and severity of parathyroid-mediated osseous abnormalities in uremia. *J Clin Endocrinol Metab 75*: 145–150.
9. Goodman WG, Coburn JW, Slatopolsky E, Salvsky IB (1996). Renal osteodystrophy in adults and children. In: *Primer on the metabolic bone diseases and disorders of mineral metabolism*, 3rd edn, ed. MJ Favus, pp. 341–360. Lippincott-Raven, New York.
10. Ritz E, Kuster S, Schmidt-Gayk H et al. (1995). Low-dose calcitriol prevents the rise in 1,84 iPTH without affecting serum calcium and phosphate in patients with moderate renal failure (prospective placebo-controlled multicentre trial). *Nephrol Dial Transplant 10*: 2228–2234.
11. Delmez JA, Slatopolsky E (1992). Hyperphosphataemia: its consequences and treatment in patients with chronic renal disease. *Am J Kidney Dis 19*: 303–317.
12. Goodman WG, Coburn JW (1992). The use of 1,25-dihydroxyvitamin D_3 in early renal failure. *Ann Rev Med 43*: 227–237.
13. Hamdy NAT, Kanis JA, Beneton MNC et al. (1995). Effect of alfacalcidol on natural course of bone disease in mild to moderate renal failure. *Br Med J 310*: 358–363.
14. Fernandez E, Borras M, Pais B, Montoliu J (1995). Low-calcium dialysate stimulates parathormone secretion and its long-term use worsens secondary hyperparathyroidism. *J Am Soc Nephrol 6*: 132–135.
15. Argiles A, Kerr PG, Canaud B, Flavier JL, Mion C (1993). Calcium kinetics and the long-term effects of lowering dialysate calcium concentration. *Kidney Int 43*: 630–640.
16. Reichel H, Szabo A, Uhl J et al. (1993). Intermittent versus continuous administration of 1,25-dihydroxyvitamin D_3 in experimental renal hypoparathyroidism. *Kidney Int 44*: 1259–1265.

17. Herrmann P, Ritz E, Schmidt-Gayk H et al. (1994). Comparison of intermittent and continuous oral administration of calcitriol in dialysis patients: a randomized prospective trial. *Nephrology 67*: 48–53.

18. Quarles LD, Yohay DA, Carroll BA, Spritzer CE, Minda SA, Lobaugh BL (1994). Prospective trial of pulse oral versus intravenous calcitriol treatment of hyperparathyroidism in ESRD. *Kidney Int 45*: 1710–1721.

19. Ritz E (1994). Earl parathyroidectomy should be considered as the first choice. *Nephrol Dial Transplant 9*: 1819–1821.

7

Transplantation Bone Disease

Juliet Compston and Cornelle Parker

Introduction • Prevalence • Pathogenesis • Immunosuppressive agents • Pathophysiology
  • Management of post transplantation bone disease • Optimization of bone mass prior to
transplantation • Prevention and treatment of peri- and post-transplantation bone loss

INTRODUCTION

Bone disease is increasingly recognized as a major complication of solid organ transplantation.[1-3] Over recent years, modification of immunosuppressant regimens, in particular the introduction of cyclosporin, has prolonged the life-span of transplanted organs. Although these changes confer indisputable advantages to transplant recipients in terms of quality and expectancy of life, these agents also have deleterious effects on bone.

After cardiac and liver transplantation, approximately one-third of patients develop fractures in the first 6 to 12 months post-operatively, often resulting in long-term pain and disability. Renal transplantation is the treatment of choice in end-stage renal failure, and multiple factors predispose transplant recipients to reduced bone mineral density. Although less well documented, osteoporotic fractures are also widespread in this population.

Although some of the pathogenetic factors responsible for bone disease are common to all types of transplantation, there are also important differences related mainly to pre-existing bone disease and the use of particular immuno-

suppressive agents. As a consequence of these differences renal transplantation bone disease is considered separately in some of the following sections.

In view of the increasing life expectancy of transplant recipients, prevention and treatment of bone disease, which otherwise may result in an increased risk of fractures, are a major priority.

PREVALENCE

Liver, cardiac and lung transplantation

Cross-sectional studies in cardiac transplant recipients report a vertebral fracture prevalence rate as high as 50%.[4] Prospective studies have shown a fracture incidence of up to 35% and 38% in the first year after liver and cardiac transplantation respectively.[5-7] Increased rates of bone loss have been demonstrated in the first few months after transplantation both in the proximal femur and spine,[8-14] although some recent data indicate lower rates of bone loss. This is possibly a result of changes in immuno-suppressive regimens, both with reduced

---

Table 7.1 Pathogenetic factors in post-transplantation bone disease.

Pre-existing osteopenia/osteoporosis

Drugs – glucocorticoids, cyclosporin and other immunosuppressive agents

Calcium and vitamin D deficiency

Hypogonadism

Reduced physical activity

Malnutrition

---

cumulative exposure to glucocorticoids and choice of agents used.[15] Nevertheless, it appears that the high fracture risk persists, even in the absence of demonstrable rapid bone loss, in the lumbar spine or proximal femur. In one study, despite the absence of significant bone loss in the lumbar spine and an annual rate of loss of 2.4% in the proximal femur, Ninkovic et al.[16] reported a 27% incidence rate of vertebral fractures in the first three months after liver transplantation.

Some studies have demonstrated a tendency for bone mineral density to recover 6 to 12 months post-transplantation,[6,10,12] but this finding has not been universal.[11,17] Low bone mass has also been reported after lung transplantation,[18] and in the only reported prospective study in this population there was a 4% reduction in spinal bone mineral density in the first six months post-operatively, while 14.2% of patients (3/21) developed fractures.[19]

Renal transplantation

Several studies have shown rapid rates of post-transplantational bone loss, which mostly occur in the 2-year period following transplantation, when doses of immunosuppressants are maximal in order to combat rejection.[20] Rates of bone loss vary considerably, but figures approximating 5% at the lumbar spine during the first 6 months after transplantation are to be expected.[21,22]

Bone loss is more pronounced in the predominantly trabecular lumbar spine when compared with cortical-rich sites such as hip and mid-radius.[23,24] These findings mirror the pattern of bone loss found secondary to glucocorticoid therapy, which characteristically affects trabecular bone.

Published data relating to fracture prevalence in the renal transplant population are sparse and restricted to cross-sectional studies. In one study, peripheral fractures occurred in 11% and vertebral fractures in a further 3% of patients,[25] whilst in a second study 33% (17/51) of female renal transplant recipients had a prevalent low-trauma fracture.[26]

PATHOGENESIS

The pathogenesis of post-transplantation bone disease is likely to be multifactorial (Table 7.1). Many patients have low bone mass before transplantation. Additional factors include glucocorticoid therapy, cyclosporin and other immunosuppressive agents, reduced physical activity, calcium and vitamin D deficiency, malnutrition and hypogonadism. Some of these factors may also contribute to bone disease prior to transplantation,[27] and several are potentially modifiable. In view of their relevance to the prevention and management of post-transplantation bone disease they are discussed in more detail below.

Pre-existing osteopenia/osteoporosis

A high prevalence of osteopenia and osteoporosis has been documented in patients prior to liver, cardiac and lung transplantation. In a study of 169 patients undergoing liver transplantation, Porayko et al.[5] reported that over one-half had bone mineral density values below the so-called fracture threshold and nearly 10% had previous fragility fractures. Other groups have also reported low bone mineral density in pre-transplant patients and fracture prevalence rates of around 10%. In contrast, Abdelhadi et al.[28] reported normal pre-transplant bone mineral density in 25 patients with chronic liver disease.

Studies of patients undergoing cardiac transplantation have produced conflicting results. Muchmore et al.[29] reported that vertebral bone mineral density, assessed by computed quantitative tomography, was approximately 20% below that of age- and sex-matched control values. In contrast, Shane et al.[4] found that bone density in the spine and hip was normal in most patients prior to cardiac transplantation, and Lee et al.[30] reported reduced hip but normal spine bone mineral density in a small group of men awaiting transplantation.

The most severe bone disease has been reported in patients with end-stage pulmonary disease prior to lung transplantation. In a study of 70 patients, osteoporosis (defined by a T score below -2.5) was present in 30% of patients at the spine and 49% at the hip. In addition, there was a high prevalence of vertebral fractures, 29% of patients with chronic obstructive pulmonary disease and 25% of those with cystic fibrosis having at least one vertebral fracture.[31]

There is considerable evidence confirming the prevalence of reduced bone mass at the time of renal transplantation,[22,24] although perhaps surprisingly this is not a universal finding.[21] One study describes Z score reductions (comparison to the age-matched mean) at both lumbar spine (mean Z -1.2 SD) and radius (mean Z -0.7 SD),[22] whereas others have only found reductions in female patients.[24]

Vitamin D deficiency

Vitamin D deficiency is known to be common in patients with chronic liver disease. In one study, low serum 25-hydroxyvitamin D levels (20 nmol/l or less) were found in 74% of patients undergoing assessment for liver transplantation.[32] In patients with end-stage pulmonary disease awaiting lung transplantation, vitamin D deficiency was reported in 36% of patients with cystic fibrosis and in 20% of patients with other chronic pulmonary disorders.[31]

In patients undergoing cardiac transplantation, normal serum 25-hydroxyvitamin D levels have been reported, although circulating 1,25-dihydroxyvitamin D concentrations were reduced in 35% of patients.[4]

Renal bone disease

The pathogenesis of post-renal transplant osteoporosis differs from that of cardiac, liver or lung transplantation because of the influence of the skeletal effects of both chronic renal failure and maintenance dialysis.

Early on in the course of renal failure, there is development of bone disease due to secondary hyperparathyroidism.[33] Adynamic bone disease, both aluminium- and non-aluminium-related forms, is widely prevalent in dialysis populations, with between one-third[34] and one-half of patients[35] being affected. Although evidence is more widespread in the dialysis population, there is growing awareness that a similar histological picture exists in the renal transplant population.[22,23,26,36]

Although renal transplantation aims to restore normal renal function, a degree of renal impairment often persists, and transplant recipients can experience varying degrees of transplant failure. In patients with declining renal function the occurrence of phosphate retention leads to hypocalcaemia and the development of secondary hyperparathyroidism.[32] This view has been challenged[37] by suggesting that since hyperparathyroid bone disease can develop in the presence of hypercalcaemia[38] the driving force for parathyroid hyperplasia is the increased set-point for calcium-regulated PTH secretion. Concomitant reduction of circulating 1,25-dihydroxyvitamin D exacerbates the condition by further stimulating parathyroid hormone secretion.

IMMUNOSUPPRESSIVE AGENTS

Glucocorticoids

The effects of glucocorticoids on bone are well characterized in other populations (for review see Lukert and Raisz).[39] Prednisolone in daily doses of 7.5 mg or greater has deleterious effects, particularly on trabecular bone;[40] and with renal impairment, accumulation of glucocorticoid enhances the adverse effects.[41]

Glucocorticoids disturb calcium metabolism through inhibition of gastrointestinal absorption, increased renal excretion, inhibition of pituitary secretion of gonadotropins leading to hypogonadism, and inhibition of 1,25-dihydroxyvitamin D action. Glucocorticoids also act to decrease synthesis of insulin-like growth factor (IGF-I) (a stimulator of collagen synthesis) and reduce levels of transforming growth factor (TGF-β) (an enhancer of osteoblast replication and bone matrix protein synthesis).[42]

At the cellular level, the effects of glucocorticoids are complex. They decrease both osteoblast and osteoclast replication. They also act to reduce matrix production through genetic effects (reducing type I collagen expression by transcriptional and post-transcriptional mechanisms) and reduce collagen synthesis by increasing MMP-13 (matrix metalloproteinase) ex-pression, an essential factor in collagen degradation.[43]

Histomorphometric changes include reduced mean wall thickness, low mineral apposition rate, elevation of bone resorption, suppression of osteoblast recruitment, and depression of mature osteoblast function.[39]

Cyclosporin

In vitro work initially suggested that cyclosporin had an anabolic effect on bone.[44] *In vivo* studies in rats however suggest that cyclosporin is highly catabolic, resulting in high-turnover osteopenia.[45] Isolating a specific influence of cyclosporin in the clinical setting is made particularly difficult in renal transplant recipients because of the almost universal tendency for co-prescription with other agents such as prednisolone and azathioprine.[46]

Tacrolimus, a recently introduced macrolide immunosuppressant, has a similar mode of action to cyclosporin. Although more potent than cyclosporin, it has a similar side-effect profile, and experiments in rats also indicate similar negative effects on bone.[47]

Azathioprine

Azathioprine is used in immunosuppressive regimens as a glucocorticoid or cyclosporin-sparing agent. *In vivo* studies in the rat model using azathioprine alone show an increase in osteoclast numbers, but no effect on bone volume.[48] The combination of cyclosporin and azathioprine does not appear to exaggerate cyclosporin-induced osteopenia. Long-term studies are awaited, but in the clinical setting it is difficult to identify a specific effect, since azathioprine is rarely used in isolation.

PATHOPHYSIOLOGY

The pathophysiology of post-transplantation bone disease has not been clearly defined. In patients undergoing liver transplantation, histomorphometric analysis of bone biopsies obtained before and at three months after transplantation demonstrated a highly significant increase in bone turnover and a trend towards an increase in the size of resorption cavities.[49] These relatively early changes provide a mechanism at the cellular and tissue level for bone loss, but are unlikely to be representative of steady state changes. In particular, although no significant disruption of cancellous bone architecture could be demonstrated three months after transplantation, such changes may develop at a later stage, resulting in increased bone fragility, which may persist despite subsequent restoration of bone mass.

Histologically, renal osteodystrophy can be classified into four categories: hyperparathyroid bone disease, adynamic bone disease, osteomalacia and mixed bone disease (hyperparathyroidism and osteomalacia in combination). Prevalence figures in the dialysis population for each category are: hyperparathyroid 47%, adynamic 32%, mixed bone disease 13%, osteomalacia 8%.[34] Any of these abnormalities can be associated with low bone mineral density as determined by dual energy X-ray absorptiometry.

In renal transplant recipients prevalence figures for each type vary considerably, and are influenced by the severity and duration of pre-existing renal failure and the time elapsed since transplantation. Julian et al.[22] found changes consistent with mild hyperparathyroidism at the time of transplantation; but 6 months later, many of the indices of increased bone turnover had reverted to normal. A study of biopsies from 26 female transplant recipients between 1 and 22 years from initial transplantation revealed 16 cases of hyperparathyroid bone disease, 8 cases of adynamic bone disease and 2 patients with osteomalacia.[26] In several small cross-sectional studies others have found a preponderance of either adynamic bone disease[36] or mixed bone disease.[23]

MANAGEMENT OF POST TRANSPLANTATION BONE DISEASE

Investigation

A thorough evaluation should be performed in all patients in whom transplantation is considered in order to document the presence of existing bone disease and to exclude conditions such as vitamin D deficiency, thyroid disease and hypogonadism. In view of the adverse effects of transplantation on bone mineral density in patients with pre-existing osteoporosis, many physicians counsel against transplantation in such cases, at least until appropriate treatment has been instituted. As a minimum, therefore, bone densitometry should be performed and spinal radiographs should be obtained for evidence of vertebral deformity; blood tests should be performed for calcium, phosphate, alkaline phosphatase, 25-hydroxyvitamin D, parathyroid hormone, thyroid function and, in men, serum testosterone.

Post-renal transplantation histological abnormalities are almost universal, and because of the different mechanisms involved and the implications for subsequent treatment these patients require additional investigation. As yet the only reliable way of identifying histological subtype in renal transplant bone disease is through bone biopsy. Because the histologic category into which a patient falls has implications for treatment, bone biopsy is now considered an essential investigation in the management of these patients.[51] Renal dialysis[50] and renal transplant[26] patients with biopsy-proven hyperparathyroid bone disease tend to have higher parathyroid hormone levels than their adynamic bone disease counterparts. There is considerable overlap, making parathyroid hormone an unreliable sole discriminator. However, serum calcium and parathyroid hormone measurements remain an important part of the assessment, as markedly elevated values in the presence of severe bone mass reduction may indicate tertiary hyperparathyroidism and the need for parathyroidectomy.

In order to facilitate classification, biopsies in patients already transplanted should include an oral double tetracycline label. In those undergoing transplantation, biopsies should ideally be taken at the time of transplantation, both to limit discomfort and to eliminate the need for further sedation. In these circumstances there is not time for a tetracycline label.

Following transplantation, bone densitometry should be repeated at 6 months, 12 months and yearly thereafter. Radiographs should be obtained when indicated clinically and since the majority of vertebral fractures are asymptomatic, vertebral morphometry should be performed one year after transplantation.

Prediction of those at high risk of post-transplantation osteoporosis

Although risk factors for post-transplantation osteoporosis have not been well established, those that predispose to osteoporosis in the general population may improve prediction of the individuals most likely to be at risk after transplantation (Table 7.2). Previous fragility fracture is a particularly strong predictor of fracture after transplantation. In one study, 46% of such patients developed vertebral fracture after liver transplantation, compared with 16.7% of those patients with no previous history of fracture – a difference that was statistically significant.[16]

OPTIMIZATION OF BONE MASS PRIOR TO TRANSPLANTATION

The importance of low bone mass prior to transplant, especially if accompanied by fracture, cannot be overemphasized as a risk factor for post-transplantation disease. Attention should be paid to lifestyle measures such as maintaining adequate levels of physical activity, stopping smoking and dietary calcium intake. Calcium supplements of at least 1 g daily in divided doses should be advised.

In view of the high prevalence of vitamin D deficiency in patients with chronic liver disease and end-stage pulmonary disease, routine vitamin D supplementation should be considered

at an oral dose of 800 IU/day or 150 000 IU every three months parenterally.

The situation is more complex in those on dialysis awaiting renal transplantation, and the importance of controlling phosphate levels in these patients may take precedence over issues regarding vitamin D supplementation.

Hormone replacement therapy in women and testosterone replacement in men should be offered when clinically indicated. In women with chronic liver disease, transdermal oestrogen preparations are preferable, because they avoid first-pass hepatic metabolism.

Liver, cardiac and lung transplantation

In patients treated with glucocorticoids for their underlying condition, prophylaxis with cyclical etidronate should be considered for the following groups:

- those on high-dose therapy (>15 mg/day oral prednisolone or its equivalent)
- those with strong risk factors for osteoporosis
- those with a bone mineral density T score below −1.5 at the lumbar spine or proximal femur.

In non-glucocorticoid treated patients with osteoporosis prior to transplantation, appropriate treatment should be given, for example bisphosphonates or hormone replacement therapy, depending on age, gender and clinical circumstances.

Table 7.2 Risk factors for post-transplantation osteoporosis.

Prevalent fracture or past history of fracture
Low body mass index
Family history of osteoporosis
Hypogonadism
Glucocorticoid therapy

Renal transplantation

The effects of bisphosphonates on adynamic bone disease in end-stage renal failure await evaluation. Because of possible adverse effects on patients with underlying undiagnosed osteomalacia they cannot be recommended as a general preventive strategy, and should be reserved for biopsy-proven hyperparathyroid bone disease.

PREVENTION AND TREATMENT OF PERI- AND POST-TRANSPLANTATION BONE LOSS

The observation that bone loss and fracture incidence appear to be maximal in the first few months after transplantation indicates that early intervention at the time of and/or soon after transplantation is likely to be most effective.

No randomized controlled studies of any treatment have yet been reported in patients undergoing any form of organ transplantation, and thus treatment decisions have to be based on data from trials in patients with other forms of osteoporosis such as postmenopausal or glucocorticoid-induced osteoporosis. However, the pathogenesis and pathophysiology of these types of osteoporosis may well differ, and it cannot be assumed that interventions that are effective in one condition necessarily have similar effects in another. In particular, although glucocorticoids are likely to play a role in transplantation bone disease, other factors are also important, and it remains to be proved that agents that prevent glucocorticoid-induced osteoporosis are effective in post-transplantation bone disease.

Liver, cardiac and lung transplantation

In view of the evidence that increased bone turnover plays an important role in bone loss in the first three months after transplantation, a case can be made for using antiresorptive therapy.

In an open, uncontrolled study Muchmore et al.[29] investigated the effects of salmon calcitonin, oestrogen or testosterone in patients who had undergone cardiac transplantation several months previously and reported some mitigation, although not prevention, of vertebral bone loss. All patients received 800 mg of calcium supplements in the form of calcium citrate, while hypogonadism was treated with testosterone (100 mg intramuscularly every 10 days) or oestrogen replacement as appropriate. Those with severe or continuing bone loss were subsequently given 50–100 IU of synthetic salmon calcitonin daily by subcutaneous injection. Treatment was started at varying intervals after transplantation and, in general, appeared to reduce vertebral bone loss. In five patients, some of whom were also receiving hormone replacement therapy, calcitonin treatment was associated with an increase in bone mineral density. However, because of the non-randomized nature of this study it is difficult to draw any firm conclusions about its efficacy.

The effects of either calcitonin (40 IU/day by intramuscular injection) or cyclical etidronate (400 mg daily for 15 days every three months) were examined in a randomized uncontrolled study of patients who had undergone liver transplantation.[52] Only those with a low bone mineral density (defined as a spinal Z score less than -2) received treatment, which was started between 1 and 74 months after transplantation. After 12 months of either treatment, a significant and similar increase in spinal bone mineral density was observed, the magnitude of which was 6.4% in the calcitonin-treated group and 8.2% in those treated with cyclical etidronate. In another open randomized study, however, Garcia-Delgado et al.[53] found that neither calcitonin therapy (100 IU/day intranasally) nor cyclical etidronate therapy (400 mg/day for 2 weeks out of every three months) prevented bone loss in patients treated immediately after cardiac transplantation, although spinal bone mineral density increased by 4.9% after 18 months' treatment with calcidiol (32 000 IU daily).

Results from the study of Riemens et al.[37] also support the view that oral cyclical etidronate therapy is ineffective in preventing bone loss after transplantation. In an open uncontrolled study of 53 patients, a combination of cyclical etidronate (90 day cycles composed of 400 mg daily of etidronate for two weeks and calcium supplements 500 mg daily for 76 days), 1 α-hydroxyvitamin D, 1 mcg daily and calcium 1 g daily was started at the time the patients were listed for liver transplantation. During the first three post-operative months, spinal bone mineral density fell by 4.5% and there was also a significant reduction in hip bone mineral density. Moreover, 25% of patients sustained new vertebral fractures during the first post-operative year.

The effects of administration of intravenous pamidronate, 60 mg, pre-operatively and every three months thereafter in patients undergoing liver transplantation was reported by Reeves et al.[54] In this study, treatment was non-randomized and allocated on the basis of low bone mineral density. The incidence of clinically symptomatic vertebral fractures was lower in patients who received pamidronate, although this difference was not statistically significant and the numbers were small (5 fractures in the 11 untreated patients and none in 6 patients treated with pamidronate). Shane et al.[55] reported the effects of an intravenous infusion of pamidronate, 60 mg, in 17 patients within two weeks of cardiac transplantation, followed by four cycles of etidronate (400 mg daily for 14 days every three months). All patients also received calcium and vitamin D supplementation and calcitriol 0.25 mcg daily. In comparison to 45 historical controls who had received only calcium and vitamin D the treatment group showed a significant reduction in bone loss (1.3% vs 7.4% in the spine and 1.6% vs 6.2% in the femoral neck). Fracture incidence at one year post-transplantation was also reduced in the treatment group (11% vs 35%).

Finally, Meys et al.[56] investigated the effects of calcium (1 g daily) and calcidiol (25 mcg daily), either alone or combined with monoflu-orophosphate (200 mg daily) in an open and uncontrolled study of patients undergoing cardiac transplantation. Patients were stratified to either treatment on the basis of bone mineral density, those with lower values (some of whom also had fragility fractures prior to trans-

plantation) receiving the latter combination. In patients receiving calcium and calcidiol alone, lumbar spine bone mineral density was maintained for up to 2 years. In those also receiving monofluorophosphate, there was a linear increase in spinal bone mineral density which averaged 12.5% at one year and 29.5% at 2 years. No further fractures were seen in this group over the 2-year study period. Nevertheless, the number of patients in this study was small, and in view of the increase in fracture rate that has been reported in other studies of sodium fluoride, despite increases in bone mineral density, this therapy cannot be recommended at present for the prevention of post-transplantation bone disease.

At present, therefore, the optimum regimen for prevention of post-transplantation bone disease is uncertain, because of the lack of a randomized controlled design in reported studies. The variable timing of treatment with respect to transplantation and the different populations studied may partly explain the conflicting results with respect to calcitonin and oral bisphosphonates. Intuitively the most attractive approach is that of intermittent infusions of a bisphosphonate, for example pamidronate, which avoids problems due to poor compliance and/or reduced intestinal absorption; but further studies are required. In particular, the importance of fracture as the primary end-point should be emphasized in view of the discrepancy in some studies between bone loss and fracture rate after transplantation. There is also the increasing recognition that anti-fracture efficacy cannot be accurately predicted from therapeutically induced changes in bone mass.

Renal transplantation

Although bone histology should direct treatment choice, there have been no histology-based clinical studies investigating the effects of any therapy. In one study in rats, alendronate has been shown to prevent the adverse effects of cyclosporin on bone remodelling.[57] It may be tempting to instigate prophylactic antiresorptive therapy in renal transplant patients in the same way that etidronate can be prescribed for glucocorticoid-induced osteoporosis. However, the effects of these agents on patients with osteomalacia may be damaging, and the effects on adynamic bone remain to be established.

As yet there is only one published clinical trial addressing treatment of the renal transplant population.[58] A total of 48 patients with reduced bone mineral density, transplanted within the previous 19 years, were randomly assigned to one of three groups: oral clodronate 800 mg daily, nasal calcitonin 200 IU daily for 2 weeks every 3 months or an untreated control group. Bone mineral density increased by 4.6% in the clodronate group ($n = 15$, $p = 0.005$), by 3.2% in the calcitonin group ($n = 16$, $p = 0.034$) and by 1.8% in the controls ($n = 15$, $p = ns$). However, the post-treatment differences in bone mineral density between the three groups were not statistically significant. There were reductions in serum calcium in all groups (4.6%), with a significant rise in parathyroid hormone in the two treatment groups (116%). Therapy was well tolerated without impact on graft function. There are real difficulties in assessing therapeutic interventions in this population because of the heterogeneity of the type and severity of bone disease, both pre- and post-transplantation. Immunosuppressive regimens vary from centre to centre and, although transplantation aims to restore normal renal function, this is always achieved. Diminished creatinine clearance also limits the use of agents that are cleared by the kidney to those patients with good renal function.

The aim of any treatment is to reduce the risk of fracture, but, since BMD does not appear to correlate well with fracture prevalence in this population, it cannot be assumed that a gain in BMD translates into a reduction in fracture incidence. In the design of clinical trials it is essential to include fracture incidence as the primary end-point.

Since treatment depends on histology, it seems logical to initiate treatment with anti-resorptive agents such as bisphosphonates in patients with the increased bone turnover typified by hyperparathyroid bone disease. It should be remembered, however, that these drugs are relatively untested in this population and are only licensed for those with relatively normal renal function. Alendronate (10 mg daily), for example, should only be used if the serum creatinine is less than 180 µmol/l. Osteomalacia should be treated with calcitriol (0.25–1.0 mcg/day), but in cases related to previous aluminium exposure this intervention may prove ineffective or actually counter-productive (Chapter 6).

Until clinical trials are undertaken to assess the impact of treatment modalities on the histology of adynamic bone disease and mixed bone disease, it must be emphasized that specific treatment recommendations cannot be endorsed for these conditions.

REFERENCES

1. Epstein S, Shane E, Bilezikian JP (1995). Organ transplantation and osteoporosis. *Curr Opin Rheumatol* 7: 255–261.
2. Epstein S, Shane E (1996). Transplantation osteoporosis. In: *Osteoporosis*, eds R Marcus, D Feldman, J Kelsey, pp. 947–957. San Diego, Academic Press.
3. Rodino MA, Shane E (1998). Osteoporosis after organ transplantation. *Am J Med* 104: 459–469.
4. Shane E, Rivas MC, Silverberg SJ, Kim TS, Staron RB, Bilezikian JP (1993). Osteoporosis after cardiac transplantation. *Am J Med* 94: 257–264.
5. Porayko MK, Wiesner RH, Hay JE, Krom RA, Dickson ER, Beaver S, Schwerman L (1991). Bone disease in liver transplant recipients: incidence, timing, and risk factors. *Transplant Proc* 23: 1462–1465.
6. Navasa M, Monegal A, Guanabens N et al. (1994). Bone fractures in liver transplant patients. *Br J Rheumatol* 33: 52–55.
7. Shane E, Rivas M, Staron RB et al. (1996). Fracture after cardiac transplantation: a prospective longitudinal study. *J Clin Endocrinol Metab* 81: 1740–1746.
8. Shane E, Rivas M, McMahon DJ et al. (1997). Bone loss and turnover after cardiac transplantation. *J Clin Endocrinol Metab* 82: 1497–1506.
9. Sambrook PN, Kelly PJ, Fontana D et al. (1994). Mechanisms of rapid bone loss following cardiac transplantation. *Osteoporosis Int* 4: 273–276.
10. Henderson NK, Sambrook PN, Kelly PJ (1995).

Bone mineral loss and recovery after cardiac transplantation. [Letter]. *Lancet 346*: 905.

11. Van Cleemput J, Daenen W, Nijs J, Geusens P, Dequeker J, Vanhaecke J (1995). Timing and quantification of bone loss in cardiac transplant recipients. *Transplant Int 8*: 196–200.

12. Eastell R, Dickson ER, Hodgson SF et al. (1991). Rates of vertebral bone loss before and after liver transplantation in women with primary biliary cirrhosis. *Hepatology 14*: 296–300.

13. Hawkins FG, Leon M, Lopez MB et al. (1994). Bone loss and turnover in patients with liver transplantation. *Hepato-Gastroenterol 41*: 158–161.

14. Meys E, Fontanges E, Fourcade N, Thomasson A, Pouyet M, Delmas PD (1994). Bone loss after orthotopic liver transplantation. *Am J Med 97*: 445–450.

15. Compston JE, Alexander GA (1997). Bone disease after liver transplantation should not be underestimated. [Letter]. *Gut 40*: 695–696.

16. Ninkovic M, Bearcroft PWP, Skingle SJ, Love S, Alexander GA, Compston JE (1998). Vertebral fractures after liver transplantation: incidence and relationship to bone loss. [Abstract]. *J Bone Miner Res 13*: 521.

17. Arnold JC, Hauser D, Ziegler R, Kommerell B, Otto G, Theilmann L, Wuster C (1992). Bone disease after liver transplantation. *Transplant Proc 24*: 2709–2710.

18. Aris RM, Neuringer IP, Weiner MA, Egan TM, Ontjes D (1996). Severe osteoporosis before and after lung transplantation. *Chest 109*: 1176–1183.

19. Ferrari SL, Nicod LP, Hamacher J et al. (1996). Osteoporosis in patients undergoing lung transplantation. *Eur Respir J 9*: 2378–2382.

20. Grotz WH, Mundinger FA, Rasenack J et al. (1995). Bone loss after kidney transplantation: a longitudinal study in 115 graft recipients. *Nephrol Dial Transplant 10*: 2096–2100.

21. Almond MK, Kwan JT, Evans K, Cunningham J (1994). Loss of regional bone mineral density in the first 12 months following renal transplantation. *Nephron 66*: 52–57.

22. Julian BA, Laskow DA, Dubovsky J, Dubovsky EV, Curtis JJ, Quarles LD (1991). Rapid loss of vertebral mineral density after renal transplantation. *New Engl J Med 325*: 544–550.

23. Carlini RG, Rojas E, Arminio A, Weisinger JR, Bellorin-Font E (1998). What are the bone lesions in patients with more than four years of functioning renal transplant? *Nephrol Dial Transplant 13*(suppl 3): 103–104.

24. Horber FF, Casez JP, Steiger U, Czerniak A, Montandon A, Jaeger P (1994). Changes in bone mass early after kidney transplantation. *J Bone Miner Res 9*: 1–9.

25. Grotz WH, Mundinger FA, Gugel B, Exner VM, Kirste G, Schollmeyer PJ (1995). Bone mineral density after kidney transplantation. A cross-sectional study in 190 graft recipients up to 20 years after transplantation. *Transplantation 59*: 982–986.

26. Parker CR, Freemont AJ, Blackwell PJ, Grainge MJ, Hosking DJ (1999). Cross sectional analysis of renal transplant osteoporosis. *J Bone Miner Res 14*: 1943–1951.

27. Monegal A, Navasa M, Guanabens N et al. (1997). Osteoporosis and bone mineral metabolism disorders in cirrhotic patients referred for orthotopic liver transplantation. *Calcif Tissue Int 60*: 148–154.

28. Abdelhadi M, Eriksson SA, Ljusk ES, Ericzon BG, Nordenstrom J (1995). Bone mineral status in end-stage liver disease and the effect of liver transplantation. *Scand J Gastroenterol 30*: 1210–1215.

29. Muchmore JS, Cooper DK, Ye Y, Schlegel V, Pribil A, Zuhdi N (1992). Prevention of loss of vertebral bone density in heart transplant patients. *J Heart Lung Transplant 11*: 959–964.

30. Lee AH, Mull RL, Keenan GF et al. (1994). Osteoporosis and bone morbidity in cardiac transplant recipients. *Am J Med 96*: 35–41.

31. Shane E, Silverberg SJ, Donovan D et al. (1996). Osteoporosis in lung transplantation candidates with end-stage pulmonary disease. *Am J Med 101*: 262–269.

32. Compston JE, Greer S, Skingle SJ et al. (1996). Early increase in plasma parathyroid hormone levels following liver transplantation. *J Hepatol 25*: 715–718.

33. Llach F, Massry SG, Singer FR, Kurokawa K, Kaye JH, Coburn JW (1975). Skeletal resistance to endogenous parathyroid hormone in patients with early renal failure. A possible cause for secondary hyperparathyroidism. *J Clin Endocrinol Metab 41*: 339–345.

34. Hernandez D, Concepcion MT, Lorenzo V et al. (1994). Adynamic bone disease with negative aluminium staining in pre-dialysis patients: prevalence and evolution after maintenance dialysis. *Nephrol Dial Transplant 9*: 517–523.

35. Sherrard DJ, Hercz G, Pei Y, Segre G (1996). The aplastic form of renal osteodystrophy. *Nephrol Dial Transplant 11*(suppl 3): 29–31.

36. Velasquez-Forero F, Mondragon A, Herrero B,

Pena JC (1996). Adynamic bone lesion in renal transplant recipients with normal renal function. *Nephrol Dial Transplant 11*(suppl 3): 58–64.

37. Riemens SC, Oostdijk A, van Doormaal JJ et al. (1996). Bone loss after liver transplantation is not prevented by cyclical etidronate, calcium and alphacalcidol. The Liver Transplant Group, Groningen. *Osteoporosis Int 6*: 213–218.

38. Epstein S (1996). Post-transplantation bone disease: the role of immunosuppressive agents and the skeleton. *J Bone Miner Res 11*: 1–7.

39. Lukert BP, Raisz LG (1990). Glucocorticoid-induced osteoporosis: pathogenesis and management. *Ann Intern Med 112*: 352–364.

40. Seeman E, Wahner HW, Offord KP, Kumar R, Johnson WJ, Riggs BL (1982). Differential effects of endocrine dysfunction on the axial and the appendicular skeleton. *J Clin Invest 69*: 1302–1309.

41. Kozower M, Veatch L, Kaplan MM (1974). Decreased clearance of prednisolone, a factor in the development of corticosteroid side effects. *J Clin Endocrinol Metab 38*: 407–412.

42. Canalis E (1996). Mechanisms of glucocorticoid action in bone: implications to glucocorticoid-induced osteoporosis. *J Clin Endocrinol Metab 81*: 3441–3447.

43. Delaney AM, Gabbitas BY, Canalis E (1995). Cortisol downregulates osteoblast alpha 1 (I) procollagen mRNA by transcriptional and post-transcriptional mechanisms. *J Cell Biochem 57*: 488–494.

44. Orcel P, Denne MA, De Vernejoul MC (1991). Cyclosporin-A in vitro decreases bone resorption, osteoclast formation, and the fusion of cells of the monocyte-macrophage lineage. *Endocrinology 128*: 1638–1646.

45. Movsowitz C, Epstein S, Fallon M, Ismail F, Thomas S (1988). Cyclosporin-A in vivo produces severe osteopenia in the rat: effect of dose and duration of administration. *Endocrinology 123*: 2571–2577.

46. Katz IA, Epstein S (1992). Posttransplantation bone disease. *J Bone Miner Res 7*: 123–126.

47. Katz IA, Takizawa M, Jaffe II, Stein B, Fallon MD, Epstein S (1991). Comparison of the effects of FK506 and cyclosporin on bone mineral metabolism in the rat. A pilot study. *Transplantation 52*: 571–574.

48. Bryer HP, Isserow JA, Armstrong EC et al. (1995). Azathioprine alone is bone sparing and does not alter cyclosporin A-induced osteopenia in the rat. *J Bone Miner Res 10*: 132–138.

49. Vedi S, Greer S, Skingle SJ et al. (1999). Mechanism of bone loss after liver transplantation: a histomorphometric analysis. *J Bone Miner Res 14*: 281–287.

50. Hutchinson AJ, Whitehouse RW, Boulton HF et al. (1993). Correlation of bone histology with parathyroid hormone, vitamin D3, and radiology in end-stage renal disease. *Kidney Int 44*: 1071–1077.

51. Malluche HH, Monier-Faugere MC (1994). The role of bone biopsy in the management of patients with renal osteodystrophy. *J Am Soc Nephrol 4*: 1631–1642.

52. Valero MA, Loinaz C, Larrodera L, Leon M, Moreno E, Hawkins F (1995). Calcitonin and bisphosphonates treatment in bone loss after liver transplantation. *Calcif Tissue Int 57*: 15–19.

53. Garcia-Delgado I, Prieto S, Gil F, Robles E, Rufilanchas JJ, Hawkins F (1997). Calcitonin, etidronate, and calcidiol treatment in bone loss after cardiac transplantation. *Calcif Tissue Int 60*: 155–159.

54. Reeves HL, Manas DM, Bassendine MF et al. (1996). Intravenous bisphosphonate pre liver transplant prevents osteoporotic vertebral collapse. [Abstract]. *Hepatology*: 178A.

55. Shane E, Thys-Jacobs S, Papadopoulos A et al. (1996). Antiresorptive therapy prevents bone loss after cardiac transplantation. [Abstract]. *J Bone Miner Res*: S340.

56. Meys E, Terreaux-Duvert F, Beaume-Six T, Dureau G, Meunier PJ (1993). Bone loss after cardiac transplantation: effects of calcium, calcidiol and monofluorophosphate. *Osteoporosis Int 3*: 322–329.

57. Sass DA, Bowman AR, Yuan Z, Ma Y, Jee WS, Epstein S (1997). Alendronate prevents cyclosporin A-induced osteopenia in the rat. *Bone 21*: 65–70.

58. Grotz WH, Rump LC, Niessen A et al. (1998). Treatment of osteopenia and osteoporosis after kidney transplantation. *Transplantation 66*: 1004–1008.

8

Osteoporosis: Primary Prevention

Pernille Ravn

Introduction • **Risk factors for osteoporosis** • Treatment modalities • **Tibolone** • **Selective oestrogen receptor modulators (SERMs)** • **Calcium** • **Bisphosphonates** • **Monitoring of treatment**

INTRODUCTION

Age-related bone loss is a universal skeletal phenomenon that results in low bone mass and architectural damage, leading in turn to an increased risk of fracture. The destruction of bone trabeculae is mostly irreversible. A woman at the age of 50 is at an estimated risk of 16% for forearm fracture, 32% for vertebral fracture, and 15% for hip fracture during her remaining lifetime.[1]

The risk of osteoporosis depends largely upon peak bone mass, attained during early adulthood, and the rate of bone loss later in life. A poor intake of calcium and vitamin D, physical inactivity, and prolonged amenorrhoea are among the factors that can severely diminish peak bone mass. Since peak bone mass cannot be influenced at the menopause, the main goal of osteoporosis prevention is therefore to reduce postmenopausal bone loss.

In theory, there are two preventive strategies, neither of which are mutually exclusive. Population-based prevention of osteoporosis by public health initiatives to reduce clinical risk factors such as physical inactivity, low intakes of calcium and vitamin D, and smoking is one option. However, these measures would require universal and long-term compliance before an effect on the prevalence of osteoporosis could be achieved. The universal use of hormone replacement therapy (HRT) in postmenopausal women would have much greater impact, but necessitates careful cost–benefit analyses because of the considerable individual and socio-economic consequences. Currently there is no evidence to substantiate the overall utility of such a strategy, which is also complicated by the fact that most women will not accept prolonged HRT. The currently accepted strategy is therefore to target prevention of postmenopausal osteoporosis at women at particular risk.

The drug of first choice in the prevention of postmenopausal osteoporosis is HRT.[2] In contrast to popular belief, physical exercise, calcium, and vitamin D are not sufficient to prevent postmenopausal osteoporosis in women at risk. They are however better than no treatment at all,[2] and have an additional effect when combined with HRT.

Before beginning an assessment of the risk of osteoporosis in an individual, it should be mutually agreed that the outcome will have an

---

Table 8.1 Risk factors for osteoporosis.

Age (×2 risk/decade)
  Previous fragility fracture (×10 risk of future
  fracture)
Endocrine
  Premature (<45 yrs) menopause – natural or
  surgical
  Thin body build (BMI <20)
  Previous amenorrhoea (>6 months duration)
Genetic
  Low trauma fracture in first-degree relative
  Caucasian or Asian ethnicity
  Female gender
Life style
  Low level of physical activity
  Poor calcium intake (<0.5 g/day)
  Alcohol excess (>14 units/week)
  Cigarette smoking

Table 8.2 Use of risk factors in management.

Target individuals for further investigation:
  Densitometry
  Bone turnover markers
Eliminate modifiable risk factors
Discuss treatment:
  Advantages
  Disadvantages

---

influence on the decision for and choice of intervention. Secondary causes of osteoporosis are outside the scope of this review, but should be considered as a part of this initial evaluation (Chapter 9).

RISK FACTORS FOR OSTEOPOROSIS

Clinical assessment of risk of osteoporosis

A number of risk factors, some of which are listed in Table 8.1, are known to be involved in the pathogenesis of osteoporosis. Some affect bone loss, others affect fracture risk by increasing bone fragility and the risk of injury, others are linked to osteoporosis without any known cause–effect relationship. The most important risk factors include female gender, caucasian or Asian ethnicity, early menopause, a personal history of low-trauma fracture, a history of low-trauma fractures in first-degree relatives, current smoking, and slim body build. A prior

fragility fracture causes an approximately 10-fold increase in the risk of fracture.[3] Additional factors include chronic illness, endocrine disorders, excessive alcohol intake, and use of certain drugs, particularly prednisolone in doses above 7.5 mg/day for more than 6 months. It is important to emphasize that none of the risk factors predict bone mass with sufficient accuracy in an individual patient. The best combination of risk factors only accounts for about 20% of the variability in bone mass.[4] Clinical risk factors thus add information about the risk of osteoporosis, which is only partly explained by variation in bone mass. They should therefore preferably be used to target individuals for further investigations (bone densitometry and biochemical markers of bone turnover) and treatment (Table 8.2). They also provide an opportunity to discuss with the patient those factors that can be eliminated or altered. This is particularly worth while as many of them also have an impact on general health and other organ systems.

Assessment of risk of osteoporosis by bone densitometry

The definition of osteoporosis developed for the World Health Organization (WHO) is based on bone densitometry. Normal bone mass is defined as a bone mineral density (BMD) above or below 1 standard deviation (SD) from the premenopausal mean value (T-score), osteopenia as a BMD below -1 SD but above -2.5 SD, and osteoporosis as a BMD below -2.5 SD.[2] The definitions are influenced by the need for clearly defined entry criteria for clinical trials, and are used to provide diagnostic labels, but not necessarily indications for intervention. The definitions do, however, reflect the fact that bone mass accounts for 75–85% of the variability in ultimate bone strength, that bone mass is considered one of the best single predictors of fracture risk, that low bone mass is an important risk factor for osteoporosis,[5] and that prevention of osteoporosis almost exclusively means intervention to prevent declining bone mass.

For each SD decrease in BMD there is an approximately two-fold increase in risk of fracture, depending on the site of measurement and the technique used.[6] Site-specific measurements do not improve the prediction of overall risk of fracture, and any measurement is better than none.[2] However, because hip fracture is the most serious osteoporotic fracture and is best estimated by measurement at the hip,[7] this skeletal site should always be measured if possible.

In the management of individual patients, bone densitometry should be used as a measure of risk, and not as an either/or diagnostic criterion. Information on bone mass should be added to information on clinical risk factors and balanced against the benefits and risks of the intervention considered.[2] Currently, there is no generally accepted nomogram using BMD and clinical risk factors to target prevention and treatment of postmenopausal osteoporosis. One suggestion for postmenopausal women might be to consider treatment whenever BMD is below -1 SD (T-score) and clinical risk factors are present. If treatment is postponed, repeated assessment of risk, including measurement of BMD, should be performed after 2 years. With decreasing BMD and an increasing number of, and length of exposure to, clinical risk factors, the indications for treatment become stronger. A BMD of -2.5 SD or below is a compelling indication for treatment even if clinical risk factors are not present (Chapter 9).

Assessment of risk of osteoporosis by biochemical markers

As was outlined above, a low bone mass is associated with an increased risk of fracture,[5,6] and the combination of low bone mass and a high rate of bone loss further increases the risk (Figure 8.1).[8] High bone turnover as estimated by biochemical markers is associated with an increased rate of bone loss,[8,9] and predicts the risk of fracture independently of BMD.[10,11] The Odds Ratio for fracture seems to be around 2 per 2 SD increase in the biochemical marker above the premenopausal mean value.[10,11] In these studies, the biochemical markers with the best predictive accuracy were urine C- and N-telopeptides of type I collagen and urine deoxypyridinoline, all known to be biochemical markers of bone resorption.[10,11] However, the biochemical markers present a diagnostic field in rapid development, and other markers may appear with similar or even better predictive accuracy. It is significant that a bone mass in the osteoporotic range (2.5 SD below the premenopausal mean value) and an increased value of a biochemical marker (more than 2 SD above the premenopausal mean) increase the Odds Ratio for hip fracture to 4–5,[10] suggesting that combined information on bone densitometry and biochemical markers improves the estimation of osteoporosis risk.

TREATMENT MODALITIES

Oestrogen and oestrogen–progestin replacement therapy

Indications for treatment
In general, the indications for postmenopausal HRT can be divided into two categories: relief of postmenopausal symptoms attributable to oestrogen deficiency and reduction of risk of diseases associated with oestrogen deficiency (osteoporosis and cardiovascular disease).

Treatment regimens
Replacement therapy with oestrogen alone is often called unopposed oestrogen therapy, and

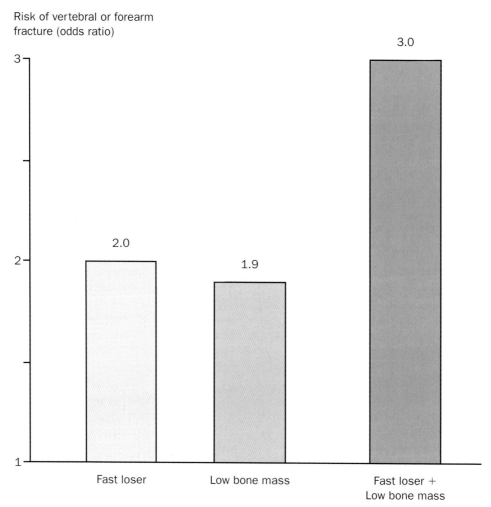

Figure 8.1 Odds ratio of having a fracture with low bone mass at menopause and/or fast rate of bone loss. Cut-off levels were: forearm bone mass $\leqslant-1$ standard deviation and/or rate of bone loss $\geqslant3\%$ per year within first 2 years of menopause. Reprinted by permission of the publisher from Bjarnason NH, Hassager C, Christiansen C (1998). Postmenopausal bone remodelling and hormone replacement. *Climacteric 1*: 72–79. Copyright by the International Menopause Society 1998.

abbreviated ERT (estrogen replacement therapy), whereas combined oestrogen–progestin therapy is abbreviated HRT (hormone replacement therapy). ERT increases the risk of endometrial hyperplasia and cancer in women with an intact uterus,[12] and should be reserved for women who have undergone hysterectomy. For women with an intact uterus, oestrogen should be combined with progestin to protect the endometrium.[13] Because most of the undesirable effects of HRT are caused by the progestin, the lowest possible dose ensuring protection of the endometrium should be used. Progestin is not needed in women without a uterus except in those who have undergone hysterectomy because of endometrial cancer or recurrent endometriosis. Replacement therapy in these women should be in the form of combined oestrogen–progestin therapy. HRT can be given in a cyclical combined or continuous combined regimen. In the cyclical combined regimen, a progestin is added for the last 10–14 days of the cycle; less than this is inadequate to protect the endometrium.[13] If the oestrogen and progestin are to be given as separate tablets then the first 10–14 days of the calendar month may be chosen for convenience; but if a calendar strip package is used, then the progestin days are fixed. The cyclical regimen mimics the natural premenopausal cycle, and provokes monthly withdrawal bleeds. In the continuous combined regimen, the progestin is given continuously with the oestrogen, which causes the endometrium to remain in an atrophic state, so that withdrawal bleeding is avoided. Spotting may occur during the first 6 months of treatment,[14] but most women (90%) experience amenorrhoea with prolonged use.[14] This regimen should be reserved for women at least 2 years, and preferably more than 5 years, past the menopause, because the endogenous oestrogen production, which is still present during the early menopause, may otherwise result in endometrial proliferation and subsequent irregular bleeding. A regimen with addition of progestin every 3 months[15] is another way to restrict withdrawal bleeding. Since most data on endometrial safety are from studies of cyclical combined regimens, this should be the first choice for women with an intact uterus. Other options should be reserved for elderly women or those who find withdrawal bleeding unacceptable.

Oestrogen definitions
The main groups of oestrogen are:

1. Synthetic oestrogen analogues without a steroid skeleton (stilboestrol derivatives).
2. Synthetic oestrogen analogues with a steroid skeleton.
3. Non-human oestrogens, produced from an equine source (conjugated equine oestrogens).
4. Native human oestrogens or compounds that are transformed to native oestrogens in the body.

Synthetic oestrogens without a steroid structure are now obsolete. Synthetic oestrogens with a steroid structure (ethinyl oestradiol) are still the most commonly used preparations in the oral contraceptive. Ethinyl oestradiol can be used for postmenopausal replacement therapy and prevention of postmenopausal osteoporosis,[16] but is associated with an increased risk of thrombosis. For postmenopausal replacement therapy, conjugated equine oestrogens are most commonly prescribed in the United States, whereas in Europe there has been a tradition of using native human oestrogens (17β-oestradiol) or oestradiol valerate.

Progestin definitions
The progestins differ greatly in their non-uterine properties but have in common the ability to cause secretory transformation of an oestrogen-primed endometrium.

Progestins may be divided into three subgroups:

1. Nortestosterone derivatives (C-19 steroids), with a relatively high androgenic effect (norethisterone acetate).
2. Progesterone derivatives (C-21 steroids), with less androgenic activity (medroxyprogesterone acetate).
3. Natural human progesterone, available in micronized form for oral therapy.

In addition, the progestins may, to a varying degree, have oestrogenic, anti-oestrogenic, androgenic, anti-androgenic, anti-gonadotropic, glucocorticoid-like, and adrenocorticotropic hormone-stimulating activities. These differences are most important in terms of adverse events, but can also be used therapeutically, as in the case of the C-21 steroid, cyproterone acetate, which has marked anti-androgenic effects. Most clinical experience has been gained with the use of norethisterone acetate, medroxyprogesterone acetate, and levonorgestrel.

Dose
Oral doses of 0.625 mg conjugated equine oestrogen or 2 mg 17β-oestradiol prevent early post-

Table 8.3 Doses of commonly used oestrogens and progestins having a bone-sparing effect and giving endometrial protection.

Oestrogens	Route	Dose
Oestradiol	oral	2 mg
	patch	50 µg
	gel	1 mg
	implants	50 mg/6 months
Conjugated equine oestrogens		0.625 mg
Oestradiol valerate		2 mg

Progestins	Sequential	Continuous combined
Medroxyprogesterone	10 mg	2.5 mg
Cyproterone acetate	1 mg	1 mg
Dydrogesterone	10–20 mg	10 mg
Megestrol	80 mg	—
Progesterone	200 mg	100 mg
Norethisterone (norethindrone)	0.7–1 mg	0.35 mg
Norgestrel	150 µg	50 µg
Levonorgestrel	75 µg	30 µg

menopausal bone loss[17,18] (Table 8.3). The oestrogenic effect on bone is dose-dependent, and lower doses of oestrogen may be sufficient to prevent postmenopausal bone loss.[16,19,20] This has substantial implications because most adverse effects, which limit compliance to HRT, are dose-related. The minimal serum oestradiol level for prevention of postmenopausal bone loss appears to be 60 pg/ml (400 µmol/l).[21] It is important to recognize that the dose that is effective in the management of menopausal complaints does not necessarily prevent bone loss.

The doses of progestin given in Table 8.2 give satisfactory bleeding control in most (80–90% of) women.

Applications
Delivery systems other than oral HRT are available. For instance, 17β-oestradiol can be given as a transdermal patch twice per week. In women with an intact uterus, the patch should be given with cyclical progestin,[22,23] or as a patch containing both oestradiol and progestin in a continuous combined regimen.[24] Recently, an oestradiol gel requiring daily skin applications has also been introduced.[25] Transdermal or percutaneous HRT prevents skeletal bone loss as effectively as oral HRT.[24,25] This confirms that the effect is independent of the route of administration, providing that the achieved serum oestradiol levels are adequate. The patch causes more stable serum oestradiol levels than oral administration or percutaneous gel application, which may be important (in women with migraine, where fluctuating levels may precipitate attacks). The liver metabolism of oestrogen is retarded by ethanol, and enhanced by smoking. Serum oestradiol levels are consequently more variable and unpredictable in smokers or in women with a regular intake of

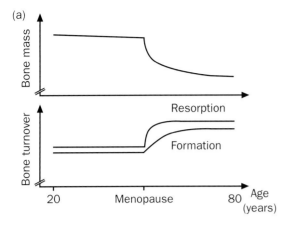

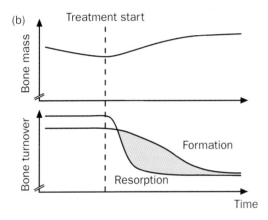

Figure 8.2 Relationship between bone mass and bone turnover before and after menopause, and showing response to antiresorptive treatment (see text for details). Reprinted by permission of the publisher from Bjarnason NH, Hassager C, Christiansen C (1998). Postmenopausal bone remodelling and hormone replacement. *Climacteric 1*: 72–79. Copyright by the International Menopause Society 1998.

alcohol. In these cases, it may be advantageous to bypass the liver with a non-oral application.

Finally, compliance should have a major influence on the choice of application.

Effects on bone remodelling

Before the onset of the menopause, rates of bone formation and resorption are approxi-

mately equal. Calcium balance is maintained, and no bone loss occurs (Figure 8.2). After the menopause, both bone formation and resorption rates increase, but the rate of bone resorption increases more rapidly, resulting in a calcium imbalance and a net loss of bone.[26] The difference between these two processes is greatest during the first few years after the menopause, when, as a consequence, bone loss is greatest (Figure 8.2). With increasing postmenopausal age, bone formation and resorption converge towards a new steady state at a higher level. In osteoporosis prevention, bone formation and resorption should ideally be maintained in balance at premenopausal levels, resulting in a stable calcium balance and bone mass.

Oestrogens

Oestrogens have a direct effect on bone mass through oestrogen receptors in bone, and this is reflected by a reduction in bone turnover and bone loss. Oestrogen receptors have been demonstrated in both osteoblasts and osteoclasts, but the precise mechanism of action of oestrogen at the cellular level is not fully understood. Their inhibition of bone resorption and perforation of bone trabeculae reduces the risk of subsequent disintegration of trabecular architecture. Treatment with oestrogen primarily decreases bone resorption and only secondary bone formation,[26,27] resulting in a temporary positive bone balance lasting 1–2 years.[24] In this period, the resorption lacunae are filled in (the size of the remodelling space decreases), resulting in an increase in bone mass. When the rates of bone formation and resorption reach a new equilibrium, the increase in bone density stabilizes and this will continue as long as treatment continues[14] (Figure 8.3).

Progestins

Because of the different qualities of the progestins, the effects on bone and calcium metabolism should ideally be studied separately. However, relatively few data are available on the individual effect of progestin on postmenopausal calcium metabolism. Norethister-

BMC arm (%)

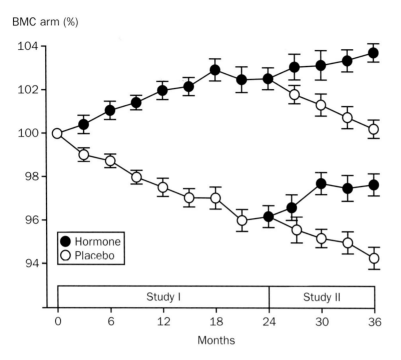

Figure 8.3 Bone mineral content at the distal forearm as a function of time and treatment in women soon after the menopause. Hormone: cyclic combined oral 17β-oestradiol/ oestriol and norethisterone (Trisequens Forte™). All women received a calcium supplement of Calcium Sandoz™ 500 mg. Reprinted by permission of the publisher from Christiansen C, Christensen MS, Transbøl I (1981). Bone mass in postmenopausal women after withdrawal of oestrogen/gestagen replacement therapy. *Lancet 1*: 459–461. Copyright by the Lancet Ltd. 1981.

one acetate when combined with oestrogen appears to prevent bone loss[14,28] through a direct reduction in bone turnover,[29] whereas medroxyprogesterone does not seem to have this additional effect on bone mass.[30] There is therefore no evidence that progestins impair the oestrogenic effect on calcium metabolism.

Effects on bone mass
ERT and HRT prevent osteoporosis in post-menopausal women[16–24,30–33] independently of chronological or menopausal age.[31,32,34] In recently postmenopausal women, a 5% increase in bone mass occurs within 1–2 years of treat-ment, followed by a plateau.[31–34] The effect of HRT is more pronounced in skeletal sites with mainly trabecular bone compared to areas with mainly cortical bone,[22,33] but an adequate dose of HRT prevents bone loss in all skeletal regions.[22,33] When HRT is stopped, bone loss resumes at a normal postmenopausal rate.[32]

Effects on fracture
From retrospective and cross-sectional studies,

it has been shown that oestrogen treatment reduces the occurrence of fractures at clinically relevant skeletal sites[35,36,38] irrespective of post-menopausal age.[36] Results from prospective studies are scarce and short term, but appar-ently correspond to the results from epidemio-logic studies.[23,37] The reduction in fracture incidence through long-term HRT (5–10 years) is estimated to be about 50–75%.[35–38] Since post-menopausal bone loss resumes after cessation of oestrogen, prolonged treatment is necessary to achieve effective results, and currently 5–10 years of treatment are recommended.[2] However, the protection against fractures decreases after cessation of treatment, and is substantially reduced after 5 years.[38] Treatment beyond 10 years is probably more effective, and should be recommended if HRT is started early after the menopause with the purpose of pre-venting osteoporotic fractures later in life. If HRT is restricted to only 5–10 years of treat-ment then it is probably more cost-effective to start much later, for example around the age of 65 years. In this way an anti-fracture effect is achieved in the seventh to eighth decade, when hip fractures have their greatest incidence and constitute a serious health care and socio-economic problem.

Non-skeletal beneficial effects

A detailed assessment of the non-skeletal risks and benefits of HRT is beyond the scope of this chapter. Notwithstanding, it is inappropriate to ignore these issues, since they have a critical impact on strategies for the prevention and treatment of osteoporosis. In general terms, the benefits outweigh the risks, and this is reflected in both morbidity and mortality.[39]

Menopausal complaints

The duration of the climacteric varies considerably from one woman to another. About 50% of menopausal women experience severe hot flushes, eventually combined with other menopausal complaints. Only 25–50% experience hot flushes for more than 5 years, but a few suffer from disturbing symptoms for up to 10 years after the menopause. Oestrogen is the most effective treatment for hot flushes, and also relieves most other menopausal complaints in a dose-related manner. Relief of postmenopausal complaints is the primary factor improving compliance with HRT in many women. Prolonged HRT for other indications challenges the physician and is complicated by the fact that atherosclerosis and osteoporosis are silent processes that, by definition, are asymptomatic during prevention.

Cardiovascular disease

Cardiovascular disease (CVD) is the major cause of death and disability in women in Western societies. After the menopause, the risk of CVD increases, partly as a result of changes in lipoprotein profiles. The favourable effect of oral ERT on serum lipoproteins is well established.[40] Progestins, especially C-19 steroids like norethisterone acetate and norgestrel, antagonize the effects of oestrogens on serum lipids and lipoproteins[41] in a dose-related manner.[42] With appropriate dosing of oestrogen and progestin, the overall effect is, however, almost neutral.[42,43]

A range of differently designed epidemiological studies have investigated the interrelationship between CVD and HRT, mostly with unopposed conjugated equine oestrogen treatment, although a few reports of combined oestrogen–progestin treatment are available. Most studies show a 35–50% reduction in the relative risk of CVD in women taking oestrogen,[40,44] with a more pronounced effect during secondary prevention. Recent results from the first large, long-term randomized trial (HER5) surprisingly showed that treatment with continuous combined oestrogen–medroxyprogesterone acetate in postmenopausal women with established CVD did not reduce the rate of CVD events in spite of a beneficial effect on the lipid profile.[45] This might be because medroxyprogesterone acetate antagonized the effect of oestrogen. This would be consistent with a recent study of oophorectomized cynomulgus macaque monkeys that showed that ERT protected against coronary atherosclerosis, whereas continuous combined oestrogen–medroxyprogesterone acetate treatment did not, in spite of a similar beneficial influence on lipid metabolism.[46] These results confirm that the lipoprotein profile is a surrogate marker for risk of CVD, which do not fully explain the anti-atherosclerotic effect of oestrogen. Before changing the general recommendations for postmenopausal HRT, results from large ongoing prospective trials should be awaited.

Cerebrovascular and central nervous systems

Stroke is the third leading cause of death in European women. Some studies have reported a 30–50% lower incidence of stroke among women using oestrogen,[47] whereas other studies have suggested that the incidence of stroke is unaffected by their use.[44,48] Again, most of currently available data are based on unopposed oestrogen treatment. Results from ongoing trials are awaited. Dementia due to Alzheimer's disease is a common disorder with enormous impact on quality of life. Recent prospective studies have suggested that use of ERT may delay the onset, and decrease the risk, of Alzheimer's disease by about 50%,[49] while cognitive function may also be better preserved.

Deleterious effects

Unfortunately, the general compliance with HRT is low, and only 25–50% of women will continue for more than one year. Compliance can be substantially increased by better information and support during treatment. The most common reasons for discontinuation are anxiety over side-effects, especially breast cancer, and dislike of withdrawal bleeding.

Breast cancer

ERT appears to be associated with an increased risk of breast cancer,[50,51] and long-term use of ERT (more than 10 years) increases the risk of breast cancer by 5–30%, which equates to an increase in lifetime risk of 13–17% relative to a non-user. The risk of breast cancer is unaffected by the use of HRT for less than 5 years, and is not influenced by the addition of progestin. The risk decreases after cessation of HRT, and has almost returned to baseline after about 5 years. Whether HRT affects the mortality of breast cancer is not clear, but most studies have suggested that the risk of death from breast cancer is only influenced to a limited extent.[50,51] It is interesting that the risk of breast cancer appears to be dose-related to the level of endogenous oestrogens,[52] and low-dose oestrogen regimens recently suggested for the prevention of osteoporosis[16,19,20] might therefore be associated with a lower risk of breast cancer.

Overall mortality has recently been reported to be reduced by 40% in current users of HRT,[39] with a major impact from the reduction in CVD mortality. Since the lifetime risk of death from CVD is far greater than the risk of death from breast cancer, the beneficial impact of even a small reduction in the risk of CVD far outweighs the negative impact of a small increase in the risk of breast cancer.

Venous thrombo-embolism

Venous thrombo-embolism (VTE) is a recognized risk of oral contraception, whereas HRT was not thought to be associated with this problem until recently. It now appears that the risk of VTE and pulmonary embolism is increased about threefold during HRT.[53] However, the absolute risk remains low, at

approximately one event/5000 woman-years, most common in the early period of HRT use.

Common adverse events

Irregular bleeding is most common during the first 3–6 months of HRT. Irregular bleeding, particularly when occurring 6 months after the start of treatment and not controllable by simple adjustments of doses (particularly of progestin) should be investigated by endometrial biopsy. Breast tenderness, leg cramps, headaches, increase in appetite, and change in libido comprise the HRT 'start-up syndrome', which is pronounced in some women, but almost absent in others. Usually, the symptoms decline substantially or even disappear within the first 3 months of treatment. Generally, HRT does not increase weight, but occasionally there may be an idiosyncratic weight gain or the development of hypertension. Undesired prolonged mood changes are usually caused by the progestin; norethisterone (C-19) derivatives may be associated with aggressiveness, and the progesterone (C-21) derivatives with depressions. Nausea can be managed by taking the treatment before bedtime or by switching to a non-oral route of administration. Finally, perimenopausal women need to be warned that HRT does not protect against pregnancy.

Starting treatment

Absolute contraindications (active breast or endometrial cancer, active significant liver disease, pregnancy or undiagnosed vaginal bleeding) should be excluded. There are several conditions where HRT is relatively, but not absolutely, contraindicated (hypertension, migraine, previous venous or pulmonary thromboembolism, diabetes, gallstones, endometriosis, uterine fibroids, and previous breast or stage 1 endometrial cancer). In these cases, HRT can be started under careful supervision, with focus on the potential problems associated with HRT in that particular patient. If HRT is started with combined oestrogen–progestin or progestin alone, lowers the frequency of irregular bleeding during the first monthly cycles. In the elderly, it is prudent to start with a small dose of oestrogen for a few months and subsequently to increase to a bone-sparing dose. The patient should be assessed 3 months after start of treatment by repeating a breast and pelvic examination, and measuring blood pressure and body weight. In most countries a mammogram every second year is recommended. Women who persist with HRT during the first year are more likely to continue on prolonged treatment. Closer supervision and support during the early phase of HRT is therefore worthwhile.

The future
Adherence to treatment is probably the greatest challenge for the future. Most of the beneficial effects of HRT, including prevention of osteoporosis, are only obtained after several years of treatment, and a short course of HRT is unlikely to have any long-term health benefits. As outlined above, compliance is mostly limited by factors that appear to be dose-related. It is therefore intriguing that recent results have shown that prevention of osteoporosis can be obtained at low doses of HRT. New combinations of oestrogen and progestin are being investigated in the search for optimal bleeding control. New means of application (nasal sprays) may increase compliance. If progestin turns out to limit the protective effect of oestrogen on CVD, systemic oestrogen combined with local applications of progestin (creams, vaginal tablets) should be further investigated.

TIBOLONE

Tibolone is a synthetic analogue of gonadal steroids with combined oestrogenic, androgenic, and progestogenic properties that is closely related to the anabolic steroids. In the endometrium tibolone is transformed to a metabolite without oestrogenic activity, so that at the recommended dose (2.5 mg/day) the endometrium is unaffected and combination with progestin is unnecessary. As with a continuous combined HRT regimen, tibolone should be reserved for women at least 2 years past the menopause. Continuous combined HRT and tibolone are similarly effective in alleviating

menopausal symptoms, but spotting during the first 6 months of treatment appears to be less frequent during tibolone treatment than with continuous combined HRT. Because of the androgenic component, tibolone treatment increases libido, and at a dose of 2.5 mg/day reduces bone turnover by 30–50%.[54] As a consequence bone loss is prevented and bone mass may increase by 2–5% during the first 2 years of treatment,[54] an effect similar to that of conventional HRT.[55] Half the recommended dose of tibolone appears to have a similar effect on bone mass and bone turnover (Figure 8.4), and may be adequate for prevention of osteoporosis in some women.[54] Tibolone reduces serum cholesterol and triglycerides, does not affect LDL-cholesterol, and decreases HDL-cholesterol and apolipoprotein A-1 by about 30%.[56] The overall effect on haemostatic factors tends towards increased fibrinolysis and unchanged coagulation. This may theoretically counterbalance the potentially negative effect of the decrease in HDL-cholesterol.[56] However, the long-term effect of tibolone on cardiovascular morbidity and mortality is at present unknown. Significantly, the effect on fracture risk remains to be determined, although studies in animal models indicate that tibolone increases bone strength.[57]

SELECTIVE OESTROGEN RECEPTOR MODULATORS (SERMs)

The selective oestrogen receptor modulators (SERMs) form a group of 'designer oestrogens' with selective, tissue-specific effects on the oestrogen receptors. These tissue-specific oestrogens were designed to preserve the beneficial effects of oestrogen, including protection against CVD and osteoporosis, but to have no undesired effects on the reproductive organs (endometrium and breast).

Tamoxifen was the first of this class of drug to be clinically evaluated. Because of its anti-oestrogenic effect on the breast tamoxifen is used in the prevention of breast cancer recurrence. Tamoxifen was later found to have an oestrogenic effect on the cardiovascular[58] and

BMD arm (%)

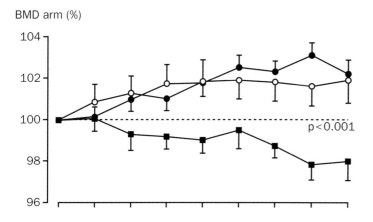

BMD spine (%)

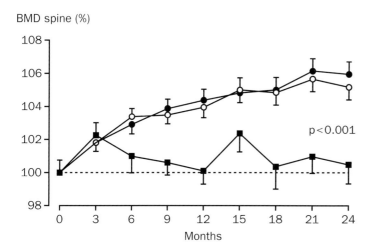

Months

Figure 8.4 Bone mineral density at the distal forearm and spine as a function of time and treatment in elderly women. Open circles: tibolone 2.5 mg; closed circles: tibolone 1.25 mg; squares: placebo. Reprinted by permission of the publisher from Bjarnason NH, Bjarnason K, Haarbo J et al. (1996). Tibolone: prevention of bone loss in late postmenopausal women. *J Clin Endocrinol Metab 81*: 2419–2422. Copyright by the Endocrine Society 1996.

skeletal[59] systems, but unfortunately, it was also found to increase the incidence of endometrial cancer.[60]

Raloxifene was initially shown in animal models to act as an oestrogen receptor antagonist in breast and endometrium, but as an oestrogen agonist in the skeletal and cardiovascular systems. In a recent large randomized study of healthy, recently postmenopausal women, raloxifene 60 mg/day was shown to be the lowest dose with significant and clinically relevant effects on bone turnover and bone mass.[61] It is now the recommended dose for the prevention of postmenopausal osteoporosis and reduces bone turnover by 25–40% (Figure 8.5), increases BMD at the spine, hip and total body by 1.2–1.6% (Figure 8.6) without stimulating uterine or breast tissue, and is generally well tolerated. A large study of raloxifene in elderly women with low bone mass and/or a prevalent vertebral fracture have revealed a similar effect on bone turnover and bone mass to that in younger women and a 30–50% reduction in the incidence of low-trauma vertebral fractures.[62] Raloxifene significantly reduces aortic atherosclerosis in cholesterol-fed rabbits,[63] and in early and late postmenopausal women it decreases serum total cholesterol, LDL-choles-

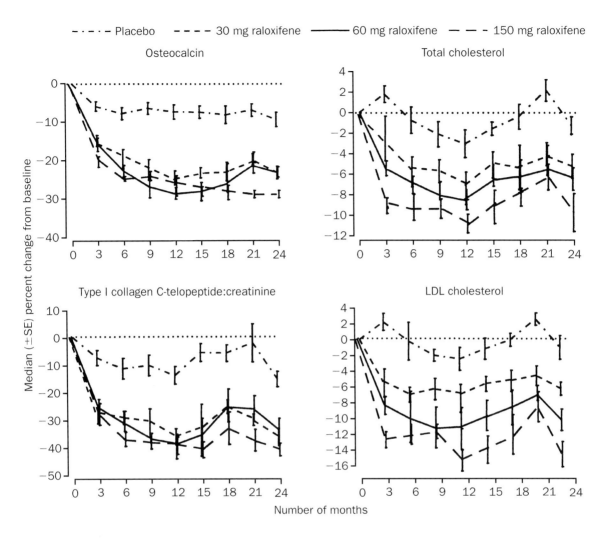

Figure 8.5 Effects of raloxifene or placebo in early postmenopausal women. Median percentage change in biochemical markers of bone turnover and serum cholesterol concentrations. Reprinted by permission of the publisher from Delmas PD, Bjarnason NH, Mitlak BH et al. (1997). Effects of raloxifene on bone mineral density, serum cholesterol concentrations, and uterine endometrium in postmenopausal women. *New Engl J Med 337*: 1641–1647. Copyright 1997 Massachusetts Medical Society. All rights reserved.

terol, and lipoprotein a, and increases HDL_2-cholesterol, but to a lesser extent than HRT (Figure 8.5).[61,64] Further clinical trials are, however, necessary to determine whether these favourable biochemical effects are associated with protection against CVD. Because of the anti-oestrogenic effect, raloxifene is expected to be associated with an increased incidence of hot flushes; but in doses of 60–120 mg/day it does not seem substantially to increase the frequency of such menopausal symptoms.[61,64] Furthermore, since hot flushes tend to decrease with time, this does not seem to result in discontinuation from raloxifene treatment.[61,64]

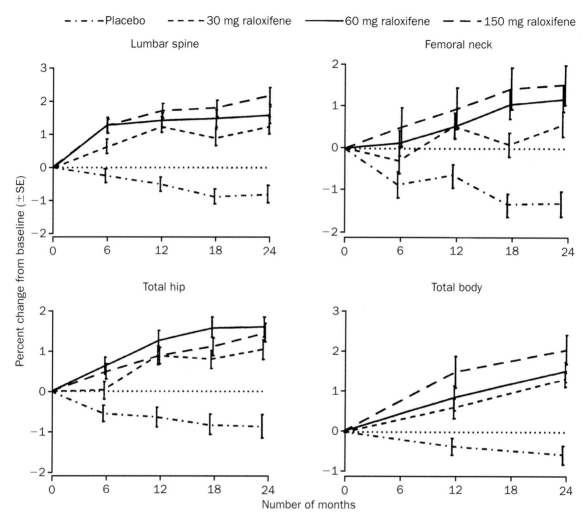

Figure 8.6 Percentage change in bone mineral density in early postmenopausal women treated with raloxifene or placebo. Reprinted by permission of the publisher from Delmas PD, Bjarnason NH, Mitlak BH et al. (1997). Effects of raloxifene on bone mineral density, serum cholesterol concentrations, and uterine endometrium in post menopausal women. *New Engl J Med 337*: 1641–1647. Copyright 1997 Massachusetts Medical Society. All rights reserved.

CALCIUM

The effect of calcium is modest in the years immediately following the menopause, when the decrease in endogenous oestrogen is driving bone loss. Although insufficient to prevent bone loss when administered alone, calcium may, however, add an effect to HRT. Thus, some studies have shown that the addition of calcium allows a dose reduction in HRT in recently postmenopausal women.[19] In contrast, other longitudinal studies have failed to reveal any additional effect on bone mass of a daily calcium supplement of up to 2000 mg.[66] Present evidence therefore indicates that calcium has a limited impact on early postmenopausal bone loss.

BISPHOSPHONATES

In women with contraindications or reservations about the use of HRT, the bisphosphonates provide an alternative option for the prevention of postmenopausal osteoporosis. Bisphosphonates inhibit bone resorption at the level of the osteoclast, and have an exclusive action on bone.[67] Treatment with a cyclical regimen of 400 mg daily of oral etidronate for 2 weeks followed by 11 weeks of calcium (500 mg/day) prevented bone loss at the spine, hip, and total body in postmenopausal women with normal bone mass,[68,69] with a safety profile comparable to that of placebo. There is also substantial evidence that daily treatment with oral alendronate prevents postmenopausal bone loss in women with normal bone mass. In two large randomized trials ($n = 2056$) treatment with oral alendronate 5 mg/day increased BMD at the spine, hip, and total body by 1–4%, and attenuated bone loss at the forearm by 2%,[70,71] again with a safety profile comparable to placebo. The effect on BMD was most pronounced within 1–2 years of the start of treatment, thereafter remaining stable. Alendronate 5 mg/day thus stabilizes rather than increases bone mass; but this is the optimal therapeutic approach in recently postmenopausal women with normal bone mass. In the placebo group, which only received 500 mg/day calcium, BMD decreased significantly in all skeletal regions and incidentally confirmed that calcium is without a clinically relevant effect in recently postmenopausal women.

MONITORING OF TREATMENT

Bone densitometry

Few women fail to respond in terms of prevention of bone loss during treatment with ade-

quate doses of HRT.[30] A rigorously cost-effective response to this might be to omit monitoring altogether. It is, however, generally accepted that an objective measure of the effect of treatment is likely to increase compliance. For treatment modalities other than HRT, the evidence of efficacy is either still uncertain or less consistent, and monitoring is therefore mandatory.

Bone densitometry constitutes the most widely accepted method of monitoring, and, while BMD can be measured at any skeletal site, the more pronounced response of trabecular bone makes the spine a common choice. Detection of a treatment response is thus easier at this skeletal sites, although the precision error of the BMD measurement is also usually greater, being in the region of 1–3%, which is of about the same magnitude as the expected annual treatment effect. This means that measurements should be delayed for about 2 years in order to detect a significant and clinically meaningful treatment effect on BMD.

Biochemical markers

Treatment in an individual patient can be monitored with both biochemical markers of bone formation (serum osteocalcin or alkaline phosphatase) and bone resorption (urine or serum degradation products of type I collagen). The biochemical markers show a pronounced response 3–6 weeks after the start of treatment. Recent studies have shown a close association between the increase in bone mass over the long term (2 years) and the decrease in biochemical markers measured after 3 months of treatment.[66,72] The potential advantage is therefore that a significant and clinically relevant response to treatment can be detected much earlier than is possible with bone densitometry. The day-to-day variability in the biochemical markers with regard to monitoring is less of an issue in the case of sensitive biochemical markers and effective treatments where there will be a clear response. A strategy could therefore be developed that would restrict monitoring by bone densitometry to women without a significant depression of biochemical markers 2–3 months after the start of treatment. Suggested cut-points indicating the need for bone densitometry are a decrease of less than about 40% in the newer biochemical markers of bone resorption (urine C- and N-telopeptides of type I collagen) and a decrease of less than about 20% in the markers of bone formation (serum osteocalcin).

If there is lack of response to treatment and the treatment is taken consistently as recommended, then measurement of serum oestradiol could be used to verify normal absorption and metabolism of HRT. There is then the remaining choice of adding calcium to the treatment[19] and/or of increasing the dose of HRT. In cases where there is no response to the biochemical markers or BMD, then compliance is more likely to be the problem than a true non-response to treatment.

REFERENCES

1. Melton LJ III, Chrichilles EA, Cooper C et al. (1992). How many women have osteoporosis? *J Bone Miner Res 7*: 1005–1010.
2. Consensus Development Statement (1997). Who are candidates for prevention and treatment for osteoporosis? *Osteoporosis Int 7*: 1–6.
3. Ross PD, Davis JW, Epstein RS, Wasnich RD (1991). Pre-existing fractures and bone mass predict vertebral fracture incidence in women. *Ann Intern Med 114*: 919–923.
4. Slemenda CW, Hui SL, Longcope C et al. (1990). Predictors of bone mass in perimenopausal women: a prospective study of clinical data using photon absorptiometry. *Ann Intern Med 112*: 96–101.
5. Ross PD, Davis JW, Vogel JM, Wasnich RD (1990). A critical review of bone mass and risk of fractures in osteoporosis. *Calcif Tissue Int 46*: 149–161.
6. Melton LJ III, Atkinson EJ, O'Fallon WM et al. (1993). Long-term fracture prediction by bone mineral assessed at different skeletal sites. *J Bone Miner Res*: 1227–1233.
7. Cummings SR, Black DM, Nevitt MC et al. (1993). The Study of Osteoporotic Fractures Research Group: bone density at various sites for prediction of hip fractures. *Lancet 341*: 72–75.
8. Riis BJ, Hansen MA, Jensen AM et al. (1996). Low bone mass and fast rate of bone loss at menopause: equal risk factors for future fracture: a 15-year follow-up study. *Bone 19*: 9–12.
9. Hansen MA, Overgaard K, Riis BJ, Christiansen C (1991). Role of peak bone mass and bone loss in postmenopausal osteoporosis: 12 year study. *BMJ 303*: 961–964.
10. Garnero P, Hausher E, Chapey MC et al. (1996). Markers of bone resorption predict hip fracture in elderly women: the EPIDOS prospective study. *J Bone Miner Res 11*: 1531–1538.
11. Melton LJ 3rd, Khosla Atkinson EJ et al. (1977). Relationship of bone turnover to bone density and fractures. *J Bone Miner Res 12*: 1083–1091.
12. Mack TM, Pike MC, Henderson BE et al. (1976). Estrogens and endometrial cancer in a retirement community. *New Engl J Med 294*: 1262–1267.
13. Voight LF, Weiss NS, Chu J et al. (1991). Progestogen supplementation of exogenous estrogens and the risk of endometrial cancer. *Lancet 338*: 274–277.
14. Christiansen C, Riis B (1990). Five years with continuous-combined oestrogen–progestogen treatment. Effects on calcium metabolism, lipoproteins, and bleeding pattern. *Br J Obstet Gynecol 97*: 1087–1091.
15. Ettinger B, Selby J, Citron JT et al. (1994). Cyclic hormone replacement therapy using quarterly progestin. *Obstet Gynecol 83*: 693–700.
16. Speroff L, Rowan J, Symons J et al. (1996). The comparative effect on bone density, endometrium, and lipids of continuous hormones as replacement therapy (CHART study): a randomized controlled trial. *JAMA 276*: 1397–1403.
17. Christensen MS, Hagen C, Christiansen C, Transbøl I (1982). Dose-response evaluation of cyclic estrogen/gestagen in postmenopausal women. Placebo-controlled trial of its gynecologic and metabolic actions. *Am J Obstet Gynecol 144*: 873–879.
18. Lindsay R, Hart CM, Clark DM (1983). The minimum effective dose of estrogen for prevention of postmenopausal bone loss. *Obstet Gynecol 63*: 759–763.
19. Ettinger B, Genant HK, Steiger P, Madvig P (1992). Low-dosage micronized 17β-estradiol prevents bone loss in postmenopausal women. *Am J Obstet Gynecol 166*: 479–488.
20. Genant HK, Lucas J, Weiss S et al. (1997). Low-dose esterified estrogen therapy: effects on bone,

plasma estradiol concentrations, endometrium, and lipid levels. *Arch Intern Med 157*: 2606–2615.

21. Reginster JY, Sarlet N, Deroisy R et al. (1992). Minimal levels of serum estradiol prevent postmenopausal bone loss. *Calcif Tissue Int 51*: 340–343.

22. Riis BJ, Thomsen K, Strøm V, Christiansen C (1987). The effect of percutaneous estradiol and natural progesterone on postmenopausal bone loss. *Am J Obstet Gynecol 156*: 61–65.

23. Lufkin EG, Wahner HW, O'Fallon WM et al. (1992). Treatment of postmenopausal osteoporosis with transdermal estrogen. *Ann Intern Med 117*: 1–9.

24. Stevenson JC, Cust MP, Gangear KF et al. (1990). Effects of transdermal versus oral hormone replacement therapy on bone density in spine and proximal femur in postmenopausal women. *Lancet 335*: 265–269.

25. Hirvonen E, Lamberg-Allardt C, Lankinen KS et al. (1997). Transdermal oestradiol gel in the treatment of the climacterium: a comparison with oral therapy. *Br J Obstet Gynecol 104*(suppl 16): 19–25.

26. Christiansen C, Rødbro P, Tjellesen L (1984). Serum alkaline phosphatase during hormone treatment in early postmenopausal women. *Acta Med Scand 216*: 11–17.

27. Prestwood KM, Pilbeam CC, Burleson JA et al. (1994). The short-term effects of conjugated estrogen on bone turnover in older women. *J Clin Endocrinol Metab 79*: 366–371.

28. Abdallah HI, Hart DM, Lindsay R, Leggate I, Hooke A (1985). Prevention of bone mineral loss in postmenopausal women by norethisterone. *Obstet Gynecol 66*: 789–792.

29. Christiansen C, Nilas L, Riis BJ et al. (1985). Uncoupling of bone formation and resorption by combined oestrogen and progestogen therapy in postmenopausal osteoporosis. *Lancet ii*: 800–801.

30. The writing group for the PEPI trial (1996). Effects of hormone therapy on bone mineral density: results from the postmenopausal estrogen/progestin interventions (PEPI) trial. *JAMA 276*: 1389–1396.

31. Lindsay R, Hart DM, Aitken JM et al. (1976). Prevention of postmenopausal osteoporosis by oestrogen. *Lancet i*: 1038–1041.

32. Christiansen C, Christensen MS, Transbøl I (1981). Bone mass in postmenopausal women after withdrawal of estrogen/gestagen replacement therapy. *Lancet i*: 459–461.

33. Munk-Jensen N, Pors Nielsen S, Obel EB, Bonne Eriksen P (1988). Reversal of postmenopausal vertebral bone loss by oestrogen and progestogen: a double blind placebo controlled study. *BMJ 296*: 1150–1152.

34. Christiansen C, Riis BJ (1990). 17β-estradiol and continuous norethisterone: a unique treatment of established osteoporosis in elderly women. *J Clin Endocrinol Metab 71*: 836–841.

35. Weiss NS, Ure CL, Ballard JH et al. (1980). Decreased risk of fractures of the hip and lower forearm with postmenopausal use of estrogen. *New Engl J Med 303*: 1195–1198.

36. Cauley JA, Seeley DG, Ensrud K et al. (1995). Estrogen replacement therapy and fractures in older women. *Ann Intern Med 122*: 9–16.

37. Lindsay R, Hart DM, Forrest C, Baird C (1980). Prevention of spinal osteoporosis in oophorectomised women. *Lancet ii*: 1151–1154.

38. Michaëlsson K, Baron JA, Farahmand BY et al. (1998). Hormone replacement therapy and the risk of hip fracture: population based case-control study. *BMJ 316*: 1858–1863.

39. Grodstein F, Stampfer MJ, Colditz GA et al. (1997). Postmenopausal hormone therapy and mortality. *New Engl J Med 336*: 1769–1775.

40. Bush TL, Barrett-Connor E, Cowan LD (1987). Cardiovascular mortality and noncontraceptive use of estrogen in women. Results from the lipid research clinics program follow-up study. *Circulation 75*: 1102–1109.

41. Hirvonen E, Malkanen M, Manninen V (1981). Effect of different progestogens on lipoproteins during postmenopausal replacement therapy. *New Engl J Med 304*: 560–563.

42. Jensen J, Christiansen C (1987). Dose–response effects on serum lipids and lipoproteins following combined oestrogen therapy in postmenopausal women. *Maturitas 9*: 259–266.

43. The writing group for the PEPI trial (1995). Effects of estrogen or estrogen/progestin regimens on heart disease risk factors in postmenopausal women. The postmenopausal estrogen/progestin interventions (PEPI) trial. *JAMA 273*: 199–208.

44. Stampfer MJ, Colditz GA, Willett WC et al. (1991). Postmenopausal estrogen therapy and cardiovascular disease. Ten-year follow-up from the nurses' health study. *New Engl J Med 325*: 756–762.

45. Hulley S, Grady D, Bush T et al. (1998). Randomized trial of estrogen plus progestin for secondary prevention of coronary heart disease in postmenopausal women. Heart and estrogen/progestin replacement study (HERS) research group. *JAMA 280*: 605–613.

46. Adams MR, Register TC, Golden DL et al. (1997). Medroxyprogesterone acetate antagonizes inhibitory effects of conjugated equine estrogens on coronary artery atherosclerosis. *Am Heart Assoc 17*: 217–221.

47. Falkeborn M, Persson I, Terent A et al. (1993). Hormone replacement therapy and the risk of stroke. *Arch Int Med 153*: 1201–1209.

48. Pedersen AT, Lidegaard Ø, Kreiner S, Ottesen B (1997). Hormone replacement therapy and risk of non-fatal stroke. *Lancet 350*: 1277–1283.

49. Tan MX, Jacobs D, Stern Y et al. (1996). Effect of oestrogen during menopause on risk and age at onset of Alzheimer's disease. *Lancet 348*: 429–432.

50. Colditz GA, Hankinson SE, Hunter DJ et al. (1995). The use of estrogens and progestins and the risk of breast cancer in postmenopausal women. *New Engl J Med 332*: 1589–1593.

51. Collaborative Group on Hormonal Factors in Breast Cancer (1997). Breast cancer and hormone replacement therapy: collaborative reanalysis of data from 51 epidemiological studies of 52 705 women with breast cancer and 108 411 women without breast cancer. *Lancet 350*: 1047–1059.

52. Toniolo PG, Levitz M, Zeleniuch-Jacquotte A et al. (1995). A prospective study of endogenous estrogens and breast cancer in postmenopausal women. *J Natl Cancer Inst 87*: 190–197.

53. Daly E, Vessey MP, Hawkins MM, Carson JL, Marsh S (1996). Risk of venous thrombo-embolism in users of hormone replacement therapy. *Lancet 348*: 977–980.

54. Bjarnason NH, Bjarnason K, Haarbo J et al. (1996). Tibolone: prevention of bone loss in late post-menopausal women. *J Clin Endocrinol Metab 81*: 2419–2422.

55. Lippuner K, Haenggi W, Birkhaeuser MH et al. (1997). Prevention of postmenopausal bone loss using tibolone or conventional peroral or trans-dermal hormone replacement therapy with 17β-estradiol and dydrogesterone. *J Bone Miner Res 12*: 806–812.

56. Bjarnason NH, Bjarnason K, Haarbo J et al. (1997). Tibolone: influence on markers of cardiovascular disease. *J Clin Endocrinol Metab 6*: 1752–1756.

57. Kasugai Y, Ikegami A, Matsuo K et al. (1998). Effects of tibolone (Org OD-14) treatment for 3 months on ovariectomy-induced osteopenia in 8-month-old rats on a low-calcium diet: preventive testing for 3 months. *Bone 22*: 119–124.

58. Love RR, Wiebe DA, Newcomb PA et al. (1991). Effects of tamoxifen on cardiovascular risk factors in postmenopausal women. *Ann Int Med 115*: 860–864.

59. Love RR, Mazess RB, Barden HS et al. (1992). Effects of tamoxifen on bone mineral density in postmenopausal women with breast cancer. *New Engl J Med 326*: 852–856.

60. van Leeuwen FE, Benraadt J, Coebergh JWW et al. (1994). Risk of endometrial cancer after tamoxifen treatment of breast cancer. *Lancet 343*: 448–452.

61. Delmas PD, Bjarnason NH, Mitlak BH et al. (1997). The effects of raloxifene on bone mineral density, serum cholesterol, and uterine endometrium in postmenopausal women. *New Engl J Med 337*: 1641–1647.

62. Ettinger B, Black DM, Mitlak BH, et al. (1999). Reduction of vertebral fracture risk in post-menopausal women with osteoporosis treated with raloxifene. Results from a 3-year random-ized clinical trial. *JAMA 282*: 637–645.

63. Bjarnason NH, Haarbo J, Byrjalsen I et al. (1997). Raloxifene inhibits aortic accumulation of choles-terol in ovariectomized, cholesterol-fed rabbits. *Circulation 96*: 1964–1969.

64. Walsh BW, Kuller LH, Wild RA et al. (1998). Effects of raloxifene on serum lipids and coagula-tion factors in healthy postmenopausal women. *JAMA 279*: 1445–1451.

65. Riis BJ, Thomsen K, Christiansen C (1987). Does calcium supplementation prevent post-menopausal bone loss; a double-blind controlled clinical study. *New Engl J Med 316*: 173–177.

66. Riis BJ, Overgaard K, Christiansen C (1995). Biochemical markers of bone turnover to monitor the response to postmenopausal hormone replacement therapy. *Osteoporosis Int 5*: 276–280.

67. Fleisch H (1998). Bisphosphonates: mechanism of action. *Endocr Rev 19*: 80–100.

68. Herd RJ, Balena R, Blake GM, Ryan PJ, Fogelman I (1997). The prevention of early postmenopausal bone loss by cyclical etidronate therapy: a 2-year, double-blind, placebo-controlled study. *Am J Med 103*: 92–99.

69. Meunier PJ, Confavreux E, Tupinon I et al. (1997). Prevention of early postmenopausal bone loss with cyclical etidronate therapy (a double-blind, placebo controlled study and 1-year folow-up. *J Clin Endocrinol Metab 82(9)*: 2784–2791.

70. McClung M, Clemmesen B, Daifotis A et al. for the Alendronate Osteoporosis Prevention Study Group (1998). Alendronate prevents post-menopausal bone loss in women without osteo-porosis. A double-blind randomized, controlled trial. *Ann Intern Med 128*: 253–261.

71. Hosking D, Chilvers CED, Christiansen et al. (1998). Prevention of bone loss with alendronate in postmenopausal women under 60 years of age. *New Engl J Med 338*: 485–492.

72. Bjarnason NH, Bjarnason K, Hassager C, Christiansen C (1997). The response in spinal bone mass to tibolone treatment is related to bone turnover in elderly women. *Bone 2*: 151–155.

9

Management of Established Osteoporosis

Roger Francis

Introduction • Bone density and fracture risk • Other risk factors for fractures • Diagnosis of osteoporosis • Investigation of osteoporosis • Management of osteoporosis

INTRODUCTION

Osteoporosis is characterized by a reduction in the amount of bone in the skeleton, associated with skeletal fragility and an increased risk of fracture after minimal trauma. The incidence of fractures of the hip, forearm, vertebra, humerus, pelvis and ankle increases with advancing age,[1] but rises particularly rapidly after the age of 75 years (Figure 9.1). The lifetime risk of symptomatic fracture for a 50-year-old white woman in the UK has been estimated to be 13% for the forearm, 11% for the vertebra, and 14% for the hip, whereas the corresponding figures for a 50-year-old man are 2%, 2%, and 3% respectively.[2] These fractures are a major cause of mortality, morbidity and health/social service expenditure in elderly people but this is particularly the case with hip fractures. The excess mortality after hip fracture is 10–20%,[2] but is generally higher in men than women. Up to 50% of patients become more dependent after hip fracture, many requiring placement in a residential or nursing home.[3] The annual cost of osteoporotic fractures in the UK has been estimated at £942 million, of which 87% is attributable to hip fractures.[4]

BONE DENSITY AND FRACTURE RISK

There is a strong inverse relationship between bone mineral density (BMD) and fracture risk, with a 2–3 fold increase in fracture incidence for each standard deviation reduction in BMD. Bone density and therefore the risk of fracture at any age is determined by peak bone mass, the age at which bone loss begins, and the rate at which it progresses. Genetic factors account for as much as 80% of the variance in peak bone mass, whilst other potential determinants of bone mass at maturity include exercise, dietary calcium intake, smoking, alcohol consumption and age at puberty.[5,6] Involutional bone loss starts between the ages of 35 and 40 in both sexes, but there is an acceleration of bone loss in the decade after the menopause in women. Overall, women lose 35–50% of trabecular and 25–30% of cortical bone mass with advancing age, whereas men lose 15–45% and 5–15% respectively. Bone loss continues into the ninth decade of life in both sexes,[7] offering the prospect of decreasing fracture risk by using treatment to prevent bone loss (Figure 9.2).

Bone loss may be influenced by genetic

(a)

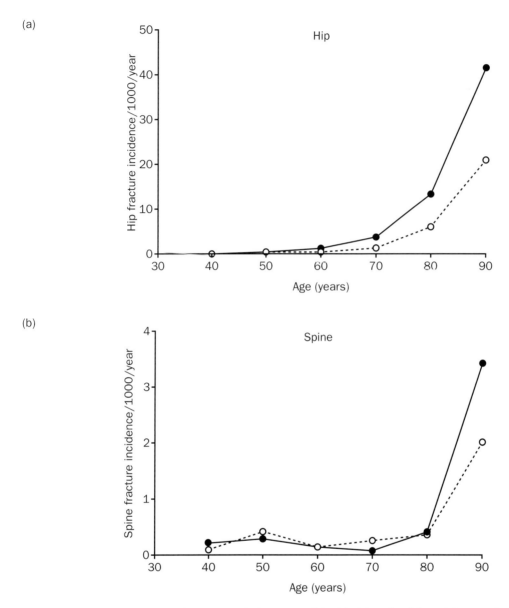

(b)

Figure 9.1 Annual incidence of symptomatic fractures of the hip (a), spine (b), and forearm/wrist (c) and upper-arm fractures (d) in women (solid circles and continuous line) and men (open circles and broken line) in the UK. Figure redrawn from *Injury* 1997; Vol. **28**: 655–660, Johansen A, Evans RJ, Stone MD, Richmond PW, Lo SV, Woodhouse KW, Fracture incidence in England and Wales: a study based on the population of Cardiff, © 1997, with permission from Elsevier Science.

factors, low body weight, smoking, excess alcohol consumption, physical inactivity, poor dietary calcium intake, reduced production and impaired metabolism of vitamin D, and declining calcium absorption.[5,6] There are also a number of secondary causes of osteoporosis, which are present in up to 30% of women and 55% of men with symptomatic vertebral crush fractures (Figure 9.3). The prevalence of secondary osteoporosis is similar in both the young and

(c)

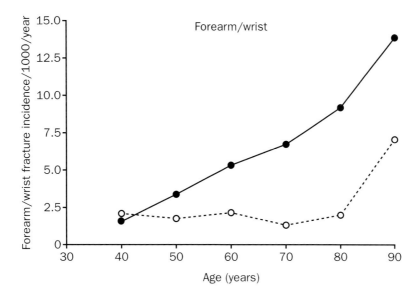

(d)

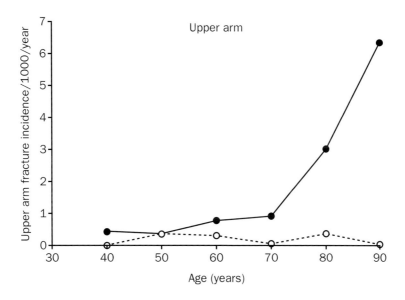

OTHER RISK FACTORS FOR FRACTURES

the old patients with vertebral fractures seen at the Bone Clinic in Newcastle. Secondary causes of osteoporosis, such as oral corticosteroid therapy, anticonvulsant treatment, thyroid disease and hypogonadism, have also been identified as risk factors for hip fractures.

Other factors affect fracture risk independently of BMD, including trabecular architecture, skeletal geometry, bone turnover, postural instability and propensity to fall. Studies from Europe, the US and Australia show that the risk of fracture is determined not only by BMD, but also by factors associated with physical frailty and an increased risk of falls.[8-10]

(a)

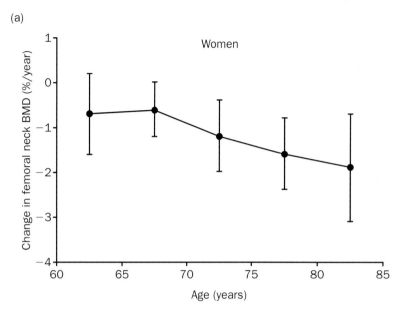

(b)

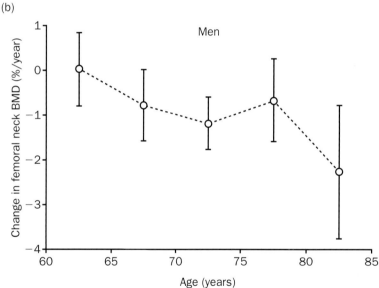

Figure 9.2 Annual change in femoral neck BMD in women (a) and men (b). Figure redrawn from the data of Jones et al.[7] This figure was first published in the *BMJ* [Jones G, Nguyen T, Sambrook P, Kelly PJ, Eisman JA. Progressive loss of bone from the femoral neck in elderly people: longitudinal findings from the Dubbo osteoporosis epidemiological study. *BMJ* 1994; **309:** 691–695] and is reproduced by permission of the *BMJ*.

A prospective study from Australia showed that BMD and body sway both predicted the risk of osteoporotic fractures (Figure 9.4), but the combination of low BMD and high body sway conferred a greater risk of fracture than either alone.[10] The Study of Osteoporotic Fractures in the US confirmed that bone density predicted the future risk of hip fracture, but identified a number of other important risk factors[9] (Table 9.1). Although women with low calcaneal BMD had a 2–3 fold higher incidence of fractures than those with high BMD, the presence of other risk factors had a major effect on the incidence of fractures. Women with five or more of these risk factors had at least a ninefold higher risk of fracture than those with 0–2 risk factors.[9]

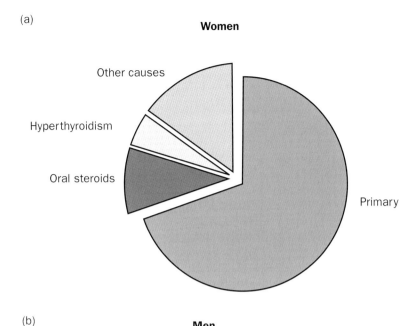

(a)

Women

Other causes

Hyperthyroidism

Oral steroids

Primary

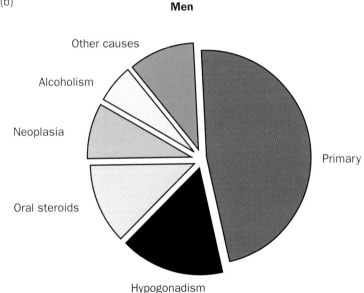

(b)

Men

Other causes

Alcoholism

Neoplasia

Oral steroids

Primary

Hypogonadism

Figure 9.3 Prevalence of secondary causes of osteoporosis in women (a) and men (b) with symptomatic vertebral fractures attending the Bone Clinic in Newcastle upon Tyne. Figure reproduced from Francis RM. Metabolic bone disease. In: Tallis RC, Fillit HM, Brocklehurst JC. (eds.), *Brocklehurst's textbook of geriatric medicine and gerontology*, 5th edn, pp. 1137–1154. Edinburgh, Churchill Livingstone, 1998, with permission of the publishers.

DIAGNOSIS OF OSTEOPOROSIS

Prior to the development of techniques that acurately measure bone density, osteoporosis was usually only diagnosed after a fracture had occurred. The term 'osteoporosis' was therefore reserved for the fracture syndrome resulting from reduced bone density. With the advent of dual energy X-ray absorptiometry (DXA), the term 'osteoporosis' is now increasingly used to describe reduced bone mineral density (BMD) before fractures have occurred. BMD measurements may be expressed as standard deviation units above or below the mean value for normal young adults (T score) or relative to the mean value for control subjects of the same age

(a)

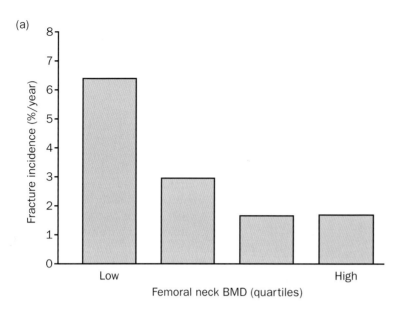

(b)

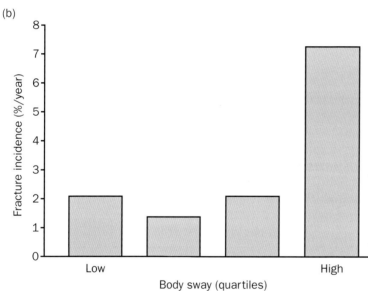

Figure 9.4 The relationship between fracture incidence and quartiles of femoral neck BMD (a) and fracture incidence and quartiles of body sway (b). Figure drawn from the data of Nguyen et al.,[10] which were first published in the *BMJ* [Nguyen T, Sambrook P, Kelly P, Jones G, Lord S, Freund J, Eisman J. Prediction of osteoporotic fractures by postural instability and bone density. *BMJ* 1993; **307:** 1111–1115]. The figure is reproduced by permission of the *BMJ*.

(Z score).[11,12] The T score reflects current fracture risk, whereas the Z score predicts lifetime fracture risk, although the relative merits of T and Z scores in clinical practice remain controversial.[12] Nevertheless, a low Z score (< -2.0) indicates that there is an underlying cause of osteoporosis other than age-related bone loss, which should be identified and modified where possible.

The World Health Organization (WHO) has defined osteoporosis as a BMD 2.5 standard deviations or more below the mean value for young adults (T score < -2.5), whereas the term severe or established osteoporosis indicates that there has also been at least one fragility fracture.[11] Although the WHO definition is useful for the diagnosis of osteoporosis, it does not necessarily represent a threshold for

---

Table 9.1 Non-BMD-related risk factors for hip fracture identified by the Study of Osteoporotic Fractures.[9]

Age above 80 years

Maternal history of hip fracture

Personal history of fracture after the age of 50 years

Fair, poor or very poor health

Previous hyperthyroidism

Anticonvulsant therapy

Current long-acting benzodiazepine therapy

Current weight less than at the age of 25 years

Height at the age of 25 > 168 cm

Caffeine intake > equivalent of two cups of coffee/day

On feet < four hours/day

No walking for exercise

Inability to rise from chair without using arms

Poor visual perception of depth

Poor visual contrast sensitivity

Resting pulse rate above 80/minute

Although precise and accurate measurements of lumbar spine and femoral neck BMD can be made using DXA, population-based bone density screening is not justified at present. A number of indications for bone density measurements have been advocated, including a past history of early menopause, oral steroid therapy, peripheral fractures after minimal trauma and apparent osteopenia on radiography,[13] but the relevance of these indications in elderly people remains uncertain. It is also important to appreciate that spine bone density measurements may be spuriously elevated in older people, because of degenerative changes and aortic calcification. Serial measurements at the lumbar spine may still be useful to assess the efficacy of treatment, as changes in bone density at this site occur more rapidly than at the hip.

Pragmatic suggestions on the indications for bone density measurements are provided in Table 9.2. The most important reason is a fracture after minimal trauma in a previously fit individual, to confirm the diagnosis of osteoporosis, assess the risk of future fractures and allow the most appropriate use of expensive treatment. This is important, as 70% of women above the age of 80 years have a T score of less than -2.5, but only a proportion of these will sustain an osteoporotic fracture.[11] For these reasons it may be more appropriate to use Z scores in interpreting BMD measurements in older people,[12] to identify individuals whose bone density is lower than expected for their age and who are at greater risk of osteoporotic fractures. A pragmatic approach in this age group might be:

1. In patients with a past history of fracture, specific treatment for osteoporosis may be unnecessary if BMD Z score > 0.
2. In patients with a past history of fracture, consider treatment for osteoporosis if BMD Z score < 0.
3. In patients with no previous fractures, consider treatment for osteoporosis if BMD Z score < -1.0, or < 0 if other risk factors are present.

Table 9.2 The use of bone density measurement.

Indications for BMD measurement:

Fractures after minimal trauma in previously fit individuals

Past history of early menopause (< 45 years) in women up to the age of 70 years

Underlying secondary causes of osteoporosis

Apparent osteopenia on radiography

To monitor response to treatment

Treatment for osteoporosis justified without BMD measurement:

Fractures after minimal trauma in frail individuals

Prolonged oral steroid therapy (>7.5 mg prednisolone/day)

treatments such as alendronate (see later). Other indications for bone density measurements in older people are a past history of an early menopause in women (up to the age of 70 years), underlying secondary causes of osteoporosis, such as hyperthyroidism, hyperparathyroidism and male hypogonadism (particularly if the results are likely to alter management) and apparent osteopenia on radiography (Table 9.2). Early menopause has not been included as an indication for measurement in women over the age of 70 years, as the impact of this risk factor appears to diminish with advancing age. Serial BMD measurements may be used to assess the efficiency of treatment for osteoporosis. We usually perform these after one, three and five years' treatment, and consider alternative therapy if significant bone loss occurs.

Bone density measurements are of limited value in the assessment of frail elderly patients with hip and other fractures, as the vast majority will have reduced bone density and the results are unlikely to influence management. Prolonged oral steroid therapy has also been excluded from the list of indications for bone density measurement, as a Consensus Group from the UK has recently recommended that all people over the

age of 65 years on 7.5 mg prednisolone daily should be offered treatment for osteoporosis.[14]

Although bone ultrasound attenuation (BUA) measurements predict the risk of hip fractures in elderly people as well as DXA measurement at the femoral neck,[15,16] there are no criteria for the diagnosis of osteoporosis using bone ultrasound measurements. Furthermore, the precision of ultrasound measurements is inferior to BMD measurements obtained using DXA, which may limit the value of ultrasound measurements in monitoring the response to treatment. Nevertheless, because of low cost and portability, ultrasound measurements may ultimately prove to be a cost-effective method of targeting specific osteoporosis treatment to those elderly people at highest risk of fractures. At present the use of ultrasound measurements for this purpose cannot be recommended.

INVESTIGATION OF OSTEOPOROSIS

In patients with symptomatic vertebral fractures, secondary causes of osteoporosis should be identified by careful history, physical examination and appropriate investigation (Table 9.3), as treatment

Table 9.3 Suggested investigations for secondary osteoporosis in people with fractures after minimal trauma or low BMD (Z score < −2.0).

Vertebral fractures	Hip and other fractures	Low BMD
Full blood count	Full blood count	Full blood count
ESR	ESR	ESR
Biochemical profile	Biochemical profile	Biochemical profile
Thyroid function tests	Thyroid function tests	Thyroid function tests
Serum testosterone (men)	Serum testosterone (men)	Serum testosterone (men)
SHBG (men)	SHBG (men)	SHBG (men)
Gonadotrophins (men)	Gonadotrophins (men)	Gonadotrophins (men)
Serum electrophoresis	? 25OHD	
Urine electrophoresis	? PTH	

ESR = Erythrocyte Sedimentation Rate.

of underlying conditions such as hyperthyroidism, hypogonadism and hyperparathyroidism decreases the rate of bone loss and may at least in part reverse the osteoporotic process.

Underlying secondary causes of osteoporosis should also be sought in men and women presenting with low-trauma hip and other non-vertebral fractures (Table 9.3). Routine biochemical profile is probably worth while, as hypocalcaemia and hypophosphataemia may indicate possible osteomalacia, although these measurements lack diagnostic specificity or sensitivity. Serum 25 hydroxyvitamin D (25OHD) and intact parathyroid hormone (PTH) measurements may be useful in the diagnosis of vitamin D deficiency in patients with limited sunlight exposure, previous gastric resection, malabsorption or anticonvulsant treatment. Serum 25OHD and PTH measurements are probably unnecessary if calcium and vitamin D supplementation is planned.

Up to 20% of elderly men with symptomatic vertebral fractures and 50% of those with hip fractures have biochemical evidence of hypogonadism. Measurement of serum testosterone should therefore be performed in men with these fractures, together with sex hormone-binding globulin (SHBG) and gonadotrophins. Our current practice is to consider testosterone replacement where there is a reduction in serum testosterone (< 10 nmol/l) or free testosterone index (testosterone/SHBG < 0.30), with abnormal gonadotrophin.

Investigations for secondary osteoporosis should also be performed in patients found to have a bone density below the normal range for their age (Z score < -2.0) so as to identify underlying causes of bone loss that may be capable of being modified (Table 9.3).

MANAGEMENT OF OSTEOPOROSIS

All patients with osteoporotic fractures should be given general advice on lifestyle measures to decrease further bone loss, including eating a balanced diet rich in calcium, moderating tobacco and alcohol consumption and, if possible, maintaining regular physical activity and exposure to sunlight. As bone loss continues into old age in both men and women, specific treatment for osteoporosis should be considered in all patients with osteoporotic fractures. Unfortunately, most studies of the treatment of established osteoporosis have only recruited women up to the age of 75 or 80 years with vertebral fractures. No secondary prevention studies of the treatment of osteoporosis in older patients with vertebral and hip fractures have yet been published, but there is no evidence of an attenuated response to treatment with advancing age. Furthermore, treatment of osteoporosis is likely to be more cost-effective in older people, because of their higher fracture rate.

Drug treatment of osteoporosis

Treatments for osteoporosis may be classified into antiresorptive agents, such as hormone relacement therapy (HRT), tibolone, selective (o)estrogen receptor modulators (SERMs), bisphosphonates, calcitonin, vitamin D and calcium supplements, and anabolic agents like anabolic steroids, sodium fluoride and PTH.[17] Although antiresorptive agents decrease bone resorption, the transient uncoupling of resorption and formation leads to a modest increase in bone density of 5–10%, predominantly in the first year of treatment. In contrast, anabolic agents increase bone density by up to 50%, although this is not necessarily associated with a decreased risk of fractures. It is therefore important that randomized controlled trials of osteoporosis treatment should have the statistical power to detect not only increases in BMD but also a meaningful reduction in fracture incidence.

HRT
The use of HRT in normal women at the menopause prevents the rapid bone loss that occurs at this time.[18] It also decreases the risk of fractures, if given for a period of five to ten years.[19] Unfortunately, the benefit of previous long-term HRT decreases progressively once treatment is stopped, and may be lost com-

pletely by the age of 75 years.[20] An alternative approach is to use HRT in older women or those with established osteoporosis, where the reduction in fracture risk may be apparent earlier. Small studies in older women with established osteoporosis (mean age 68 and 65 years respectively) show that HRT increases spine density by 5%[21,22] and decreases the risk of further vertebral fractures by 60%.[22]

HRT is the treatment of choice in younger women with osteoporosis, as it also has a beneficial effect on climacteric and urogenital symptoms. It may also potentially decrease the risk of ischaemic heart disease, Alzheimer's disease and osteoarthritis. HRT may be given orally, transdermally using skin patches or gel, or by implantation of oestradiol pellets into the abdominal wall. It is our usual practice to start with oral treatment, using a continuous oestrogen preparation with cyclical progestogen (such as Prempak C 0.625: conjugated oestrogen 0.625 mg daily continuously and norgestrel 150 mcg g daily for 12 days each cycle) in women within a year or two of the menopause if the uterus is present.

Long-term compliance with HRT is often poor, however, because of the return of menstruation and concern about the risks of breast cancer and thromboembolic disease. The advent of continuous combined oestrogen/ progestogen preparations such as Kliofem (oestradiol 2 mg and norethisterone acetate 1 mg daily by mouth) and Premique (conjugated oestrogen 0.625 mg and medroxyprogesterone acetate 5 mg daily by mouth) may improve the situation, as they offer the benefits of HRT without the need for a regular monthly bleed, and so might be more acceptable to the older woman with osteoporosis. Furthermore, there is evidence that continuous combined oestrogen/progestogen preparations have a better effect on bone density than conventional sequential HRT, owing to the effects of the continuous progestogen treatment. Patchy vaginal bleeding may occur during the first few months of continuous combined treatment, but this is less common in older women. About 90% of women on continuous combined oestrogen/ progestogen treatment are amenorrhoeic within a year.

Breast tenderness can be a problem in older women starting HRT; but this may be avoided by using a low-dose preparation on alternate days during the first few weeks of treatment. The relationship between HRT and the development of breast cancer remains contentious, although there is evidence of a small increase in risk after ten years' use. Women on HRT should therefore be encouraged to have regular mammography as part of any national breast cancer screening campaign. In older women excluded from such screening on the basis of age (>64 years in the UK), mammography should be requested in long-term HRT users. The use of HRT is also associated with an increased risk of venous thromboembolism, but the absolute risk is still relatively low at 3/10 000 patient years.

Our own experience in the Bone Clinic in Newcastle suggests that few women over the age of 70 years are prepared to start HRT unless they have previously undergone hysterectomy, and so are able to take unopposed oestrogen treatment such as Premarin (conjugated oestrogen 0.625 mg daily by mouth). Nevertheless, all postmenopausal women with osteoporosis should be given information about the potential risks and benefits of HRT, in order to make an informed decision about treatment.

Tibolone

Tibolone (Livial: 2.5 mg daily by mouth) has weak oestrogenic, progestogenic and androgenic actions. It prevents bone loss in normal postmenopausal women and older women with osteoporosis, although there is no information on its effect on fracture incidence.[3] Tibolone is now licensed in the UK for the control of menopausal symptoms and the prevention of osteoporosis, but is also an option for the management of older women with established osteoporosis. It is generally well tolerated, but may cause vaginal bleeding at the onset of treatment.

SERMs

Tamoxifen is the prototype SERM, with oestrogen agonist and antagonist actions on different tissues. Although tamoxifen is used in the management of breast cancer because of its action as an oestrogen antagonist, it acts as a partial oestrogen agonist on the skeleton and cardiovascular system in postmenopausal women, reducing bone loss and decreasing the risk of ischaemic heart disease. Raloxifene (Evista: 60 mg daily by mouth) is the first SERM to be licensed for the prevention of osteoporosis. It has been shown to prevent bone loss from the lumbar spine and hip and to improve the lipid profile in normal women who have been postmenopausal for between two and eight years, without stimulating the endometrium.[23] Preliminary results suggest that raloxifene decreases the incidence of new vertebral fractures by 44% in older women (mean age 67 years) with osteoporosis,[24] as well as reducing the incidence of breast cancer by 53% after 2.5 years' treatment. Potential adverse effects of raloxifene include vasomotor symptoms, leg cramps and an increased risk of venous thromboembolism, comparable to that seen with HRT. There is no current evidence that raloxifene reduces the incidence of non-vertebral fractures. Raloxifene is therefore most useful in the management of older postmenopausal women at increased risk of osteoporosis and vertebral fractures.

Bisphosphonates

These are analogues of naturally occurring pyrophosphate, which, although poorly absorbed from the bowel, localize preferentially in bone, where they bind to hydroxyapatite crystals. Bisphosphonates decrease bone resorption by reducing osteoclast recruitment and function. As they persist in the skeleton for many months, their duration of action is prolonged beyond the period of administration.

Intermittent cyclical etidronate therapy (Didronel PMO: disodium etidronate 400 mg daily by mouth for two weeks, followed by 500 mg elemental calcium daily by mouth for 11 weeks) and continuous alendronate (Fosamax: 10 mg daily by mouth) both increase spine bone density in women with osteoporosis by 5–8% over two to three years and decrease the incidence of further vertebral fractures by about 60%.[25-29] Alendronate also increases

femoral neck bone density by 4.1–5.9% over three years, compared with 1.4% with cyclical etidronate.[27-29] Results from the large Fracture Intervention Trial show that alendronate treatment in women with low hip bone density and at least one vertebral fracture significantly increases bone density in the forearm, spine and femoral neck and decreases the incidence of fractures at these sites by 48%, 55% and 51% respectively.[29]

Randomized controlled trials of bisphosphonates in the management of established osteoporosis have included women up to the age of 75 years in the case of cyclical etidronate[25-27] and 80 years with alendronate,[28,29] with no apparent attenuation of effect with advancing age. The Fracture Intervention Trial shows that alendronate decreases the incidence of hip fractures in women with established osteoporosis,[29] but there are no published studies on the effect of alendronate in women over the age of 80 years or those with hip fractures. There are no interventional studies showing a reduction in hip fracture incidence with cyclical etidronate, but retrospective data from the GP Research Database show a 44% reduction in hip fractures with cyclical etidronate in women over the age of 76 years.[30] Bisphosphonates may therefore be useful in the management of older patients with hip fractures, provided they are able to follow the instructions on administration.

Bisphosphonates are generally well tolerated, but commonly cause mild gastrointestinal disturbance. More severe erosive oesophagitis has been reported with aminobisphosphonates such as alendronate, although, in the majority of cases, patients were not complying with the recommended instructions on administration or had a past history of upper gastrointestinal disease.[31] Although high-dose or continuously administered etidronate may impair bone mineralization, no clinical evidence of osteomalacia has been found with intermittent cyclical etidronate therapy.

In order to ensure optimal absorption, etidronate should be taken in the middle of a 4-hour fast, whereas alendronate should be ingested after an overnight fast, which should be continued for a further 30 min after administration. Alendronate should be taken with 250 ml water and recumbency avoided for 30 min, to decrease the risk of oesophageal reflux and irritation.

Calcitonin

Calcitonin is a potent antiresorptive agent, with a rapid but short-lived effect on osteoclast function. A dose-response study of intranasal calcitonin (100–400 IU daily) in the treatment of women (mean age 70 years) with reduced forearm bone density showed significant increases in spine bone density of 1–3% over 2 years, associated with a reduction in the number of vertebral fractures of 64–68%.[32] Another study in postmenopausal women with vertebral fractures (mean age 68 years) demonstrated that cyclical IM calcitonin (100 IU daily) and oral calcium supplements (500 mg elemental calcium daily) for 10 days every 4 weeks decreased the incidence of vertebral fractures by 60% over 2 years, compared with an increase in 35% in a group receiving calcium alone.[33] Preliminary results from the Prevent Recurrence of Osteoporotic Fractures (PROOF) study in women with established osteoporosis show only marginal benefits on bone density with calcitonin, with a reduction in new vertebral fractures with doses of 200 IU/day, but not with 100 or 400 IU/day.[34]

Calcitonin is expensive and associated with side effects such as flushing, nausea, vomiting, diarrhoea, dizziness and headache, although these side effects may be less with the intranasal route of administration. Calcitonin cannot currently be advocated for the long-term management of osteoporosis, because of its high cost, side-effect profile and doubts about efficacy. It may be useful however in the short-term treatment of acute vertebral fractures (as salmon calcitonin in a dose of 100 IU daily by IM or subcutaneous injection) because of its analgesic properties.

Calcium supplements

Although calcium supplements were previously used alone in the treatment of osteoporosis, this is probably no longer appropriate, as more effective agents are now available.

Oral calcium supplements (500–1000 mg daily) decrease bone loss, but not to the same extent as other antiresorptive agents. There is limited evidence that calcium supplements (500 mg daily) alone may decrease the risk of vertebral fractures by 55%, as shown in a study in vitamin D-replete people with a mean age of 72 years.[35]

Calcium and vitamin D

Calcium and vitamin D supplementation may be the most appropriate treatment for frail elderly patients with osteoporosis, as vitamin D deficiency and secondary hyperparathyroidism cause bone loss with advancing age. A French study in women (mean age 84 years) living in nursing homes and apartment blocks for the elderly, showed that 800 IU vitamin D_3 and 1.2 g elemental calcium daily decreased PTH, increased femoral neck BMD and reduced the risk of hip fracture by 27%.[36] A smaller American study of older men and women (mean age 70 years) living at home demonstrated that 700 IU vitamin D_3 and 500 mg elemental calcium daily had a modest beneficial effect on bone density and decreased the incidence of non-vertebral fractures by 54%.[37] It is unclear if the benefits of treatment seen in these studies were due to vitamin D, calcium or the combination of both. A Finnish study showed that an annual IM injection of 150 000–300 000 IU vitamin D decreases the risk of fractures in elderly people by 25%.[38] In contrast, a Dutch study showed a small increase in hip bone density with 400 IU vitamin D_3 daily, but no effect on the incidence of hip fractures in elderly people.[39]

The UK Medical Research Council has recently agreed to fund a multi-centre study of the secondary prevention of osteoporotic fractures in elderly people. Over 6000 men and women over the age of 70 years presenting with an osteoporotic fracture will be randomized to receive calcium, vitamin D, calcium and vitamin D, or double placebo. This study will examine the effect of treatment on the incidence of subsequent fractures, and will hopefully establish if supplementation with both calcium and vitamin D is required. Meanwhile, it may be prudent to use a combination of calcium and vitamin D in the management of frail elderly patients with osteoporosis, although there is little information on the effect on vertebral bone loss and fracture incidence. Measurement of serum 25OHD and PTH may identify individuals with vitamin D insufficiency and secondary hyperparathyroidism, who might be expected to benefit particularly from calcium and vitamin D supplementation: the cost-effectiveness of such a strategy remains unclear.

Vitamin D metabolites

There may also be a role for the vitamin D metabolites (calcitriol and alfacalcidol) in the management of osteoporosis in the elderly. Patients with vertebral fractures have lower calcium absorption than age-matched control subjects, which may be due to reduced serum $1,25(OH)_2D$ or to relative resistance to the action of vitamin D metabolites on the bowel. Malabsorption of calcium in osteoporosis does not usually respond to physiological doses of vitamin D (500–1000 IU daily), but may be corrected by low doses (0.5 mcg g daily) of the vitamin D metabolites, calcitriol and alfacalcidol.[40] Studies of the effect of treatment with vitamin D metabolites on bone loss and fractures in established osteoporosis have produced conflicting results.[40] A study comparing oral calcitriol 0.25 mcg g twice daily with calcium 1 g daily in women with vertebral fractures (mean age 64 years) showed a significantly lower incidence of new vertebral fractures with calcitriol, although this was mainly due to an increase in fracture rate with calcium rather than a reduction with calcitriol.[41] Subsequent analysis of this study suggests that the beneficial effect of calcitriol on vertebral fractures is only seen in women over the age of 65. This study also showed a significant reduction in non-vertebral fractures with calcitriol compared with calcium supplements.

Treatment with calcitriol (Rocaltrol) or alfacalcidol (One-Alpha) in doses of 0.5 mcg g daily is associated with an increased risk of hypercalcaemia. Plasma calcium and renal function should therefore be checked after one, three and six months' treatment and at six-monthly intervals thereafter. The presence of hypercalciuria will give early warning of impending hypercalcaemia, but accurate 24-hour urine collections are difficult to obtain in elderly patients. Although they are considerably more potent than vitamin D, the half life of calcitriol and alfacalcidol is much shorter, so that hypercalcaemia reverses more rapidly after intoxication than with vitamin D. The hydroxylated metabolites should be reserved as a second-line therapy for patients who have failed to respond to, or have been unable to tolerate, hormonal agents or bisphosphonates.

Anabolic steroids

Anabolic steroids such as stanozolol (Stromba: 5 mg daily by mouth) and nandrolone (Deca-Durabolin: 50 mg IM every three weeks) increase bone mass in women with established osteoporosis by 5–10%.[42,43] These increases in bone mass are modest and may be due to a decrease in bone resorption, rather than an increase in new bone formation. Anabolic steroids are associated with fluid retention and androgenic side effects such as acne, weight gain and hirsuitism. Prolonged administration may lead to abnormal liver function tests and even hepatocellular tumours. Their use in the management of osteoporosis cannot be advocated, particularly as there is no evidence of a reduction in fracture incidence.

Testosterone

Testosterone replacement in hypogonadal men with osteoporosis increases spine bone density by up to 15%, particularly if the epiphyses are still open. Treatment may also increase muscle mass and improve well-being. Osteoporotic men with evidence of hypogonadism should therefore be offered testosterone replacement therapy, after discussion of the potential risks and benefits. Side effects of testosterone treatment include increased libido, mild truncal acne, weight gain, a rise in haematocrit and azospermia in 50–70% of cases. Although it has been suggested that testosterone treatment has an adverse effect on glucose tolerance and serum lipids, the overall impact on cardiovascular risk factors is probably neutral.[44] The long-term risk of testosterone treatment in prostatic disease remains uncertain, however. In older men with hypogonadism, we usually start treatment with monthly IM injections of Sustanon 100 mg. The dose and frequency of injections are then adjusted after six months' treatment, according to patient tolerability and serum testosterone, SHBG and gonadotrophin measurements obtained 7 and 28 days after administration. We also monitor the safety of treatment by performing full blood count, biochemical profile, glucose, serum lipids and prostate-specific antigen (PSA) basally and at six-monthly intervals.

Preliminary studies suggest that testosterone supplementation (Sustanon 250 mg IM every two weeks) also increases spine bone density by 5% in eugonadal men (age range 34–73 years) with osteoporosis,[44] but there are currently no data to show if this is associated with a reduction in fracture risk. Further studies are required to evaluate the safety and efficacy of testosterone supplementation in eugonadal men.

Fluoride salts

Early studies showed that sodium fluoride (75 mg daily by mouth) increased spine bone density by up to 35% over four years in women with vertebral osteoporosis but this appeared to be at the expense of cortical bone loss.[17] There was no reduction in vertebral fracture incidence, whereas the number of non-vertebral fractures increased. These studies also showed that sodium fluoride is potentially toxic, causing nausea, vomiting, indigestion and lower-extremity bone pain.[17] A more recent study using lower-dose, slow-release sodium fluoride (25 mg twice daily by mouth) in women with vertebral osteoporosis (mean age 68 years) showed smaller increases in spine and hip bone density, without adverse effects on forearm bone mass.[45] This study also showed a significant reduction in vertebral fracture incidence, without the side-effect profile described with the higher-dose treatment. The beneficial effect of treatment on vertebral fracture incidence was less apparent in women with more severe osteoporosis,[45] suggesting that treatment may be ineffective in elderly people.

Fluoride salts are not widely available, and are only licensed in the US and some European countries. The therapeutic window for fluoride appears to be narrow, limiting its potential use in the management of elderly patients with osteoporosis. Fluoride salts may be useful as a second-line treatment in patients unresponsive to, or unable to tolerate, HRT, bisphosphonates and vitamin D metabolites.

PTH

Initial studies with PTH showed large increases in trabecular bone density, but these were accompanied by cortical bone loss. Recent work suggests that the combination of PTH with calcitonin or HRT increases spine bone density without adverse effects on cortical bone mass. A randomized controlled trial in 34 HRT treated postmenopausal women with osteoporosis (mean age 62 years) demonstrated that the addition of three years' treatment with PTH (400 IU daily by subcutaneous injection) increased BMD by 13% at the spine and 2.7% in the hip.[46] Although this study lacked the statistical power to assess accurately the effect of treatment on fracture incidence, there was a significant reduction in new vertebral deformities. Pending the results of larger studies examining the effect of PTH on fracture incidence, this treatment should be regarded as promising but experimental.

Reducing the incidence of falls

All patients with hip and other non-vertebral fractures should ideally undergo a falls assessment. Risk factors for falling are divided into intrinsic factors, including poor vision, neurological disease and medication, and extrinsic or environmental factors, such as trailing wires, loose carpets and ill-fitting footwear. Intrinsic causes should be sought by history, examination and review of medication, whereas extrinsic or environmental causes may be identified from the history and a home visit. In elderly patients with unexplained falls or syncope, tilt testing may also be useful.

A number of randomized controlled trials

have assessed the effect of modifying risk factors for falling. A standard geriatric assessment of elderly people with recurrent falls led to significantly fewer admissions to hospital, but a non-significant 9% reduction in falls.[47] An English study investigated whether health visitors could reduce the number of fractures in elderly people by giving advice on nutrition, modification of physical fitness and the modification of intrinsic and extrinsic risk factors for falling.[48] Over the four years of the study, there was no significant difference in the prevalence of fractures in the intervention group (5%) and the control group (4%).

The most important study of the prevention of falls was a randomized controlled study in over 300 elderly patients above the age of 70 years, each with an apparent risk factor for falling. The intervention group underwent geriatric assessment, with modification of risk factors for falling, whereas the control group had the usual health care and social visits. Over the 12-month follow-up period, 35% of the intervention group had falls, compared to 47% in the control group.[49] Although the difference in the two groups was statistically significant, the study was too small to detect an effect on fracture incidence. It is important that drugs that increase the risk of falls should generally be avoided in elderly people with osteoporosis.

Reducing the incidence and impact of falls

An alternative approach to fracture prevention is to decrease the impact of falls using external hip protectors, which are incorporated into specially designed underwear. A Danish study randomized elderly residents of nursing homes to receive external hip protectors or to serve as controls.[50] Over the 12-month study there was a reduction in hip fracture risk of over 50% in those using the hip protectors. In the group randomized to receive hip protectors, the only patients who fractured were not using hip protectors at the time. Although this is potentially one of the most promising interventions for the prevention of hip fractures, external hip protectors are generally bulky and uncomfortable,

and so may be unacceptable to many older people at risk of hip fracture.[51] External hip protectors (such as SafeHip in the UK, Robinsons, Chesterfield) are now available in Europe, generally costing less than £50 for a pair.

Management of the individual patient with osteoporosis

Decisions about the management of the individual patient with osteoporosis will depend on a number of factors, including chronological and biological age, fractures at presentation, physical and mental state and risk of falling. In the younger woman with osteoporosis and vertebral fractures it is important to consider drug treatments that reduce the risk of further fractures. In frail elderly patients with peripheral fractures it may be just as important to consider measures to decrease the risk and impact of falls. Furthermore, drug treatments that are effective in younger women may have less effect in older people, because of different mechanisms of bone loss. HRT and other hormonal treatments are therefore the treatment of choice in younger postmenopausal women with osteoporosis where bone loss may be due to oestrogen deficiency. However calcium and vitamin D supplementation may be more appropriate in frail elderly people who are likely to have vitamin D insufficiency and secondary hyperparathyroidism. Bisphosphonates appear to be effective in patients across a wide age range, but may be inappropriate in individuals with cognitive impairment because of difficulties in coping with the complex instructions for safe and effective administration. The use of alendronate in particular may be precluded in older patients with hiatus hernia, oesophageal disease and peptic ulcers because of concern about the risk of oesophagitis.

Although treatments for osteoporosis increase bone density and decrease the risk of fracture, neither return to normal. It is therefore our usual practice to continue treatment indefinitely, considering changes in therapy according to the clinical situation. A woman who has taken HRT for five to ten years may therefore change to a bisphosphonate, because of the increasing risk of breast cancer. Older people (> 80 years) who have taken a bisphosphonate for five years might instead start calcium and vitamin D supplementation, particularly if they have become frail or housebound.

Patients with vertebral fractures

Vertebral fractures may be associated with considerable back pain, so that adequate analgesia is necessary to limit loss of function. The use of opiates may be required when pain is severe. We tend to prescribe dihydrocodeine in the early stages, with aperients as required to prevent constipation, followed by paracetamol once symptoms abate. Non-steroidal anti-inflammatory drugs (NSAIDs) are effective in the control of bone pain, but their adverse side-effect profile in the elderly renders them unsuitable for long-term use. Short courses of NSAIDs may be of benefit, however. The use of a TENS machine also decreases back pain in about 50% of patients with symptomatic vertebral fractures.

There are a number of treatments that have been shown to decrease the incidence of vertebral fractures in patients with established osteoporosis (Table 9.4). In younger women HRT or some other hormonal agent is usually the treatment of choice, but bisphosphonates may be more appropriate in older patients or those unable or unwilling to take HRT (Figure 9.5).

Cyclical etidronate may be preferred in patients with predominantly vertebral osteoporosis, because of its lower cost, whereas alendronate is more appropriate in patients who also have low bone density at the hip. Although it is unclear whether calcium and vitamin D supplementation decreases vertebral bone loss and fracture incidence, this treatment is probably the most appropriate option in frail elderly people, who are at high risk of vitamin D deficiency and hip fractures. It is also uncertain whether calcium and vitamin D supplementation is as effective in elderly patients who are vitamin D-replete, so that hormonal preparations or bisphosphonates are usually the preferred choice.

Patients with hip fractures

The management of hip fractures has recently been reviewed by physicians interested in osteoporosis in the North-East of England.[52] They suggest that patients with hip fractures fall into two broad groups. The first comprises mainly elderly, frail patients, many of whom were immobile or housebound before fracture. The second group are generally younger, and were previously mobile and independent.

Patients in the first group have limited life expectancy, so that it is probably inappropriate to perform extensive investigations to exclude secondary causes of osteoporosis or to request bone density measurements. These patients are

---

Table 9.4   Summary of interventional studies showing a significant reduction in vertebral fracture incidence in women with osteoporosis.

Studies	Treatment	Fracture reduction (%)
Lufkin et al.[22]	HRT	60
Storm et al., Watts et al.[25,26]	Etidronate	58–53
Liberman et al., Black et al.[28,29]	Alendronate	63–47
Overgaard et al., Rico et al.[32,33]	Calcitonin	64–60
Tilyard et al.[41]	Calcitriol	69
Pak et al.[45]	Sodium fluoride	69

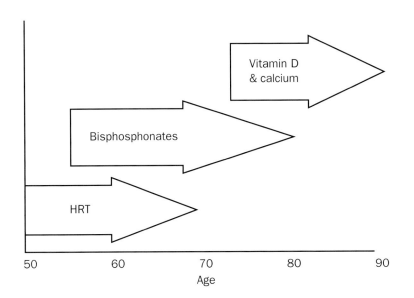

Figure 9.5 Schematic representation of the major treatment choices in patients of different ages with osteoporosis.

more likely to benefit from calcium and vitamin D supplementation than other therapeutic interventions (Figure 9.6).

Patients in the second group would benefit from more active investigation and intervention, as life expectancy and quality of life could be improved by decreasing the risk of further fractures. It is therefore recommended that investigations to exclude secondary causes of osteoporosis are performed and bone density measurements considered (Figure 9.6). Although no secondary prevention studies have been performed in patients with hip fractures, interventional studies in women with osteoporosis or institutionalized elderly women show a reduction in hip fracture incidence with alendronate and calcium and vitamin D supplementation.[29,36] However epidemiological studies suggest that HRT,[53] cyclical etidronate,[30] calcitonin[53] and calcium supplements[53] may also be

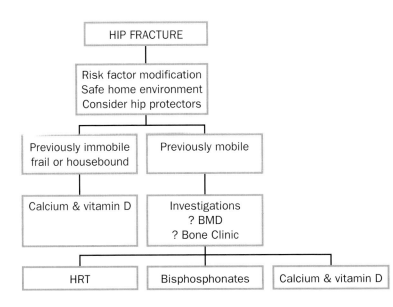

Figure 9.6 Management of patients with hip fractures. Figure redrawn from the Guidelines of the North East Osteoporosis Regional Advisory Board,[52] with permission.

Table 9.5 Summary of interventional[29,36] and epidemiological[30,53] studies showing a significant reduction in hip fracture incidence in patients receiving treatment for osteoporosis.

Studies	Treatment	Fracture reduction (%)
Kanis et al.[53]	HRT	45
van Staa et al.[30]	Etidronate	34
Black et al.[29]	Alendronate	51
Kanis et al.[53]	Calcitonin	31
Kanis et al.[53]	Calcium	25
Chapuy et al.[36]	Calcium and vitamin D	27

effective (Table 9.5). The choice of treatment depends on the individual patient, but includes HRT in younger women, bisphosphonates in older people and women unwilling or unable to tolerate HRT, and calcium and vitamin D supplementation in those with vitamin D deficiency.

REFERENCES

1. Johansen A, Evans RJ, Stone MD, Richmond PW, Lo SV, Woodhouse KW (1997). Fracture incidence in England and Wales: a study based on the population of Cardiff. *Injury 28*: 655–660.
2. Cooper C (1996). Epidemiology and definition of osteoporosis. In: *Osteoporosis, New Perspectives on Causes, Prevention and Treatment*, ed. JE Compston, pp. 1–10. Royal College of Physicians of London, London.
3. Francis RM (1998). Metabolic bone disease. In: *Brocklehurst's Textbook of Geriatric Medicine and Gerontology*, 5th edn., eds RC Tallis, HM Fillit, JC Brocklehurst, pp. 1137–1154. Churchill Livingstone, Edinburgh.
4. Dolan P, Torgerson DJ (1998). The cost of treating osteoporotic fractures in the United Kingdom female population. *Osteoporosis Int 8*: 611–617.
5. Compston JE (1992). Risk factors for osteoporosis. *Clin Endocrinol 36*: 223–224.
6. Scane AC, Francis RM (1993). Risk factors for osteoporosis in men. *Clin Endocrinol 38*: 15–16.
7. Jones G, Nguyen T, Sambrook P, Kelly PJ, Eisman JA (1994). Progressive loss of bone from the femoral neck in elderly people: longitudinal findings from the Dubbo osteoporosis epidemiological study. *Br Med J 309*: 691–695.
8. Dargent-Molina P, Favier F, Grandjean H et al. (1996). Fall-related factors and risk of hip fracture: the EPIDOS prospective study. *Lancet 348*: 145–149.
9. Cummings SR, Nevitt MC, Browner WS et al. for the Study of Osteoporotic Fractures Research Group (1995). Risk factors for hip fracture in white women. *New Engl J Med 332*: 767–773.
10. Nguyen T, Sambrook P, Kelly P et al. (1993). Prediction of osteoporotic fractures by postural instability and bone density. *Br Med J 307*: 1111–1115.
11. *Assessment of fracture risk and its application to screening for postmenopausal osteoporosis*, report of a WHO Study Group (1994). World Health Organization, Geneva.
12. Peel N, Eastell R (1993). Measurement of bone mass and turnover. In: *Baillière's Clinical Rheumatology – 7: Osteoporosis*, ed. DM Reid, pp. 479–498. Baillière Tindall, London.
13. Barlow DH (Chairman) (1994). *Report of the Advisory Group on Osteoporosis*. Department of Health, London.
14. Eastell R, Reid DM, Compston J et al. (1998). A UK consensus group on the management of glucocorticoid-induced osteoporosis: an update. *J Int Med 244*: 271–292.
15. Hans D, Dargent-Molina P, Schott AM (1996). Ultrasonographic heel measurements to predict hip fractures in elderly women: the EPIDOS prospective study. *Lancet 348*: 511–514.

16. Ross P, Huang C, Davis J et al. (1995). Predicting vertebral deformity using bone densitometry at various skeletal sites and calcaneus ultrasound. *Bone 16*: 325–332.

17. Francis RM (1998). Management of established osteoporosis. *Br J Clin Pharmacol 45*: 95–99.

18. Riis B, Thomsen K, Christiansen C (1987). Does calcium supplementation prevent postmenopausal bone loss? A double blind controlled study. *New Engl J Med 316*: 173–177.

19. Kiel DP, Felson DT, Anderson JJ, Wilson PWF, Moskovitz MA (1987). Hip fractures and the use of estrogen in postmenopausal women. *New Engl J Med 317*: 1169–1174.

20. Felson DT, Zhang Y, Hannan MT, Kiel DP, Wilson PWF, Anderson JJ (1993). The effect of postmenopausal estrogen therapy on bone density in elderly women. *New Engl J Med 329*: 1141–1146.

21. Lindsay R, Tohme J (1990). Estrogen treatment of patients with established postmenopausal osteoporosis. *Obstet Gynecol 76*: 1–6.

22. Lufkin EG, Wahner HW, O'Fallon WM et al. (1992). Treatment of postmenopausal osteoporosis with transdermal estrogen. *Ann Intern Med 117*: 1–9.

23. Delmas PD, Bjarnason NH, Mitlak BH et al. (1997). Effects of raloxifene on bone mineral density, serum cholesterol concentrations, and uterine endometrium in postmenopausal women. *New Engl J Med 337*: 1641–1647.

24. Ettinger B, Black D, Cummings S et al. (1998). Raloxifene reduces the risk of incident vertebral fractures: 24-month interim analysis. *Osteoporosis Int 8* (suppl 3): 11.

25. Storm T, Thamsborg G, Steinich T, Genant HK, Sorensen OH (1990). Effect of intermittent cyclical etidronate therapy on bone mass and fracture rate in women with postmenopausal osteoporosis. *New Engl J Med 322*: 1265–1271.

26. Watts NB, Harris ST, Genant HK et al. (1990). Intermittent cyclical etidronate treatment of postmenopausal osteoporosis. *New Engl J Med 323*: 73–79.

27. Harris ST, Watts NB, Jackson RD et al. (1993). Four-year study of intermittent cyclic etidronate treatment of postmenopausal osteoporosis: three years of blinded therapy followed by one year of open therapy. *Am J Med 95*: 557–567.

28. Liberman UA, Weiss SR, Broll J et al. (1995). Effect of oral alendronate on bone mineral density and the incidence of fractures in postmenopausal osteoporosis. *New Engl J Med 333*: 1437–1443.

29. Black DM, Cummings SR, Karpf DB et al. (1996). Randomised trial of effect of alendronate on risk of fracture in women with existing vertebral fractures. *Lancet 348*: 1535–1541.

30. van Staa TP, Abenhaim L, Cooper C (1998). Use of cyclical etidronate and prevention of non-vertebral fractures. *Br J Rheumatol 36*: 1–8.

31. de Groen PC, Lubbe DF, Hirsch LJ et al. (1996). Esophagitis associated with the use of alendronate. *New Engl J Med 335*: 1016–1021.

32. Overgaard K, Hansen MA, Jensen SB, Christiansen C (1992). Effect of Salcatonin given intranasally on bone mass and fracture rates in established osteoporosis: a dose-response study. *Br Med J 305*: 556–561.

33. Rico H, Henandez ER, Revilla M, Gomez-Castresana F (1992). Salmon calcitonin reduces vertebral fracture rate in postmenopausal crush fracture syndrome. *Bone Miner 16*: 131–138.

34. Chesnut C, Baylink DJ, Doyle D et al. (1998). Salmon-calcitonin nasal spray prevents vertebral fractures in established osteoporosis. Further interim analysis of the PROOF study. *Osteoporosis Int 8* (suppl 3): 13.

35. Chevalley T, Rizzoli R, Nydegger V et al. (1994). Effects of calcium supplements on femoral neck bone mineral density and vertebral fracture rate in vitamin D replete elderly patients. *Osteoporosis Int 4*: 245–252.

36. Chapuy MC, Arlot ME, Delmas PD, Meunier PJ (1994). Effect of calcium and cholecalciferol treatment for three years on hip fractures in elderly women. *Br Med J 308*: 1081–1082.

37. Dawson-Hughes B, Harris SS, Krall EA, Dallal GE (1997). Effect of calcium and vitamin D supplementation on bone density in men and women 65 years of age and older. *New Engl J Med 337*: 670–676.

38. Heikinheimo RJ, Inkovaara JA, Harju EJ et al. (1992). Annual injection of vitamin D and fractures of aged bones. *Calcif Tissue Int 51*: 105–110.

39. Lips P, Graafmans WC, Ooms ME, Bezemer PD, Bouter LM (1996). Vitamin D supplementation and fracture incidence in elderly persons. A randomized, placebo-controlled clinical trial. *Ann Intern Med 124*: 400–406.

40. Francis RM, Boyle IT, Moniz C et al. (1996). A comparison of the effects of alfacalcidol treatment and vitamin D_2 supplementation on calcium absorption in elderly women with vertebral fractures. *Osteoporosis Int 6*: 284–290.

41. Tilyard MW, Spears GFS, Thompson J, Dovey S

(1992). Treatment of postmenopausal osteoporosis with calcitriol or calcium. *New Engl J Med 326*: 357–362.

42. Chesnut CH, Ivey JL, Gruber HE et al. (1983). Stanozolol in postmenopausal osteoporosis: therapeutic efficacy and possible mechanisms of action. *Metabolism 32*: 571–580.

43. Need AG, Chatterton BE, Walker CJ, Steurer TA, Horowitz M, Nordin BEC (1986). Comparison of calcium, calcitriol, ovarian hormones and nandrolone in the treatment of osteoporosis. *Maturitas 8*: 275–280.

44. Anderson FH, Francis RM, Faulkner K (1996). Androgen supplementation in eugonadal men with osteoporosis – effects of six months' treatment on bone mineral density and cardiovascular risk factors. *Bone 18*: 171–177.

45. Pak CYC, Sakhaee K, Adams-Huet B, Piziak V, Peterson RD, Poindexter JR (1995). Treatment of postmenopausal osteoporosis with slow release sodium fluoride. *Ann Intern Med 123*: 401–408.

46. Lindsay R, Nieves J, Formica C et al. (1997). Randomised controlled study of effect of parathyroid hormone on vertebral-bone mass and fracture incidence among postmenopausal women on oestrogen with osteoporosis. *Lancet 350*: 550–555.

47. Rubenstein LZ, Robbins AS, Josephson KR, Schulman BL, Osterweil D (1990). The value of assessing falls in an elderly population. A randomized clinical trial. *Ann Intern Med 113*: 308–316.

48. Vetter NJ, Lewis PA, Ford D (1992). Can health visitors prevent fractures in elderly people? *Br Med J 304*: 888–890.

49. Tinetti ME, Baker DI, McAvay G et al. (1994). A multifactorial intervention to reduce the risk of falling among elderly people living in the community. *New Engl J Med 331*: 821–827.

50. Lauritzen JB, Petersen MM, Lund B (1993). Effect of external hip protectors on hip fractures. *Lancet 341*: 11–13.

51. Villar MTA, Hill P, Inskip H, Thompson P, Cooper C (1998). Will elderly rest home residents wear hip protectors? *Age Ageing 27*: 195–198.

52. Francis RM, Baillie SP, Chuck A et al. (1998). *New Guidelines for Hip Fracture.* North East Osteoporosis Regional Advisory Board, Newcastle.

53. Kanis JA, Johnell O, Gullberg B et al. (1992). Evidence for efficacy of drugs affecting bone metabolism in preventing hip fracture. *Br Med J 305*: 1124–1128.

10

Drugs for the Treatment of Osteoporosis

Peter Burckhardt

Introduction • Inhibition of bone resorption • Stimulation of bone formation • Adjuvant treatments • Duration of treatment • Combined treatments • Nutritional measures • Physical measures

INTRODUCTION

Since the major outcome of osteoporosis is the occurrence of a fracture, management can be divided into three phases. Primary prevention is indicated for those patients with a normal bone mass who are exposed to the risk of bone loss such as occurs with the onset of the menopause or the introduction of corticosteroids. The management of these patients is discussed in Chapters 8 and 11. Secondary prevention is appropriate for those who have lost substantial bone but who have not yet sustained a low-trauma fracture. Treatment is required for those who have already experienced a fracture and who need both symptom control and measures to prevent further fractures.

Since osteoporosis results in an increased risk of low-trauma fractures, any treatment aimed at preventing such fractures is in fact a measure of primary prevention. In established osteoporosis, where fractures have already occurred, treatment is first required to alleviate symptoms and then should be directed to avoid further fractures. The alleviation of the symptoms due to a fracture mostly consists of surgi-cal or physical measures in addition to analgesia. Although secondary prevention and treatment share many similarities, there are important differences in their management. The most important is that in established osteoporosis, where there is an urgency caused by the fact that every additional fracture multiplies the risk of future events and provides the justification for long-term and relatively costly treatment.

In an individual patient, the result of these efforts can be monitored through the increase in BMD but in order to justify treatment it has to be shown that it also decreases fracture incidence. The evidence can only be provided by large clinical trials performed over at least three years, but not all drugs have been tested this way. Although some increase BMD to such an extent that an effect on fracture incidence seems likely, this is only an assumption, and requires proof from an appropriately constructed clinical trial. This is particularly important when drugs with different structures are compared, because a gain in BMD does not necessarily correspond to an increase in mechanical resistance. For instance, fluoride increases trabecular BMD more than bisphosphonates, but its antifracture efficacy is less. On the other hand, the reduction in fracture incidence may be greater than that predicted by the increment in BMD, as is seen with the studies of alendronate and salmon calcitonin.

Currently available drugs have rarely been compared to one another; they have usually been compared to placebo, calcium, or vitamin D. Since these latter agents have some clinical benefit, the efficacy of new therapies will tend to be underestimated. Furthermore the increments in BMD are often reported as a percentage change from baseline, while they should be given in terms of difference from the control group, since the true effect is the sum of the bone gained and the bone loss prevented. For instance, alendronate was reported to cause a larger gain in BMD in elderly patients compared to early postmenopausal women, simply because the loss of BMD was greater in the control group of early postmenopausal women than in the control group in the study of the elderly. In reality the difference between treated patients and controls was the same at both ages.

The recommendation for the use of a drug in osteoporosis should include a gain in BMD as well as a confirmed effect on fracture incidence. The purpose of this chapter is to review the evidence provided by recent large clinical trials where there were sufficient patients to allow valid statistical conclusions, and where BMD was measured with DXA. However, it has to be admitted that the published therapeutical successes are mainly based on the results of group responses rather than on individual patient evaluation. An average increase of BMD by 3% inevitably includes individuals who lost bone with the treatment; but the percentage of patients who did not respond usually remains unknown. As a general principle it can be assumed that this will be of the order of 20% for any drug, unless a smaller figure is given.

Recommended doses of the drugs that are reviewed will be found in an appendix at the end of the chapter.

INHIBITION OF BONE RESORPTION

Bisphosphonates

Pharmacology

Bisphosphonates are the most powerful inhibitors of bone resorption available for treatment (Figure 10.1). They were derived from pyrophosphate, which has a P–O–P backbone that binds to calcium phosphate and also inhibits crystal growth and dissolution. Bisphosphonates are P–C–P compounds, and they too bind avidly to calcium phosphate crystals, and because of this characteristic act specifically on bone by adhering to the bone surface. At very high concentrations, exceeding the antiresorptive dose, bisphosphonates can inhibit bone formation.

The potency (decrease in osteoclast activity and number) and the duration of effect of an individual bisphosphonate depend on the radicals attached to the central carbon atom. Bisphosphonates with side chains containing amino-groups (pamidronate, alendronate) have been shown to be more effective and to act for longer than simpler compounds such as etidronate. The addition of further side chains to the nitrogen molecule enhances lipophilicity and activity (ibandronate), while a further increment in biological activity is achieved by including a basic ring structure (zoledronate).

Bisphosphonates are poorly absorbed from the gastrointestinal tract (1–3% of the administered dose) and only then if taken in the fasting state. After absorption 20–50% of the dose is rapidly deposited in bone, preferentially at sites of active bone formation and/or resorption. The remainder of the dose is almost totally eliminated, unchanged by the kidneys.

The osteoclast resorbs bone by sealing itself to the bone surface and secreting hydrogen ions and proteases into the cavity so formed under the cell (Figure 10.2). Since bisphosphonates are soluble in an acid medium they move off the bone surface and are taken up by the osteoclast. The nitrogen-containing bisphosphonates prevent protein prenylation and induce apoptosis, while etidronate and clodronate are metabolized to a toxic ATP analogue that inhibits

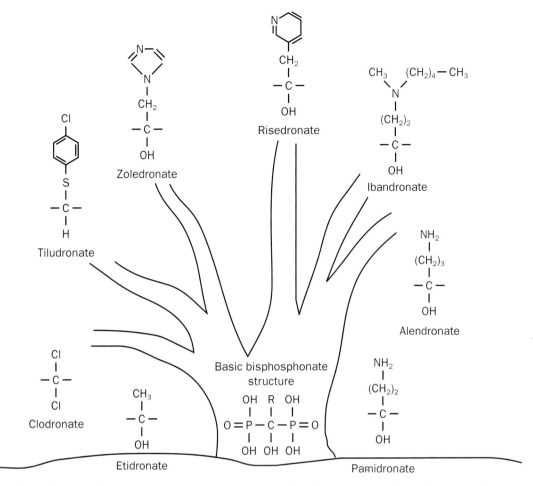

Figure 10.1 The basic bisphosphonate structure is common for all compounds which differ only with respect to the radicals attached to the carbon molecule. The figure shows these side chains for all currently available bisphosphonates.

osteoclast function. As osteoblasts move into the resorption cavity and begin to lay down new bone the bisphosphonate becomes buried and is only released by a future phase of resorption. For this reason, half life in bone is long (several months to years), depending on the rate of bone turnover. Biological half life is shorter, since only bisphosphonate on the bone surface in contact with the osteoclast inhibits resorption. Bisphosphonates are generally safe, but when given orally the aminobisphosphonates can cause mucosal irritation and damage.

Only when given in extremely high doses intravenously can they compromise renal function. Minor side effects vary from compound to compound.

The first effect of bisphosphonate treatment is to decrease bone resorption, which is then followed by an increase in BMD due to infilling of the resorption space on the bone surface. At first bone formation is unaffected, but then it declines owing to the effect of coupling. The final result is a lowering of bone turnover, both resorption and formation, which leads

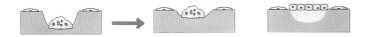

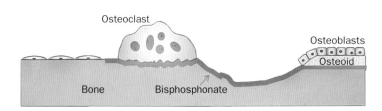

Figure 10.2 Mechanism of bisphosphonate action.

either to a further slow rise in BMD, or at least to a steady state. As a consequence the increase in BMD is most marked during the first year of treatment, with the rate decreasing subsequently. This phenomenon is common to all antiresorptive drugs, as is the pattern of reduction in fracture incidence, which is often small during the first 12 months and becomes more evident in the second and subsequent years of treatment.

Etidronate

Pharmacology

Etidronate, like all bisphosphonates, is poorly absorbed (about 2% of administered dose), and has to be taken in the fasting state with pure water, 2 hours before or after eating. It is given orally, in a dose of 400 mg/day for 2 weeks, followed by calcium 500 mg daily for 76 days. Continuous treatment and higher doses can cause mineralization defects, but this is not a problem with intermittent treatment. The effect is diminished by vitamin D deficiency[1] and combination with vitamin D or calcitriol has been advocated because of additional benefit.[2] The drug has been given for up to 7 years without significant problems, but there may be occasional transient adverse effects, which mainly consist of abdominal pains[3] and foot or leg cramps.[4]

Clinical efficacy

Etidronate increases BMD at the lumbar spine by 3–8% and at the femoral neck by about 2% over 2 to 3 years, when compared to controls[3–7] (Figure 10.3). The combination of etidronate with hormone replacement therapy has been shown to have an additive effect.[8]

During treatment the incidence of vertebral fractures decreases progressively over time, and is most obvious in patients with the longest exposure to the drug.[3] After 2 to 3 years of treatment fracture risk is reduced by about one-third, and after longer treatment by about half. With an absolute reduction in fracture risk of 3.2% over two years,[6] the numbers needing to be treated (NNT) to prevent one fracture equate to about 30 patients. In patients with a high risk (several vertebral fractures and a low BMD) prolonged treatments over 5 to 7 years reduce the NNT.[3,4,9] None of the prospective etidronate studies have shown a beneficial effect on hip fracture.

Alendronate

Pharmacology

Alendronate is the most extensively studied bisphosphonate, and has been shown to inhibit bone resorption, reduce bone turnover, and increase bone mass and bone strength. As an inhibitor of bone resorption, it is several hun-

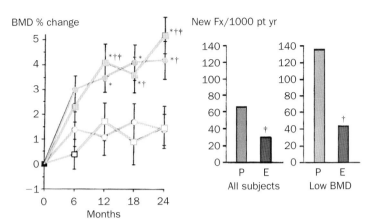

Etidronate in established osteoporosis

dred times more potent than etidronate. It does not affect bone mineralization or bone formation, and clinical studies have extended up to 5 years. After initiation of treatment, bone resorption markers decrease, reaching a nadir at about 6–12 weeks, while formation markers decrease over about 3 months.

The recommended dose is 10 mg per day, and since intestinal absorption is about 1%, the drug has to be taken in the fasting state, 30 minutes before breakfast. It should also be taken with a large glass of pure water, and the patients should remain upright for 30 minutes to prevent oesophageal reflux. If these recommendations are not followed, the drug may irritate the oesophageal mucosa and cause ulceration. For this reason, patients with a hiatus hernia or upper gastrointestinal reflux need to be monitored carefully, and may need to avoid this treatment.

Adverse events appear to vary in both frequency (up to about 25%) and severity, depending on the source of information. The main adverse events include abdominal pain and other upper gastrointestinal symptoms,[10] but they may not necessarily result in withdrawal of treatment. When patients with a history of gastrointestinal symptoms are excluded, gastrointestinal adverse effects are rare.[11] All studies with alendronate have compared calcium alone with the combination of bisphosphonate and calcium, and for this reason logic would dictate co-prescription. A pragmatic approach would be to give supplemental calcium to those patients with a poor dietary intake of calcium.

Clinical efficacy

Alendronate, when given over 2–3 years, increases the BMD at the lumbar spine by 6–10% compared with controls and at the femoral neck by 3–6%.[10-13] Although BMD mainly increases during the first two years of treatment, it continues to rise at a lower rate when the treatment is maintained, with current experience extending to over 5 years. It is effective in early postmenopausal women as well as in the elderly, where the increment in BMD between treated patients and controls appears essentially independent of age. The effect on BMD is maintained after the withdrawal of treatment for at least one year. Even when BMD starts to decline, it does so at a physiological rate, so that the relative increment compared to untreated patients is maintained.[14]

The incidence of clinical vertebral fractures decreases by about half, from 5% to 2.3% over 3 years of treatment.[11] This means that for the prevention of one clinical vertebral fracture, about 35 patients have to be treated for 3 years (Table 10.1). Alendronate, unlike etidronate, has

Table 10.1 Summary of effects of oral bisphosphonates on BMD and fracture incidence.

Bisphosphonate	Dose	Controls	Duration (years)	Vertebral fractures at baseline	% Increase of BMD at LS compared to . . .		% Increase of BMD at FN compared to . . .		Vertebral fracture incidence				Hip fracture incidence				Reference
					Baseline	Controls	Baseline	Controls	Treatment	Controls	Difference	RR	Treatment	Controls	Difference	RR	
Etidronate	400 mg/d 14 d/3 mo	0.5 g Ca	3	1–4	+5.1	+4.1	+1.4	+2.1	14.3%	17.4%	3.1%					0.82*	Harris et al.[4]
Etidronate	400 mg/d 14 d/3 mo	0.5 g Ca	2	1–4	+4.7	+3.3	+2.6	+1.7	3.0	6.3	3.3					0.48	Watts et al.[6]
Pamidronate	150 mg/d	1 g Ca	2	≥1 (average 2.5–3)	+7.0	+8.2	+1.0	+2.1	7	10	3					n.s.	Reid et al.[16]
Alendronate	5–10 mg/d	0.5 g Ca + Vit.D	3	≥1	+8.0	+6.2	+3.5	+4.1	2.3%	5.0%	2.7%		2.2%	1.1%	1.1%	0.50	Black et al.[11]
Alendronate	(5)10 mg/d	0.5 g Ca	3	0 or more	+8.0	+8.8	+4.7	+5.9	3.2%	6.2%	3.0%	0.46	0.2%	0.8%	0.6%	0.25	Liberman et al.[10]

*Lower in high risk patients
LS – Lumbar spine
FN – Femoral neck

also been shown to decrease the incidence of peripheral (appendicular) fractures in patients with at least one vertebral fracture at the start of treatment. Over a 3 year period, clinical non-vertebral fractures decreased by 28% overall including those of the wrist (4.1 to 2.2%) and hip (2.2 to 1.1%).[11] This means that, for the prevention of one hip fracture, about 90 patients have to be treated for 3 years. This number is lower when elderly patients with a higher risk of hip fracture are treated, but exceeds 150 for patients at lower risk.[10] In women with a low BMD (femoral neck T score below −2.5) but without a vertebral fracture, alendronate reduced vertebral fractures by 50% (RH 0.50, 95% CI 0.31–0.82) and clinical fractures by 36% (RH 0.64, 95% CI 0.50–0.82)[15] (Figure 10.4).

Pamidronate

Pharmacology

The aminobisphosphonate pamidronate is a powerful inhibitor of bone resorption with a prolonged action, being several hundred times more active than etidronate. It does not inhibit bone mineralization at clinically effective doses. It is given either as continuous oral therapy (150 mg daily with water 30 minutes before food) or as an intravenous infusion every 3 months (30–60 mg in 500–1000 ml saline or glucose over 1 to 2 hours). The addition of oral calcium is indicated, as for all bisphosphonates in patients with a calcium-deficient diet.

Tolerance of oral treatment may be a problem, since it causes oesophageal and gastric lesions when given in a rapidly absorbed

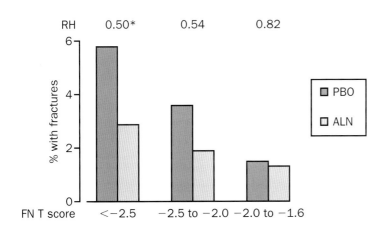

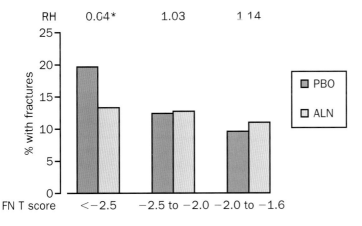

Figure 10.4 Vertebral and clinical fractures after alendronate treatment (Fracture Intervention Trial).[15]

preparation rather than in an enteric-coated form. With this latter preparation tolerance seems to be as acceptable as for other bisphosphonates.[16] Following the first intravenous infusion, a transient acute phase reaction may be observed in about 20% of the patients. Its frequency decreases by half after each new infusion, and it rarely affects compliance. The lymphocyte count may fall transiently, but with no clinical consequences, and this does not need to be monitored.

Clinical efficacy

Treatment with oral pamidronate results in a significant increase in vertebral BMD of about 8% over 2 years when compared with controls,[16] with an approximately 2% gain at the femoral neck. The drug has been given over a period of several years, and, as with other bisphosphonates, the rate of bone gain slows with time. There is a trend towards a decrease in vertebral fractures by 40%, but published studies have been too small to achieve statistical significance. After treatment for at least 5 years, the increase in BMD persists beyond the withdrawal of treatment by at least 2 years.[17] Although bone turnover returns to pretreatment values within 6 months, it is uncertain whether BMD remains elevated in the long term.[18] Currently pamidronate has been studied in a variety of disease states for 5 years, including cortisone-induced and post-transplantation osteoporosis, with beneficial effects. The drug is not marketed for osteoporosis, which accounts for the lack of large fracture studies.

When given intravenously, at a dose of 30 mg every 3 months for 2 years, pamidronate increases vertebral BMD by 10% compared witih controls, and femoral neck BMD by about 5%:[19,20] there are no fracture data available.

Clodronate

Clodronate has mainly been used in the prevention of bone metastases in myeloma and breast cancer. Its use in the treatment of osteoporosis relies on a study of intravenous administration (200 mg given IV every 3 weeks over 6 years) that increased vertebral BMD by 7% when compared to controls. There was a progressive decrease in vertebral fracture incidence by almost 50% after 4 years of treatment.[21]

Ibandronate
Pharmacology

Ibandronate is several thousand times more powerful at suppressing bone resorption than etidronate. It is effective in such small amounts that it can be given as an intravenous bolus injection. It has no adverse effect on bone mineralization or formation. Dose-response studies suggest that the drug can be given as a continuous oral treatment at a dose of 2.5 mg daily, or as a bolus intravenous injection of 1–2 mg every 3 months. Orally, it has to be taken on an empty stomach with pure water, and the only adverse effect seems to be slight diarrhoea.[22] Tolerance of, and compliance with, the intravenous regimen is excellent, and acute phase reactions are rare.[23] Oral calcium may be added, as for other bisphosphonates.

Clinical efficacy

Over one year of treatment, oral therapy increased lumbar spine BMD by almost 5%, and femoral neck BMD by more than 2%. The equivalent results obtained with 2 mg intravenously are 5% at the lumbar spine (Figure 10.5) and less than 2% at the femoral neck (n.s.). More prolonged studies are under way, but no fracture data are currently available, and ibandronate is not yet licensed for the treatment of osteoporosis.

Risedronate

Risedronate, a new bisphosphonate in clinical development, is as powerful as ibandronate in terms of antiresorptive effect. At the oral dose of 5 mg daily it has been effective in the prevention and the treatment of corticosteroid-induced bone loss and in decreasing the incidence of associated vertebral fracture. Its effect in postmenopausal osteoporosis is currently being tested in large ongoing trials, at the dose of 2.5 and 5 mg daily.

Four large trials have examined the efficacy of risedronate in the prevention of fractures. Two of these, from which data are not yet available, were designed to examine the effect on

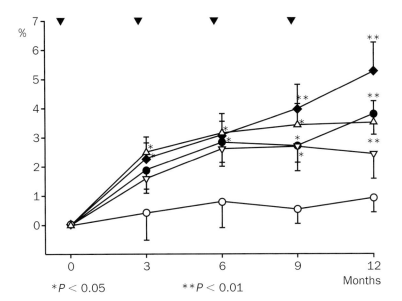

Figure 10.5 Effect of intravenous ibandronate on lumbar spine BMD in postmenopausal women. Changes (% ± SEM) in BMD of lumbar spine (L2–L4), before, 3, 6, 9 and 12 months after placebo (○) or IV bolus injections of 0.25 mg (▽), 0.5 mg (△), 1 mg (●) and 2 mg (◆) of ibandronate given every 3 months. The arrows (▼) indicate the time of IV bolus injections of study drug[23].

*P < 0.05   **P < 0.01

hip fractures, while the other two trials focused on vertebral fractures. Four other Phase III trials have examined the efficacy of risedronate in preventing bone loss or increasing BMD in postmenopausal women. All women in these trials received 1000 mg of supplemental calcium per day.

The data described here (including the vertebral fracture trials) have only been published in the form of abstracts (*Calcified Tissue International* 1999, Supplement 1, S42–43, S69–70). In a North American trial of 2458 postmenopausal women with a low spinal bone mass (T- score ≤ −2) and at least one prevalent vertebral fracture, risedronate 5 mg/day reduced the risk of new vertebral fractures by 41% (P = 0.003) and the risk of non-vertebral fractures by 39% (P = 0.02) over 3 years. Similar results were obtained in a European/Australian trial of 1226 women with at least 2 prevalent vertebral fractures. Vertebral fracture risk was reduced by 49% over 3 years (P < 0.001) and there was a trend towards a reduction in non-vertebral fracture risk (33%; P = 0.063). In both studies there were significant increases in BMD at the femoral neck, femoral trochanter and lumbar spine.

The efficacy of risedronate, in terms of its

effect on BMD, has also been examined in 541 postmenopausal women with a low bone mass (T- score ≤ −2), of whom 29% had prevalent vertebral deformities. Risedronate 5 mg/day significantly increased BMD at the lumbar spine (+3.5%), femoral neck (+1.2%) and femoral trochanter (+2.4%) with respect to baseline after 12 months of therapy. These increases were maintained up to the end of the study at 24 months, and were significantly greater than those in the placebo group at 12, 18 and 24 months.

The efficacy of risedronate 5 mg/day in preventing bone loss was also examined in a trial including 383 early postmenopausal (6–36 months) women. BMD at the lumbar spine, femoral neck and femoral trochanter increased significantly compared to both baseline and control after only 3 months. After 24 months BMD at these sites had significantly declined by 1.9–2.5% in the control group, but had increased by 0.8–2.5% in the risedronate group.

Overall, in all the postmenopausal osteoporosis studies, risedronate was well tolerated and, with the exception of a higher incidence of abdominal pain and nausea in the early postmenopausal trial, had an adverse-event profile that was similar to the control group's. The favourable gastrointestinal safety profile may be due, at least in part, to the formulation as a cellulose-film-coated tablet. This has a shorter oesophageal transit time than conventional gelatin capsules (3.3 seconds vs. 23.8 seconds) and reduces the chances of local-contact-related gastrointestinal problems.

The intravenous approach

The use of oral bisphosphonates may be limited by poor compliance caused either by gastrointestinal side effects, or by the need to take the drug each morning with pure water on an empty stomach. The intravenous route of administration avoids these problems, although it has other disadvantages, such as phlebitis and acute phase reactions. It may give rise to practical difficulties, such as the organization of facilities for regular bolus injections. For many patients the intravenous route appears to be an attractive alternative, particularly in terms of a bolus injection.

Experience with the intravenous administration of bisphosphonates has been obtained with etidronate, clodronate, alendronate, pamidronate and ibandronate; but in the treatment of osteoporosis by this route pamidronate and ibandronate have been the drugs most commonly investigated.

Administration of the drugs at intervals of 3 months is based on the observation that a single IV dose inhibits bone resorption for many weeks in healthy subjects,[24] offering the potential for long-term control of BMD. This approach was supported by a study showing that bone resorption was inhibited for 2 years after high-dose intravenous alendronate therapy in postmenopausal osteoporotic women.[25]

Pamidronate 30 mg IV or ibandronate 2 mg IV, given every 3 months to patients with established osteoporosis, has been shown to increase BMD by comparable amounts to those obtained with oral treatment.[19,23] The intravenous approach has also been tested in the prevention of postmenopausal bone loss, and this showed that clodronate was more effective than etidronate.[26]

Calcitonin

Pharmacology

Calcitonin inhibits osteoclast function for a relatively short period of time (about 12 hours after the administration of 50 IU subcutaneously or 100–200 IU intranasally), as indicated by a transient decrease of resorption markers. This mechanism is the basis for its effect of increasing mainly trabecular bone BMD. The most potent preparations are salmon and eel calcitonin; the most studied being the human and salmon peptides, of which the latter has been more commonly used in clinical trials. In the treatment of osteoporosis the recommended dose of salmon calcitonin is 200 IU intranasally per day. The co-prescription of calcium is essential, while the addition of vitamin D is recommended.

Calcitonin is absolutely safe and causes only mild and reversible side effects, the most frequent being flushing, dizziness, and headache after parenteral administration and rhinitis when given intranasally. Calcitonin was initially administered by subcutaneous injection, daily or every second day, but it was subsequently shown that the nasal spray has good bioavailability. Nasal administration needs about 4 times the dose used for subcutaneous injection. The development of antibodies to exogenous calcitonin is common, but neutralizing antibodies are relatively rare, and occur in about 20% of cases.

Clinical efficacy

Calcitonin leads to an increase in bone density or a reduction of bone loss, with an average increase of 2% at the spine, but less than 1% gain at the radius,[27] and no measurable effect at the femoral neck. The gain in BMD is more impressive when the difference from controls is taken into account in some, but not all studies.[28] When evaluated by radiogrammometry, calcitonin has also been shown to increase cortical bone.[29] The effect on BMD is transient, since the gains were eroded when treatment was discontinued, as is also seen with fluoride and oestrogens.

The effect on fracture incidence is uncertain.

Table 10.2 Summary of effects of intravenous bisphosphonates on BMD and fracture incidence.

Bisphosphonate	Dose	Controls	Duration (years)	Vertebral fractures present at baseline	Increase of BMD (in %) at LS compared to . . . Baseline	Controls	Increase of BMD (in %) at FM compared to . . . Baseline	Controls	Reference
Clodronate	200 mg IV /3 weeks		6		+5.7	+6.2			Filipponi et al.[21]
Pamidronate	10 mg /3 months	1 g Ca	1	1 or more	+8.9*	+11	—	—	Passeri et al.[20]
Pamidronate	30 mg /3 months	1 g Ca	2	none or several	+10.1	versus fluoride	+4.8	versus fluoride	Thiébaud et al.[19]
Ibandronate	2 mg /3 months	1 g Ca	1	none or several	+5.2	+4.3	+1.4	+1.1	Thiébaud et al.[23]

*Measured by DPA
LS – Lumbar spine
FN – Femoral neck

Reduction in vertebral fracture rate has been reported, but most studies have been too small to demonstrate a statistically significant effect.[29-32] A meta-analysis has suggested that calcitonin leads to a decrease in the incidence of vertebral fractures in the second year of treatment.[33] Preliminary analysis of an ongoing fracture trial shows a significant (37%) decrease of vertebral fractures after 3 years of treatment with a daily dose of 200 IU given by nasal spray. A smaller (100 IU) or higher (400 IU) dose was not effective, the latter perhaps because of inappropriate PTH stimulation.[34] This effect on vertebral fractures is greater than that which could be expected from the modest increase in BMD. The same discrepancy between the increase in BMD and decrease in fracture incidence is observed following alendronate or raloxifene therapy, although to a lesser extent. These results suggest that treatment increases bone quality independently of the gain in mineralized bone. The use of calcitonin is restricted to vertebral osteoporosis, since no effect on appendicular fractures has been found.

Oestrogens

Pharmacology

Oestrogen replacement therapy (ERT) alone or in combination with progestogens (hormone replacement therapy, HRT) reduces bone resorption, overall bone turnover and bone loss. It increases intestinal calcium absorption and renal calcium conservation and improves calcium balance. It can be given orally, transdermally, or as subcutaneous depot; vaginal application usually delivers insufficient for an action on bone. The doses used for treatment are the same as those for prevention.

Clinical efficacy

Oestrogen replacement therapy is the most commonly recommended prophylactic measure against postmenopausal bone loss.[35] For this reason, it is discussed in the chapter on prevention but it also has a proper place in the treatment of osteoporosis. On average ERT or HRT increases BMD at the lumbar spine by 3–6% over a period of several years (and to a greater extent when compared to controls); corresponding changes at the femoral neck are about 2% (4% when compared to controls).[36,37] It increases BMD even when started many years after menopause, and is also effective in preventing bone loss in elderly women.[38]

Used for prevention, ERT/HRT decreases fracture risk at the spine, the proximal femur, and the forearm.[39-41] After 5 years' treatment the relative risk of a vertebral fracture is decreased by 50–80% and that of hip and other non-vertebral fractures by 25%. In elderly current oestrogen users the incidence of all new fractures is reduced by 50–75%, after 10 years of treatment, an extraordinary high figure.[42] The problem is that so few elderly women continue on ERT/HRT for a sufficient length of time that this impressive figure derives from only a very small residual sample.

The antifracture effect takes several years to become evident[43] and is lost when ERT/HRT is discontinued.[42] For this reason current oestrogen users, but not past users (> 5 years), are protected. However, long-term compliance is low, and the treatment is usually abandoned in about half the women after one year, once the menopausal symptoms of oestrogen deficiency, the main motivation for accepting ERT/HRT, have declined in importance. For this reason, the full effectiveness of ERT/HRT in the treatment of osteoporosis is rarely achieved.

There are only a few studies describing the effects in established osteoporosis, but they seem impressive. ERT/HRT increases BMD by 5–10% over 3 years, and reduces vertebral fracture risk by two-thirds after 1 year of treatment.[44-46]

In order to achieve sustained compliance in women with osteoporosis and an intact uterus, including elderly patients, treatment is best prescribed as combined (oestrogen and progestogen) so as to avoid menstrual bleeding.

Tibolone

An alternative to HRT is treatment with tibolone, an oestrogen analogue that provides two main metabolites, one oestrogenic in action, the other progestogenic. Its effect on BMD in postmenopausal women is comparable to that of HRT. Its advantage lies in the very low incidence of endometrial bleeding, making it attractive for use in the treatment of osteoporosis. In studies over 2 years, treatment with tibolone increased lumbar spine BMD by 6.9% and femoral neck BMD by 4.5%.[47,48] Fracture data are not available.

SERMs

SERMs (Selective Estrogen Receptor Modulators) have an oestrogen-like effect on bone and an oestrogen antagonist effect on breast and uterus. Raloxifene is the best studied compound, and has been used in the treatment of established osteoporosis. In combination with calcium and vitamin D, raloxifene in a dose of 60 or 120 mg/day for 2 years lowered the risk of a new vertebral fracture by almost 50%, from 2.9% (placebo) to 1.6% in the treated group. In patients who already had a vertebral fracture, raloxifene reduced the incidence of new fractures from 14.3% (placebo) to 7.6%,[49] but had no effect on non-vertebral fractures. Although there are no published studies, it is theoretically possible that elderly patients and male patients might also respond to raloxifene.

STIMULATION OF BONE FORMATION

Fluoride

Pharmacology
Fluoride stimulates osteoblasts and the formation of new bone. It increases trabecular bone mass and density, but without a noticeable effect on cortical bone. The concern that fluoride would produce poor-quality bone, which would be prone to fracture, does not seem to be a problem with low-dose or intermittent treatment.

Fluoride can be given as either uncoated sodium fluoride, as an enteric-coated or a slow-release preparation (bioavailability decreased by about 40%), in combination with calcium citrate (bioavailability 25–30%), or as monofluorophosphate (bioavailability only slightly less than Na-fluoride). It should be prescribed as 15–20 mg

fluoride ion per day, and should be given in combination with calcium and vitamin D.

Fluoride may lead to a rapid increase in BMD, and this can cause microfractures, particularly at the ankle, leading to painful swelling. This occurs in about 10% of patients given high doses. Interruption of treatment, with calcium and vitamin D being continued, leads to rapid improvement. Fluoride can then be reintroduced, but at half the previous dose.

Gastrointestinal side effects may develop in 20–30% of patients, particularly with non-enteric-coated preparations; but this is less common with monofluorophosphate (MFP). Fluoride cannot be given in chronic renal failure, because of toxic accumulation, and must be avoided in osteomalacia.

It is necessary to add calcium and vitamin D or its metabolites in order to achieve an increase in bone formation and avoid defective mineralization.[50]

Clinical efficacy
When given in moderate doses (15–20 mg F ion/day) vertebral BMD increases by about 5% per year over several years, with no effect on cortical bone. Higher doses increase hip BMD slightly, but reduce BMD and BMC at the radius. About 20% of patients do not respond to fluoride for unknown reasons, though in some this will be due to poor absorption. The increase in spinal BMD is not maintained after therapy is discontinued, particularly in those patients with high bone turnover.

Fluoride has been investigated in large clinical trials in postmenopausal osteoporosis without showing an effect on vertebral fracture rate,[51–53] but in smaller studies there have been positive effects. Relatively low doses of sodium fluoride,[54] slow-release sodium fluoride,[55,56] intermittent therapy,[57,58] or MFP all have been reported to be effective in decreasing the incidence of new vertebral fractures by about 50% provided that BMD does not increase by more than 4–6% p.a.[59] This positive effect applies to women with established postmenopausal osteoporosis,[57,60] to osteoporotic men with no previous fractures, and to women on HRT.[61]

The failure of some large trials to show an

antifracture effect is probably due to the high doses used, to a beneficial effect of vitamin D when given as placebo, and to the absence of oestrogen replacement therapy in the postmenopausal women studied. Fluoride markedly increases the thickness of trabeculae, but does not improve their connectivity. As a consequence fluoride might not improve mechanical resistance where trabeculae have already been interrupted, as in patients who have already fractured a vertebra, although it will increase BMD. Until more data is available fluoride should be restricted to patients without, or with only a few, vertebral fractures. It is indicated in postmenopausal oestrogen-replete women with osteoporosis, and also seems to be effective in the treatment of vertebral osteoporosis in men, provided that relatively small doses are used.

The fear of increasing hip fractures with fluoride has been excluded by careful retrospective analyses. However, an unexpected rise in alkaline phosphatase calls for interruption of treatment in case this indicates an impending fracture. Fluoride is currently only available in some, but not all, European countries.

Strontium

In preliminary studies, strontium has been shown to increase lumbar spine BMD in postmenopausal women by about 3% per year and to decrease vertebral deformities. The effect on BMD has to be interpreted with caution, since the bone content of strontium alters the densitometric values. Strontium preparations are not currently available for clinical use.

PTH

Human PTH 1-84 and its active fragment, 1-34 hPTH, have been shown to stimulate bone formation, increase trabecular and cortical bone mass, trabecular thickness and connectivity. When hPTH 1-34 was injected daily for one month every quarter for 2 years in postmenopausal women with osteoporosis, lumbar spine BMD increased by about 8%, independent of the concurrent administration of calcitonin.[62] When hPTH 1-34 (400 IU/day) was given subcutaneously to oestrogen-replete osteoporotic women for 3 years (Figure 10.6), BMD increased by 13% at the lumbar spine, and by 2.7% at the hip, with a trend to a decrease in vertebral fracture rate.[63] PTH is not currently commercially available, and would probably need the development of analogues that could be given by more convenient routes of administration than daily injections.

Growth factors

Growth hormone has not yet been shown to be effective in the treatment of osteoporosis, although it has a positive effect on bone metabolism and increases BMD in patients with growth hormone deficiency. Insulin-like growth factor (IGF) has also been tested, with some positive effects in the elderly; but clinical development of these peptides will be restricted as long as they have to be administered parenterally. Other bone-stimulating peptides are in preclinical development.

Anabolic steroids

The effect of anabolic steroids has hardly been tested in osteoporosis. As stimulators of muscle strength they could be effective in osteoporosis as adjuvant treatment. Nandrolone decanoate is the most utilized preparation, and can be injected IM in a dose of 50 mg every 4 weeks. Its virilizing side effects are relatively frequent, and limit its use in postmenopausal women. In osteoporosis, it increases BMC at the forearm and BMD at the lumbar spine by about 3% after 1–2 years, with no significant effect on the femoral neck.[64–66] Its effect on BMD is uncertain, because it increases bone marrow fat, which in turn influences the measurements of BMD.

Nandrolone decanoate could be used as an adjuvant treatment in elderly women and in male osteoporosis, although controlled studies proving its effectiveness in this situation are

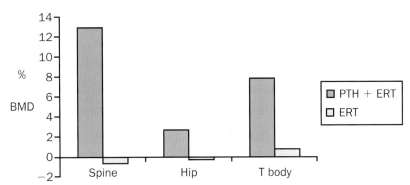

Figure 10.6 Effect of hPTH 1-34 on spine, hip and total body BMD in oestrogen-replete postmenopausal women (redrawn from ref. 63).

lacking. The combination with calcitonin showed negative results,[66] and its place in the current management of osteoporosis is limited.

ADJUVANT TREATMENTS

Calcium

Pharmacology
Calcium, although a component of the natural diet and necessary for bone health, has an additional effect on bone metabolism when given as a supplement of 0.5–1.0 g daily. The small increase in plasma calcium over a period of hours lowers PTH secretion, and in a dose of 1 g daily decreases bone resorption by up to 20%.

Another reason for using supplements relates to the relatively low absorption of calcium in some osteoporotics, particularly those who are older. Such patients may lose the adaptive ability to increase intestinal calcium absorption when intake falls, and therefore become calcium-deficient. The optimization of calcium intake is therefore important in elderly osteoporotic patients.

Clinical efficacy
Calcium supplementation reduces the age-related decline of BMD in the elderly by 2–4% per year,[67] and, provided that bone turnover is not elevated, it also slightly increases vertebral BMD through infilling of the remodelling space. It may also act in the long term[68,69] to decrease fracture incidence,[70] and together with vitamin D lowers the incidence of hip fractures in the elderly.[71,72] These preventive effects may also be seen in women with vertebral fractures, where calcium may also decrease fracture rate.[73]

For these reasons, calcium together with vitamin D can be regarded as an adjuvant treatment for osteoporosis. Since all bone-forming or antiresorptive therapies aim to increase bone density or mass, a positive calcium balance together with an appropriate calcium intake is essential. Indeed, all major therapeutic trials of new therapies for osteoporosis have included calcium supplements in both treatment and placebo groups.

The optimal intake, as defined by the NIH, is 1500 mg/day for patients over 65 years.[74] Although these amounts correspond to the requirement calculated on the basis of known obligatory losses and fractional absorption rates, they are difficult to achieve in practice. They are probably too high, since they have not been established in vitamin D-replete subjects. Vitamin D-deficiency is frequent, even in the healthy population, and, since vitamin D- supplementation is recommended for all patients with established osteoporosis, the optimal intake of calcium might be significantly lower. Clearly, it is difficult to achieve a daily intake of over 1000 mg of calcium without calcium supplementation.

Vitamin D and its metabolites

Pharmacology

Vitamin D and its metabolites enhance intestinal calcium absorption, regulate the differentiation of several cell types, are necessary for the mineralization of bone matrix, and may also stimulate osteoblast function. Vitamin D is derived both from the diet and endogenous production. Nutritional intake is only important when it has to compensate for insufficient production by the skin or reduced activation (hydroxylation) by liver or kidney.

The theoretical reasons for prescribing vitamin D or its metabolites in elderly patients with osteoporosis are the age-related decline in the skin's ability to produce vitamin D and reduced exposure to ultraviolet light. There may also be a deficiency of vitamin D 1α-hydroxylase in the kidney owing to oestrogen lack and ageing, as well as decreased responsiveness to PTH. Since nutritional intake is usually low in this age group, it rarely compensates for these deficiencies.

Subclinical vitamin D deficiency is frequent, not only in the institutionalized or housebound elderly, but also in many healthy, free-living elderly or even middle-aged people.[75,76] Subclinical deficiency has therefore to be suspected, and vitamin D supplementation should be considered for every patient with osteoporosis.

Vitamin D deficiency is defined by low plasma levels of 25 hydroxyvitamin D (< 20 nmol/l), which increase PTH secretion, contribute to the decrease in BMD, particularly of the femoral neck, and impose an additional risk of hip fracture.[77] Vitamin D therapy will reverse this secondary hyperparathyroidism, which may also be driven by antiresorptive drugs such as bisphosphonates or calcitonin. Attempts to increase the nutritional intake of vitamin D are often unsuccessful, because the main dietary sources, such as oily fishes and fish liver oil, are expensive and unattractive to many elderly people. Moreover, supplementation of milk or margarine with vitamin D does not provide an adequate intake under normal circumstances. Vitamin D seems to have a positive effect on muscle strength and decreases the risk of falling, and may therefore provide an additional protection from osteoporotic fracture.[78]

Clinical efficacy

Since the aim of treatment for osteoporosis is to prevent further fractures and arrest the decline in bone fragility, there is a place for vitamin D in the correction of dietary insufficiency as part of a broader approach to treatment. Its role as sole treatment for established osteoporosis is less certain. Vitamin D can be given in its native form, which is the most economical preparation, or as 1α hydroxylated metabolites (alfacalcidol or calcitriol). The dose of native vitamin D is between 600 and 1000 IU per day, and in one study 800 IU plus 1–2 g calcium/day decreased hip fracture incidence.[71] Larger doses can be given parenterally once or twice per year,[79] but these doses run the risk of causing hypercalciuria, and might even increase bone resorption in extreme cases. Vitamin D supplementation in the elderly reduces bone loss at the femoral neck by half[80] and, when given with calcium, enhances the effect on BMD.[81] It also decreases the risk of hip fractures by 37 to 55%,[72,78,82,83] an effect that has not been observed with vitamin D alone.[69]

The effect of vitamin D metabolites as sole treatment for osteoporosis is uncertain, because the results of controlled studies have been inconclusive. The recommended dose of alphacalcidol is 0.5–1.0 mcg g, and for calcitriol is 0.5 mcg g per day. Alfacalcidol was shown to increase BMD,[84] but not at the femoral neck, and there was no decline in fracture rate,[85] except in some studies in Japan,[86,87] where calcium intake is very low. Calcitriol reduced vertebral fractures in one study,[88] but other trials have shown no effect.[89–91] It is conceivable that the positive results could also have been obtained with calcidiol (25 hydroxyvitamin D) or with parent vitamin D. The use of parent vitamin D or its hydroxylated metabolites in vitamin D-replete subjects is currently uncertain.

DURATION OF TREATMENT

Most clinical trials of new therapeutic agents for the treatment of osteoporosis have been of 2–3 years' duration. Those with HRT, bisphosphonates and fluoride have all shown that bone loss increases once treatment is discontinued. Most therapies therefore have to be targeted at patients most at risk, with the prospect either of continuous long-term treatment or short periods of cyclical therapy that maintain the bone-protective effect.

COMBINED TREATMENTS

In most clinical trials of new therapies the placebo groups have been treated with calcium, and sometimes also with vitamin D. Little is known about the efficacy of other combinations, but recent reports using HRT have been encouraging.

Combination with oestrogen replacement

The combination of monofluorophosphate with ERT or with HRT had a synergistic effect.[61] The combination of etidronate with HRT was additive,[8] in that those who received combined therapy had significantly greater gains in BMD at the spine and hip than those treated with HRT or etidronate alone. Combination of calcitonin with HRT also showed additive effects,[92] as did the combination of PTH and HRT.[63]

Combination with vitamin D and its metabolites

Fluoride should be combined with vitamin D or calcitriol, since the former increases the need for absorbed calcium.[50] The combination of vitamin D with bisphosphonates is currently being tested in corticosteroid-induced osteoporosis. Treatment of osteoporosis with alendronate in combination with calcitriol showed additive effects at a variety of skeletal sites,[93] but the combination of calcitonin with calcitriol showed no advantage.[94]

NUTRITIONAL MEASURES

Although nutrition influences bone mass by only a few percentage points, it has a place in the general management of osteoporosis. Calcium and vitamin D are of course the most important nutrients; but new information on proteins and salt intake needs to be incorporated into current management.

Protein

Adequate protein intake lowers bone loss, while an insufficient intake is a pathogenetic factor for osteoporosis at all ages. Protein deficiency increases the risk of hip fracture by decreasing muscle strength and increasing the risk of falls, as well as through an effect on femoral neck BMD.[95] It also adversely influences the clinical outcome of elderly patients with hip fractures,[95,96] and, although rarely diagnosed, is characteristic of the ill elderly patient with osteoporosis.[97,98]

An intake of 0.8 g per kg body weight is considered to be adequate for adults of all ages. Although protein requirements seem to decline with age,[99] they are often unmet. Protein and calcium supplementation accelerates the recovery of elderly patients with hip fractures[100] and decreases their mortality. Supplementation with protein alone leads to an increase of BMD at the hip in elderly patients with osteoporosis.[101] This positive effect should not be confused with the adverse effects of a diet high in animal proteins, which, because of its acid load buffered by bone, leads to a negative bone calcium balance and increased urinary calcium excretion. Soya proteins do not have this disadvantage.

Salt

High intake of salt should also be avoided, since it increases urinary calcium excretion[102] and enhances the development of osteoporosis.[103] Chronic use of thiazides, which lowers urinary sodium and calcium excretion, is associated with a decreased incidence of hip fractures. For these reasons a low salt diet or a thiazide diuretic might reasonably be included as an adjuvant treatment in those patients who are also hypertensive.

Vitamin K

Vitamin K is a co-factor for the gamma-carboxylation and activation of osteocalcin. It has been found to be relatively deficient in osteoporotics; but although supplementation with vitamin K increases plasma levels of osteocalcin, the effect on BMD is uncertain.

Fibres

There is no need to avoid nutrients rich in oxalate or fibre because of their reported inhibitory effect on calcium absorption. Oxalate is rarely taken in amounts that become relevant for calcium homeostasis, and the positive effect of fibre of preventing constipation and colon cancer is convincing.

Calcium

Dietary calcium supplementation, particularly in the elderly, is an important adjuvant to the treatment of osteoporosis. It offsets any tendency to hypocalcaemia and secondary hyperparathyroidism that might occur with the use of inhibitors of bone resorption. The addition of 1 g of calcium above the normal intake reduces bone loss[68] and fracture rate;[70,104] but it remains uncertain how far dietary sources can cover this need. The NIH recommend[74] a dietary intake of 1.5 g for men below 65 years, 1 g for postmenopausal women on HRT (1.5 g when not on HRT), and 1.5 g for both sexes over the age of 65 years. These recommendations are high, and hard to follow. Calcium from dairy products, the main nutritional source, is as well absorbed as that from commercial supplements. Absorption is about 20% in postmenopausal women when the intake is 1 g and about 30% when the intake is 0.5 g.[105] The amount of low-fat dairy products that provides 1000–1500 mg calcium contains only about 100 mg cholesterol, a third of the total permissible intake; and this does not increase plasma cholesterol.[106] Other calcium-rich nutrients, such as nuts, vegetables, sardines, are rarely taken in amounts large enough to provide 1000 mg; but calcium-rich mineral waters may also contribute to the total intake.

Vitamin D

Only those patients spending at least 30 minutes/day outdoors might produce enough vitamin D to maintain calcium homeostasis. If the plasma level of 25(OH)vitamin D falls below 10 nmol/l, then PTH rises above the upper limit of normal, and increases bone turnover and loss.[107,108] Nutritional sources of vitamin D, mainly oily fish, are insufficient to compensate for the lack of UV exposure, and vitamin D supplementation rather than nutritional measures is indicated in the management of osteoporosis.

PHYSICAL MEASURES

Intense physical exercise increases BMD in the loaded bone in both young and postmenopausal women, at least transiently; but controlled studies in osteoporotic patients are lacking. In the prevention of vertebral fractures, extension exercises of the back are more effective than those of flexion.[109] Physiotherapy in established osteoporosis allows the mobilization of the fracture patient and also increases stability and mobility, which may prevent falls. In symptomatic patients, it not only improves balance and strength and decreases pain and analgesic requirement, but also improves the level of daily function and the quality of life beyond the training period.[110]

APPENDIX		
Drug	Dose	Regimen
Etidronate	400 mg/day orally for 2 weeks followed by 500 mg calcium/day for 76 days	Take in the fasting state with pure water, 2 hours before or after eating
Alendronate	10 mg/day	Take in the fasting state, 30 minutes before eating together with a glass of pure water The patients must remain upright after taking the drug for 30 minutes to prevent oesophageal reflux
Pamidronate	150 mg/day orally 30–60 mg IV/3 months in 500–1000 saline or glucose over 1 to 2 hours	Take with water 30 minutes before meal
Ibandronate	2.5 mg/day orally 1–2 mg IV/3 months	On an empty stomach over 5 minutes
Salmon calcitonin	50 IU IM or SC/day or 200 IU IM or SC/every 2nd day or 200 IU as nasal spray/day	
Fluoride: – NaF uncoated – NaF coated – Monofluorophosphate	40 mg (= 18 mg F^-)/day 40 mg (= 12 mg F^-)/day 100 mg (= 13.2 mg F^-)/day	During or after a meal
Vitamin D	800–1000 IU/day 150 000 IU IM/6 monthly	At any time
Alfacalcidol Calcitriol Calcium	0.5—1.0 µg/day orally 0.5 µg/day orally 500–1000 mg/day orally	At any time At any time With or after meals

REFERENCES

1. Koster JC, Hackeng WHL, Mulder H (1996). Diminished effect of etidronate in vitamin D deficient osteopenic postmenopausal women. *Eur J Clin Pharmacol 51*: 145–147.
2. Masud T, Mulcahy B, Thompson AV et al. (1998). Effects of cyclical etidronate combined with calcitriol versus cyclical etidronate alone on spine and femoral neck bone mineral density in postmenopausal women. *Ann Rheum Dis 57*: 346–349.
3. Miller PD, Watts NB, Licata AA et al. (1997). Cyclical etidronate in the treatment of postmenopausal osteoporosis: efficacy and safety after seven years of treatment. *Am J Med 103*: 468–476.
4. Harris ST, Watts NB, Jackson RD et al. (1993). Four-year study of intermittent cyclic etidronate treatment of postmenopausal osteoporosis: three years of blinded therapy followed by one year of open therapy. *Am J Med 95*: 557–567.
5. Storm T, Thamsborg G, Genant HK, Steiniche T, Sorensen OH (1990). Effect of intermittent cyclical etidronate therapy on bone mass and fracture rate in women with postmenopausal osteoporosis. *New Engl J Med 322*: 1265–1271.
6. Watts NB, Miller PD, Licata AA et al. (1995). Seven years of cyclical etidronate: continued improvement in spine BMD and progressive decline in vertebral fracture incidence. *Bone 17*: abstract 617.
7. Montessori MLM, Scheele WH, Netelenbos JC, Kerkhoff JF, Bakker K (1997). The use of etidronate and calcium versus calcium alone in the treatment of postmenopausal osteopenia: results of three years of treatment. *Osteoporosis Int 7*: 52–58.
8. Wimalawansa SJ (1998). A four-year randomized controlled trial of hormone replacement and bisphosphonate, alone or in combination, in women with postmenopausal osteoporosis. *Am J Med 104*: 219–226.
9. Storm T, Kollerup G, Thamsborg G, Genant HK, Sorensen OH (1996). Five years of clinical experience with intermittent cyclical etidronate for postmenopausal osteoporosis. *J Rheumatol 23*: 1560–1564.
10. Liberman UA, Weiss SR, Bröll J et al. (1995). Effect of oral alendronate on bone mineral density and the incidence of fractures in postmenopausal osteoporosis. *New Engl J Med 333*: 1437–1443.
11. Black DM, Cummings SR, Karpf DB et al. (1996). Randomized trial of effects of alendronate on risk of fracture in women with existing vertebral fractures. *Lancet 348*: 1535–1541.
12. Chesnut CH III, McClung MR, Ensrud KE et al. (1995). Alendronate treatment of the postmenopausal osteoporotic woman: effect of multiple dosages on bone mass and bone remodeling. *Am J Med 99*: 144–152.
13. Devogelaer JP, Broll H, Correa-Rotter R et al. (1996). Oral alendronate induces progressive increases in bone mass of the spine, hip and total body over 3 years in postmenopausal women with osteoporosis. *Bone 18*: 141–150.
14. Stock JL, Bell NH, Chesnut CH III et al. (1997). Increments in bone mineral density of the lumbar spine and the hip and suppression of bone turnover are maintained after discontinuation of alendronate in postmenopausal women. *Am J Med 103*: 291–297.
15. Cummings SR, Black DM, Thompson DE et al. (1998). Effect of alendronate on risk of fracture in women with low bone density but without vertebral fractures. *JAMA 280*: 2077–2082.
16. Reid IR, Wattie DJ, Evans MC, Gamble GD, Stapleton JP, Cornish J (1994). Continuous therapy with pamidronate, a potent bisphosphonate, in postmenopausal osteoporosis. *J Clin Endocrinol Metab 79*: 1595–1599.
17. Landman JO, Hamdy NAT, Pauwels EKJ, Papapoulos SE (1995). Skeletal metabolism in patients with osteoporosis after discontinuation of long term treatment with oral pamidronate. *J Clin Endocrinol Metab 80*: 3465–3468.
18. Orr-Walker B, Wattie DJ, Evans MC, Reid IR (1997). Effects of prolonged bisphosphonate therapy and its discontinuation on bone mineral density in postmenopausal osteoporosis. *Clin Endocrinol 46*: 87–92.
19. Thiébaud D, Burckhardt P, Melchior J et al. (1994). Two years effectiveness of intravenous pamidronate (APD) versus oral fluoride for osteoporosis occurring in the postmenopause. *Osteoporosis Int 4*: 76–83.
20. Passeri M, Baroni MC, Pedrazzoni M et al. (1991). Intermittent treatment with intravenous 4-amino-1-hydroxybutylidene-1,1-bisphosphonate (AHBuBP) in the therapy of postmenopausal osteoporosis. *Bone Miner 15*: 237–248.
21. Filipponi P, Cristallini S, Rizello E et al. (1996). Cyclical intravenous clodronate in postmenopausal osteoporosis. *Bone 18*: 179–184.

22. Ravn P, Clemmesen B, Riis BJ, Christiansen C (1996). The effect on bone mass and bone markers of different doses of ibandronate: a new bisphosphonate for prevention and treatment of postmenopausal osteoporosis. A 1-year, randomized, double-blind, placebo-controlled dose-finding study. *Bone 19*: 527–533.

23. Thiébaud D, Burckhardt P, Kriegbaum H et al. (1997). Three-monthly intravenous injections of ibandronate in the treatment of postmenopausal osteoporosis. *Am J Med 103*: 298–307.

24. Netelenbos JC, van Ginkel FC, Lips P et al. (1991). Effect of a single infusion of aminohydroxypropylidene on calcium and bone metabolism in healthy volunteers monitored during 2 months. *J Clin Endocrinol Metab 72*: 223–228.

25. Khan SA, Kanis JA, Vasikaran S et al. (1997). Elimination and biochemical responses to intravenous alendronate in postmenopausal osteoporosis. *J Bone Miner Res 12*: 1700–1707.

26. Heikkinen JE, Selander KS, Laitinen K, Arnala I, Vaanen HK (1997). Short-term intravenous bisphosphonates in prevention of postmenopausal bone loss. *J Bone Miner Res 112*: 103–110.

27. Cardona JM, Pastor E (1997). Calcitonin versus etidronate for the treatment of postmenopausal osteoporosis: a metaanalysis of published clinical trials. *Osteoporosis Int 7*: 165–174.

28. Thamsborg G, Jensen JEB, Kollerup G, Hauge EM, Melsen F, Sorensen OH (1996). Effect of nasal salmon calcitonin on bone remodeling and bone mass in postmenopausal osteoporosis. *Bone 18*: 207–212.

29. Rico H, Revilla M, Hernandez ER, Villa LF, Alvarez de Buergo M (1995). Total and regional bone mineral content and fracture rate in postmenopausal osteoporosis treated with salmon calcitonin: a prospective study. *Calcif Tissue Int 556*: 181–185.

30. Gennari C, Chiericetti SM, Bigazzi S et al. (1985). Comparative effects on bone mineral content of calcitonin, and calcium plus salmon calcitonin given in two different regimens in postmenopausal osteoporosis. *Curr Ther Res 38*: 455–464.

31. Rico H, Hernandez ER, Revilla M, Gomez-Gastresana F (1992). Salmon calcitonin reduces vertebral fracture rate in postmenopausal crush fracture syndrome. *Bone Miner 16*: 131–138.

32. Overgaard K, Hansen MA, Jensen SB, Christiansen C (1992). Effect of salcatonin given intranasally on bone mass and fracture rates in established osteoporosis: a dose-response study. *Br Med J 305*: 556–561.

33. Burckhardt P, Burnand B (1993). The effect of treatment with calcitonin on vertebral fracture rate in osteoporosis. *Osteoporosis Int 3*: 24–30.

34. Stock JL, Avioli LV, Baylink DJ et al. (1997). Calcitonin-salmon nasal spray reduces the incidence of new vertebral fractures in postmenopausal women: three-years interim results of the PROOF study. *J Bone Miner Res 12* (suppl 1): S149.

35. WHO Study Group (1994). *Assessment of fracture risk and its application to screening for postmenopausal osteoporosis: report of a WHO study group*, WHO technical report series ©843. World Health Organization, Geneva.

36. Eriksen EF, Kassem M, Langedeh B. (1996). European and North American experience with HRT for the prevention of osteoporosis. *Bone 19*: (Suppl 5) 179S–183S.

37. PEPI (1996). The Writing Group of the PEPI Trial. Results from the postmenopausal estrogen/progestin interventions (PEPI) trial. Effects of hormone therapy on bone mineral density. *JAMA 276*: 1389–1396.

38. Quigley ME, Martin PL, Burnier AM, Brooks P (1987). Estrogen therapy arrests bone loss in elderly women. *Am J Obstet Gynecol 156*: 1516–1523.

39. Maxim P, Ettinger B, Spitalny GM (1995). Fracture protection by long-term estrogen treatment. *Osteoporosis Int 5*: 23–29.

40. Eddy DM, Johnston CC, Cummings SR et al. (1998). Osteoporosis: review of the evidence for prevention, diagnosis, and treatment and cost–effectiveness analysis. Status report developed by the National Osteoporosis Foundation. *Osteoporosis Int 8* (suppl 4).

41. Grady D, Rubin SM, Petitti DB et al. (1992). Hormone therapy to prevent disease and prolong life in postmenopausal women. *Ann Intern Med 117*: 1016–1037.

42. Cauley JA, Seeley DG, Ensrud K, Ettinger B, Black D, Cummings SR (1995). Estrogen replacement therapy and fractures in older women. *Ann Intern Med 122*: 9–16.

43. Felson DT, Zhang Y, Hannan MT, Kiel DP, Wilson PWF (1993). The effect of postmenopausal estrogen therapy on bone density in elderly women. *New Engl J Med 329*: 1141–1146.

44. Lindsay R, Tohme JF (1990). Estrogen treatment

of patients with established postmenopausal osteoporosis. *Obstet Gynecol 72*: 290–295.

45. Christiansen C, Riis BJ (1990). 17-estradiol and continuous noresthisterone: an unique treatment for established osteoporosis. *J Clin Endocrinol Metab 71*: 836–841.

46. Lufkin EG, Wahner HW, O'Fallon WM et al. (1992). Treatment of postmenopausal osteoporosis with transdermal oestrogen. *Ann Intern Med 117*: 1–9.

47. Geusens P, Dequeker J, Gielen J, Schot LP (1991). Non-linear increase in vertebral density induced by a synthetic steroid (Org OD 14) in women with established osteoporosis. *Maturitas 13*: 155–162.

48. Studd J, Arnala I, Kicovic PH, Zamblera D et al. (1998). A randomized study of tibolone on bone mineral density in osteoporotic postmenopausal women with previous fractures. *Obstet Gynecol 92*: 574–579.

49. Ensrud K, Black D, Harris S et al. (1998). The effect of 2 and 3 years of raloxifene on vertebral and non-vertebral fractures in postmenopausal women with osteoporosis. [Abstract.] *J Bone Miner Res 1105*: S174.

50. Dure-Smith BA, Farley SM, Linkhart SG, Farley JR, Baylink DJ (1996). Calcium deficiency in fluoride-treated osteoporotic patients despite calcium supplementation. *J Clin Endocrinol Metab 81*: 269–275.

51. Riggs BL, Hodgson SF, O'Fallon WM et al. (1990). Effect of fluoride treatment on the fracture rate in postmenopausal women with osteoporosis. *New Engl J Med 322*: 802–809.

52. Kleerekoper M, Peterson EL, Nelson DA et al. (1994). A randomized trial of sodium fluoride as a treatment for postmenopausal osteoporosis. *Osteoporosis Int 9*: 265–275.

53. Meunier PJ, Sebert JL, Reginster JY et al. (1998). Fluoride slats are no better at preventing new vertebral fractures than calcium–vitamin D in postmenopausal osteoporosis: the FAVO study. *Osteoporosis Int 8*: 4–12.

54. Riggs BL, O'Fallon WM, Lane A et al. (1994). Clinical trial of fluoride therapy in postmenopausal osteoporotic women: extended observations and additional analysis. *J Bone Miner Res 9*: 265–274.

55. Farrerons J, Rodriguez de la Serna A, Guanabens N et al. (1997). Sodium fluoride treatment is a major protector against vertebral and nonvertebral fractures when compared with other common treatments of osteoporosis:

56. Pak CYC, Sakhaee K, Rubin CD, Zerwkh JE (1997). Sustained release sodium fluoride in the management of established postmenopausal osteoporosis. *Am J Med Sci 313*: 23–32.

57. Ringe JD, Kipshoven C, Coster A, Umbach R (1999). Therapy of established postmenopausal osteoporosis with monofluorophosphate plus calcium: dose related effects on bone density and fracture rate. *Osteoporosis Int 9*: 171–178.

58. Pak CYC, Sakhaee K, Adams-Hue B et al. (1995). Treatment of postmenopausal osteoporosis with slow-release sodium fluoride. Final report of a randomized controlled trial. *Ann Intern Med 123*: 401–408.

59. Farley SM, Wergedal JE, Farley JR et al. (1992). Spinal fractures during fluoride therapy for osteoporosis: relationship to spinal bone density. *Osteoporosis Int 2*: 213–218.

60. Reginster JY, Meunmans L, Zegels B et al. (1997). Sodium monofluorophosphate reduces vetebral fractures in moderate postmenopausal osteoporosis. *J Bone Miner Res 12* (suppl 1): S104.

61. Alexandersen P, Hassager C, Sandholdt I, Riis B, Christiansen C (1997). Synergistic effect of hormone replacement (HRT) combined with monofluorophosphate (MFP) on bone mass in late postmenopausal women. *J Bone Miner Res 12* (suppl 1): S104.

62. Hodsman AB, Fraher LJ, Watson PH et al. (1997). A randomized controlled trial to compare the efficacy of cyclical parathyroid hormone versus cyclical parathyroid hormone and sequential calcitonin to improve bone mass in postmenopausal women with osteoporosis. *J Clin Endocrinol Metab 82*: 620–628.

63. Lindsay R, Nieves J, Formica C et al. (1997). Randomised controlled study of effect of parathyroid hormone on vertebral bone mass and fracture incidence among postmenopausal women on oestrogen with osteoporosis. *Lancet 350*: 550–555.

64. Lyritis GP, Androulakis C, Magiasis B, Charalambaki Z, Tsakalakos N (1994). Effect of nandrolone decanoate and 1α-hydroxycalciferol on patients with vertebral osteoporotic collapse: a double-blind clinical trial. *Bone Miner 27*: 209–217.

65. Gennari C, Agnus Dei D, Gonnelli S, Nardi P (1989). Effects of nandrolone decanoate therapy on bone mass and calcium metabolism in

women with established postmenopausal osteoporosis: a double-blind placebo-controlled study. *Maturitas 11*: 187–197.

66. Flicker L, Hopper JL, Larkins RG, Lichtenstein M, Buirski G, Wark JD (1997). Nandrolone decanoate and intranasal calcitonin as therapy in established osteoporosis. *Osteoporosis Int 7*: 29–35.

67. Cumming RC (1990). Calcium intake and bone mass: a quantitative review of the evidence. *Calcif Tissue Int 47*: 194–201.

68. Devine A, Dick IM, Heal SJ, Criddle RA, Prince RL (1997). A 4-year follow-up study of the effects of calcium supplementation on bone density in elderly postmenopausal women. *Osteoporosis Int 7*: 23–28.

69. Lips P, Graafmans WC, Ooms ME, Bezemer PD, Bouter LM (1996). Vitamin D supplementation and fracture incidence in elderly persons. *Ann Intern Med 124*: 400–406.

70. Reid IR, Ames RW, Evans MC, Gamble GD, Sharpe SJ (1995). Long-term effect of calcium supplementation on bone loss and fracture in postmenopausal women: a randomized controlled trial. *Am J Med 98*: 331–335.

71. Chapuy MC, Arlot MF, Duboeuf F et al. (1992). Vitamin D3 and calcium to prevent hip fractures in elderly women. *New Engl J Med 327*: 1637–1642.

72. Chapuy MC, Arlot ME, Delmas PD, Meunier PJ (1994). Effect of calcium and cholecalciferol treatment for three years on hip fractures in elderly women. *Br Med J 308*: 1081–1082.

73. Recker RR, Hinders S, Davies KM et al. (1996). Correcting calcium nutritional deficiency prevents spine fractures in elderly women. *J Bone Miner Res 11*: 1961–1966.

74. NIH Consensus Statement (1994). Optimal calcium intake. *NIH 12* (4).

75. Chapuy MC, Schott AM, Garnero P, Hans D, Delmas PD, Meunier PF and Epidos Study Group (1996). Healthy elderly French women living at home have secondary hyperparathyroidism and high bone turnover in winter. *J Clin Endocrinol Metab 81*: 1129–1133.

76. Chapuy MC, Preziosi O, Maamer M et al. (1997). Prevalence of vitamin D insufficiency in an adult normal population. *Osteoporosis Int 7*: 439–443.

77. Ooms ME, Lips P, Roos JC et al. (1995). Vitamin D status and SHBG: determinants of bone turnover and BMD in elderly women. *J Bone Miner Res 10*: 1177.

78. Grady D, Halloran B, Cummings S et al. (1991). 1,25-dihydroxyvitamin D3 and muscle strength in the elderly: a randomized controlled trial. *J Clin Endocrinol Metab 73*: 1111–1117.

79. Heikinheimo RJ, Inkovaara JA, Harju EJ et al. (1992). Annual injection of vitamin D and fractures of aged bones. *Calcif Tissue Int 51*: 105–110.

80. Dawson-Hughes B, Harris SS, Krall EA, Dallal GE, Falconer G, Green CL (1995). Rates of bone loss in postmenopausal women randomly assigned to one of two dosages of vitamin D. *Am J Clin Nutr 61*: 1140–1145.

81. Peacock M (1998). Effects of calcium and vitamin D insufficiency on the skeleton. *Osteoporosis Int 8* (suppl 2): S45–51.

82. Ranstan J, Kanis JA (1995). Influence of age and body mass on the effects of vitamin D on hip fracture risk. *Osteoporosis Int 5*: 450–454.

83. Dawson-Hughes B, Harris SS, Krall EA, Dallal GE (1997). Effect of calcium and vitamin D supplementation on bone density in men and women 65 years of age or older. *New Engl J Med 337*: 670–676.

84. Menczel J, Foldes J, Steinberg R et al. (1994). Alfacalcidol (alpha D3) and calcium in osteoporosis. *Clin Orthop Rel Res 300*: 241–247.

85. Fujita T, Orimo H, Inoue T et al. (1993). Double-blind multicenter comparative study of alfacalcidol with etidronate disodium (EHDP) in involutional osteoporosis. *Clin Eval 21*: 261–302.

86. Orimo H, Skiraki M, Hayashi T, Nakamura T (1987). Reduced occurrence of vertebral crush fractures in senile osteoporosis treated with 1α (OH) vitamin D. *Bone Miner 3*: 47–52.

87. Orimo H, Shiraki M, Hayashi Y et al. (1994). Effects of 1α-hydroxyvitamin D3 on lumbar bone mineral density and vetebral fractures in patients with postmenopausal osteoporosis. *Calcif Tissue Int 54*: 370–376.

88. Tilyard MW, Spears GFS, Thomson J, Dovey S (1992). Treatment of postmenopausal osteoporosis with calcitriol or calcium. *New Engl J Med 326*: 357–362.

89. Gallagher JC, Goldgar D (1990). Treatment of postmenopausal osteoporosis with high doses of synthetic calcitriol. *Ann Intern Med 113*: 649–655.

90. Ott SM, Chesnut CH (1989). Calcitriol is not effective in postmenopausal osteoporosis. *Ann Intern Med 110*: 267–274.

91. Falch JA, Odergaard OR, Finnanger AM,

Matheson I (1987). Postmenopausal osteoporosis: no effect of three years treatment with 1,25-dihy-droxycholecalciferol. *Acta Med Scand 221*: 199–204.

92. Meschia M, Brincat M, Barbacini P, Crossignani PG, Albisetti W (1993). A clinical trial and the effects of a combination of Elcatonin (carbocal-citonin) and conjugated estrogens on vertebral bone mass in early postmenopausal women. *Calcif Tissue Int 53*: 17–20.

93. Frediani B, Allegri A, Bisogno S, Mardolongo R (1998). Effects of combined treatment with cal-citriol plus alendronate on bone mass and bone turnover in postmenopausal osteoporosis – two years of continuous treatment. *Clin Drug Invest 15*: 235–244.

94. Eriksson SA, Lindgren JU (1993). Combined treatment with calcitonin and 1,25-dihydroxy-vitamin D3 for osteoporosis in women. *Calcif Tissue Int 53*: 26–28.

95. Geinoz G, Rapin CH, Rizzoli R et al. (1993). Relationship between bone mineral density and dietary intakes in the elderly. *Osteoporosis Int 3*: 242–248.

96. Paterson BM, Cornell CN, Carbone B, Levine B, Chapman D (1992). Protein depletion and metabolic stress in elderly patients who have a fracture of the hip. *J Bone Joint Surg 74A*: 251–260.

97. Bistrian BR, Blackburn GL, Vitale J, Cochran B, Naylor G (1976). Prevalence of malnutrition in general medical patients. *JAMA 235*: 1567–1570.

98. Sullivan DH, Moriarty MS, Chernoff R, Lipschitz DA (1989). Patterns of care: an analy-sis of the quality of nutritional care routinely provided to elderly hospitalized veterans. *J Parenter Enteral Nutr 13*: 249–254.

99. Morley JE (1986). Nutritional status of the elderly. *Am J Med 81*: 679–695.

100. Delmi M, Rapin CH, Bengoa JM et al. (1990). Dietary supplementation in elderly patients with fractured neck of the femur. *Lancet 335*: 1013.

101. Schürch MA, Rizzoli R, Vadas L, Slosman D,

Bonjour JP (1996). Protein supplements in elderly with a recent hip fracture increase serum IGF-1, decrease urinary deoxypiridino-line, and prevent proximal femur bone loss. *J Bone Miner Res 11* (suppl 1): S139.

102. Breslau NA, NcGuire JL, Zerweh JE, Pak C (1982). The role of dietary sodium on renal excretion and intestinal absorption of calcium and on vitamin D metabolism. *J Clin Endocrinol Metab 55*: 369.

103. Nordin BEC, Need AG, Morris HA, Horowitz M (1991). Sodium, calcium, and osteoporosis. In: *Nutritional Aspects of Osteoporosis* (Serono Symposia), eds P Burckhardt, RP Heaney, p. 279. Raven Press.

104. Holbrook TL, Barret-Connor E, Wingard DL (1998). Dietary calcium and risk of hip fracture: a 14 year prospective population study. *Lancet ii*: 1046.

105. Heaney RP, Recker RR, Stegman MR, Moy AJ (1989). Calcium absorption in women: relation-ships to calcium intake, estrogen status and age. *J Bone Miner Res 4*: 469.

106. Baran D, Sorensen A, Grimes et al. (1990). Dietary modification with dairy products for preventing vetebral bone loss in pre-menopausal women: a three-year prospective study. *J Clin Endocrinol Metab 70*: 264.

107. Chapuy MC, Chapuy P, Meunier PJ (1987). Calcium and vitamin D supplements: effects on calcium metabolism in the elderly. *Am J Clin Nutr 46*: 324.

108. Rosen CJ, Morrison T, Zhou H et al. (1994). Seasonal bone loss in elderly women from a rural New England community. *J Bone Miner Res 5*: 83.

109. Sinaki M, Mikkelsen BA (1984). Postmenopausal spinal osteoporosis: flexion versus extension exercises. *Arch Phys Med Rehabil 65*: 593–596.

110. Malmros B, Mortensen L, Jensen MB, Charles P (1998). Positive effects of physiotherapy on chronic pain and performance in osteoporosis. *Osteoporosis Int 8*: 215–221.

11

Corticosteroid-induced Osteoporosis

Ian Reid

Introduction • Pathogenesis • Effects on bone density • Identification of those at risk • Treatment • Choice of interventions

INTRODUCTION

Glucocorticoids were introduced into clinical practice nearly 50 years ago and have become pivotal to the management of a large number of conditions. They are life-saving in illnesses such as asthma, and substantially reduce morbidity in inflammatory conditions such as rheumatoid arthritis, temporal arteritis and inflammatory bowel disease. Despite the development of other immunomodulatory drugs, they still remain of substantial importance in organ transplantation.

Their therapeutic potential is limited to some extent by their high incidence of side-effects. With chronic use, one of the principal unwanted sequelae is the development of osteoporosis, and this was described within a few years of the introduction of these drugs to clinical practice in the 1950s. It should be emphasized, however, that this is only a problem with chronic steroid use. The use of these drugs, even in high doses, over a period of days to weeks will seldom result in clinically significant skeletal changes, and any bone loss produced is likely to be reversible as the patient returns to good health.

PATHOGENESIS

Because of the widespread distribution of the glucocorticoid receptor, these agents are able to impact on bone and calcium metabolism at many levels (see Figure 11.1). These effects have recently been reviewed in detail.[1]

Osteoblasts

The most consistently demonstrated effects of glucocorticoids on bone are on the osteoblast, whether studied *in vivo* or *in vitro*. Animal and human studies of bone histomorphometry demonstrate impaired bone formation. Both the rate of bone production within each bone modelling unit and the duration of activity of each unit are reduced.

In vitro, glucocorticoids have been characterized as modulating gene expression in osteoblast precursor cells to produce a more differentiated phenotype, whereas in the mature osteoblast, cell proliferation and matrix synthesis are reduced by glucocorticoids. These effects may be biphasic with respect to both dose and time, inhibition of proliferation and

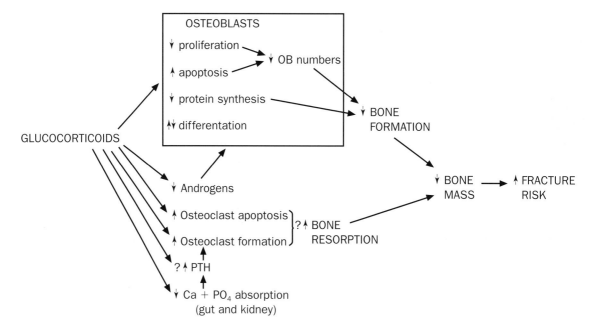

Figure 11.1 Mechanisms by which glucocorticoids result in bone loss. Copyright © 1998 IR Reid, used with permission.

synthetic activity predominating at high hormone concentrations and with long exposure periods. The differentiating effect may result from potentiation of the actions of bone morphogenic proteins, although it has recently been found that the glucocorticoids reduce expression of the transcription factor CBFal, which is intimately involved in the expression of the osteoblast phenotype. This appears to be linked to reduced expression of the TGFβ type I receptor and a resulting diminution of TGFβ-induced protein synthesis. There is also evidence for direct glucocorticoid regulation of a number of important osteoblastic genes (including those for type I collagen, osteocalcin, the insulin-like growth factors and their binding proteins) and for glucocorticoid stimulation of apoptosis in osteoblasts and osteocytes.

Osteoclasts

The effects of glucocorticoids on osteoclasts are contradictory. There is evidence that glucocorticoids increase osteoclast formation from precursor cells in bone marrow but also that they lead to apoptosis of mature osteoclasts. These opposing effects may account for the findings in organ culture that glucocorticoids can either increase or decrease bone resorption, depending on the culture conditions. In organ culture, glucocorticoid effects may be contributed to by their inhibition of production of local osteolytic cytokines such as interleukins-1 and -6, the tumour necrosis factors, and leukaemia inhibitory factor, and their stimulation of macrophage-colony stimulating factor production by osteoblasts.

Animal and human studies are also difficult to interpret, showing an increase in the eroded bone surface but a decrease in the number of osteoclasts. These findings could be accounted for by a reduced rate of recruitment of osteoblasts to the sites at which bone has been resorbed, leaving eroded surfaces unfilled for a greater time than normal. Thus, they do not necessarily imply increased rates of bone resorption. Most of the human studies of biochemical markers of bone resorption would be consistent with this conclusion.

Intestinal and renal handling of calcium and phosphate

Studies have consistently demonstrated an inhibition of calcium absorption associated with glucocorticoid treatment. This is not mediated by changes in vitamin D metabolites and is therefore likely to represent a direct effect on the calcium transport system in the small intestine.

Within weeks of glucocorticoid treatment there is a substantial rise in urine calcium excretion, which is not accounted for by changes in the serum ionized calcium or the glomerular filtration rate. This suggests that glucocorticoids directly regulate tubular resorption of calcium. There is also evidence for malabsorption of phosphate in both the gut and renal tubule associated with glucocorticoid use.

Vitamin D

There is little evidence to support the contention that changes in vitamin D metabolism contribute significantly to the development of steroid osteoporosis. Prospective studies of patients or normal subjects beginning steroid therapy have shown no changes in 25-hydroxyvitamin D or 24,25-dihydroxyvitamin D, but significant increases in 1,25-dihydroxyvitamin D have been observed 2–15 days after initiation of therapy. These are likely to be secondary to changes in parathyroid hormone and/or serum phosphate concentrations. There is no evidence for glucocorticoid effects on concentrations of vitamin D-binding protein.

Parathyroid hormone

A number of groups have found increases in circulating concentrations of parathyroid hormone within minutes to weeks of the initiation of steroid therapy, although this has not been universal. The same heterogeneity of findings occurs in cross-sectional studies of patients receiving chronic glucocorticoid therapy, some showing elevations of parathyroid hormone levels of 50–100% above those of control subjects, but others not. *In vitro* studies of parathyroid tissue from rats, cattle and humans suggest that glucocorticoids directly stimulate parathyroid hormone secretion, although *in vivo* it is possible that calcium malabsorption in both the gut and the renal tubule also contribute. There is also evidence that osteoblast sensitivity to parathyroid hormone is increased after glucocorticoid treatment, possibly as a result of increased G-protein expression.

Sex hormones

Sex hormones are important regulators of bone metabolism, and hypogonadism in either sex is associated with the development of osteoporosis. Glucocorticoids acutely depress plasma levels of testosterone in men, and their chronic use is associated with a dose-dependent reduction in free testosterone concentrations of approximately 50%. These changes appear to result from inhibition of gonadotropin secretion and a reduction in numbers of gonadotropin-binding sites in the testis. High-dose steroid therapy is associated with oligomenorrhoea in women, suggesting a similar effect on the pituitary–gonadal axis.

EFFECTS ON BONE DENSITY

Bone loss is evident within months of the start of steroid therapy. Laan et al.[2] demonstrated an

---

Table 11.1 Medical conditions associated with osteoporosis.

Hypogonadism	**Chronic inflammation**
Athletic amenorrhoea	Rheumatoid arthritis
Haemochromatosis	Inflammatory bowel disease
Turner's syndrome	Cystic fibrosis
Klinefelter's syndrome	**Bone marrow disorders**
Post-chemotherapy	Multiple myeloma
Hypopituitarism	Mastocytosis
Low body weight	Leukaemia
Anorexia nervosa	**Immobilization**
Type 1 diabetes mellitus	Parkinson's disease
Malabsorption	Poliomyelitis
Coeliac disease	Cerebral palsy
Post-gastrectomy	Paraplegia
Liver disease	Ankylosing spondylitis
Total parenteral nutrition	**Drugs**
Connective tissue disorders	Glucocorticoids
Osteogenesis imperfecta	Alcohol
Marfan's syndrome	Caffeine
Homocystinuria	Medroxyprogesterone acetate
Endocrine disorders	Anti-convulsants
Cushing's syndrome	Methotrexate
Thyrotoxicosis	Heparin
?Hyperparathyroidism	Cyclosporin

---

average loss of 8% of trabecular bone density and 2% of cortical bone density in the lumbar spine over a 20-week period in response to treatment with a mean dose of prednisone of 7.5 mg/day. The rate of loss may be less subsequently, but is still greater than that of normal subjects, even after many years of steroid treatment. Continuing bone loss is particularly likely in subjects requiring more than 10 mg/day of prednisone. As a result, bone density in steroid-treated subjects studied cross-sectionally is related both to the duration of their steroid treatment and to the average dose of these drugs. It is also dependent on the factors that influence the patient's pretreatment density, such as sex, body weight and age. The condition for which glucocorticoids are prescribed may also contribute to bone loss. Many chronic inflammatory conditions are themselves associated with bone loss, possibly because cytokine release stimulates osteoclast activity. A summary of many of the conditions that are associated with osteopenia is provided in Table 11.1.

Cross-sectional studies of patients treated for periods of five years show that integral bone density of the lumbar spine and proximal femur is about 20% below control values. However, the more rapid loss of trabecular bone results in decrements approaching 40% when lumbar spine density is assessed by quantitative computed tomography (QCT) or by dual-energy X-ray absorptiometry (DXA) in the lateral projection. The more rapid loss in the vertebrae is probably a reflection of the greater surface-to-volume ratio of trabecular bone. Since bone remodelling takes place only at bone surfaces, this bone type responds more rapidly to either positive or negative changes in bone balance. This pattern of bone loss results in fractures predominantly in trabecular bone, particularly the vertebrae and ribs. These are found in about one-third of patients after 5–10 years of glucocorticoid treatment. The risk of hip fracture is also increased nearly threefold in patients taking glucocorticoids. Fracture risk is related to the duration of glucocorticoid use, age, body weight (inversely) and gender (female).

IDENTIFICATION OF THOSE AT RISK

Most individuals using glucocorticoid drugs in doses greater than the equivalent of prednisone 5 mg/day will experience bone loss and may be at risk of fractures. The clinical risk factors cited above are of some value in identifying such patients, but are only poorly correlated with bone density, which must therefore be measured directly.

Since vertebral bodies are a common site of bone loss and fracture, they are the logical place at which to measure bone density. Techniques that focus on the vertebral body and exclude the cortical bone of the posterior processes (such as lateral scanning or quantitative computed tomography) are likely to be more sensitive in detecting steroid-induced bone loss. When selecting a method of bone density measurement in an individual patient, however, other factors need to be considered. The presence of vertebral deformities, vertebral osteophytes or aortic calcification can artefactually elevate spinal bone density measurements.

Lateral scans of the vertebral bodies, particularly in the decubitus position, are significantly less precise than antero-posterior (AP) scans, and therefore are less satisfactory for showing changes in bone mass prospectively.

My own practice in assessing steroid-treated patients is first to measure spinal bone density in the AP projection. If this is clearly low, then I advise the patient to take prophylaxis against further bone loss, and I usually remeasure their AP spinal bone density one year later to assess progress. In the individual in whom the AP spinal bone density is in the lower part of the normal range, I also perform a lateral spine scan, and base my decision regarding intervention on this value. However, in these patients I monitor therapeutic response using the AP density measurement because of its much greater precision. In a patient whose AP spine bone density is in the upper part of the young normal range (in the absence of deformity or other artefacts) the lateral density will also be within the normal range in most individuals, making the additional performance of this measurement unnecessary.

In patients in whom there is marked osteophytosis or scoliosis of the spine, proximal femoral densitometry should be carried out. Ward's triangle is the most trabecular-rich part of the proximal femur, and generally shows the most marked reduction in steroid-treated patients; but, like the lateral spine scan, it has a low precision. It is therefore unsuitable for monitoring a patient longitudinally, and the femoral trochanter or the 'total femur' region are the most suitable for this purpose.

Ultrasound measurement at the heel has also been investigated as a method of assessing bone loss in steroid-treated patients. The data are very limited at the present time, but suggest that it is about as sensitive as the femur or AP spine scans by DXA. The calcaneus is likely to be a useful site for assessing steroid-induced bone loss, because it is rich in trabecular bone. Confirmation of these findings is required before ultrasound can be used in routine clinical practice for such assessments.

The development of biochemical markers of bone turnover has been substantially driven by the hope that these would be useful in assessing an individual's fracture risk. There is little convincing evidence that this is so in steroid-treated subjects, although the available data are few. Baseline levels of osteocalin and other markers, or their changes in the early months of therapy, have generally not been found to relate to subsequent bone loss in either adults or children receiving steroids. Recently, Pearce et al. reported a modest relationship between the change in serum osteocalin and that in bone density in men starting on glucocorticoids; but this was no more accurate in predicting bone loss than was the average steroid dose used.[3]

TREATMENT

Indications

A determination of the level of bone density at which intervention is appropriate is arbitrary, and depends to some extent on the cost and potential side-effects of the available interventions. In the absence of evidence on which to base guidelines, it is reasonable to follow the practice established in postmenopausal osteoporosis, and offer treatment to those whose bone density is more than 1–2 standard deviations below the young normal mean value. In an individual beginning steroid therapy, it can be predicted that their bone density will drop a further 1–2 standard deviations below its current level in the first year of treatment, and this should be factored into the decision-making process. A past history of fracture after minimal trauma is also a major reason for weighting the balance in favour of intervention, since it implies that the individual's skeleton is already of marginal adequacy to withstand the trauma of daily living.

Available therapies

The general measures that would be considered in all osteoporotic patients (mobilization, attention to nutrition, cessation of smoking, moderation of alcohol intake) are also appropriate in those receiving steroids, whatever their bone density. In those with low bone density as defined above, pharmacological intervention is usually also necessary.

Calcium

Calcium and vitamin D have been used for several decades as an empiric therapy for osteoporosis of various aetiologies. Their use together is not necessarily logical, and the performance of trials using combinations of various doses of the two agents leaves unanswered the question as to whether any beneficial effects come from the one or the other, or from their combination. This problem should be borne in mind as the data are reviewed.

There is extensive observational data on the effect of calcium supplementation on steroid-induced bone loss, in that the 'control' groups in trials of most other agents have been given calcium.[4,5] The conclusion from these studies is that calcium alone does not completely prevent bone loss. However, it probably does have some effect, since it reduces biochemical indices of bone resorption.[6] Nilsen et al.[7] conducted a small trial in which hydroxyapatite appeared to slow forearm bone loss. More recently, Buckley et al. have reported a study in patients with rheumatoid arthritis receiving low-dose prednisone, who were randomized to receive placebo or calcium 500 mg/day plus vitamin D 500 IU/day.[8] Although the vitamin D status of these subjects was not assessed, vitamin D deficiency is apparently uncommon in the population from which they were drawn. This study demonstrated a 2% difference between the groups in the rate of bone loss, those receiving calcium and vitamin D showing more positive changes than those receiving placebo. In the absence of vitamin D deficiency, it is likely that the calcium supplement was the greatest contributor to this therapeutic effect.

Until further data are available it seems reasonable to provide calcium supplementation to those whose dietary intake is less than 1–1.5 g/day, and in whom there are no contraindications, such as a history of renal calculi. The major source of dietary calcium is dairy products, and an average serving contributes 200–250 mg of calcium.

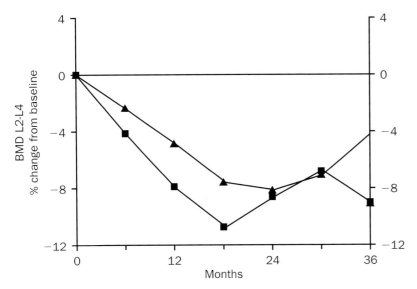

Figure 11.2 The effects of vitamin D 50 000 units/week plus calcium 1000 mg/day (triangles) compared with those of placebo in the prevention of corticosteroid-induced osteoporosis. There was no difference between the treatments in this randomized controlled trial of 62 subjects. From Adachi et al. (1996), *J Rheumatol 23*: 995,[10] used with permission.

Vitamin D

The role of vitamin D is also unresolved. There is increasing awareness of the high prevalence of vitamin D deficiency in the frail elderly population, and this is also likely to be present in frail steroid-treated patients who seldom go outdoors. Therefore, assessment of vitamin D status by a measurement of serum 25-hydroxy-vitamin D and correction with vitamin D itself (calciferol 500–1000 IU/day or 20 000–50 000 IU/month or 300 000–500 000 IU annually) is appropriate for steroid-treated patients at risk. The annual dose regimen can be administered orally or parenterally.

The case for using supraphysiological doses of calciferol with a view to increasing intestinal calcium absorption is much less persuasive, both on theoretical and practical grounds. High doses of vitamin D are likely to increase bone resorption as well as intestinal calcium absorption, thus potentially increasing bone loss as well as placing the patient at risk of hypercalcaemia. Hahn and Hahn demonstrated significant increases in forearm bone density from the use of calciferol 50 000 units three times per week plus calcium 500 mg/day.[9] However, the

recent randomized controlled trial reported by Adachi et al.[10] failed to show any benefit on lumbar spine density from the use of calciferol 50 000 IU/week plus calcium 1000 mg/day (Figure 11.2). Thus, vitamin D is probably best restricted to the treatment of demonstrable vitamin D deficiency (25-hydroxyvitamin D concentrations at or below the lower limit of normal).

Vitamin D metabolites

Metabolites of vitamin D have also been studied. Two small studies have demonstrated benefit from the use of 25-hydroxyvitamin D, but this agent is not widely available.[11,12] Since much of a dose of calciferol is converted to 25-hydroxyvitamin D, it is not clear that the effects of these two agents would be expected to be different.

Calcitriol has been assessed in two randomized controlled trials. Dykman et al.[13] found no difference between calcitriol 0.5 mcg/day and placebo in their effects on forearm bone density. Sambrook et al.[5] have reported a large study in which patients beginning glucocorticoid therapy were randomly assigned to receive calcium, calcium plus calcitriol (mean dose 0.6 mcg/day) or these two agents combined with calcitonin over a twelve-month period. Bone loss from the lumbar spine was 4.3%, 1.3% and 0.2% in the respective groups. There was a similar, non-significant trend in distal radial bone loss, but no evidence whatsoever of reduced bone loss in the proximal femur (3% in all groups). Other studies with potent vitamin D analogues have been reported by Braun et al., who demonstrated a beneficial effect of alpha-calcidol (2 mcg/day) on trabecular bone volume over a six-month period, and by Bijlsma who, in a 2-year study, failed to show any benefit from the use of dihydrotachysterol.

The relatively small number of studies with each agent and the variability of their outcomes make it difficult to determine the optimal course with respect to the vitamin D metabolites in the prevention of steroid osteoporosis. They do not have a major role as a monotherapy, since other classes of drugs, such as the bisphosphonates, produce more consistently positive outcomes in trials. The present author tends to use them as adjunctive therapy to either sex hormone replacement or bisphosphonates in the patient with severe steroid osteoporosis, or as a second-line therapy in patients for whom these other agents are not acceptable. Suitable preparations for this role are calcitriol 0.25 mcg twice daily or alfacalcidol 2 mcg daily.

Bisphosphonates

Bisphosphonates are an attractive therapy for steroid osteoporosis, offering the potential to redress directly the imbalance between bone formation and resorption. They can be used in virtually all steroid-treated patients, including the young and sex hormone-replete. The bisphosphonate nucleus consists of two phosphate groups joined through a central carbon atom, the individual members of the group differing only in the side-groups attached to that carbon atom. The clinically relevant difference between individual bisphosphonates is their anti-resorptive potency, though most of the newer agents appear to achieve a comparable maximal inhibition of bone resorption.

Pamidronate

The bisphosphonates are now becoming widely used in the management of postmenopausal osteoporosis, but their efficacy was first demonstrated in the treatment of steroid osteoporosis.[4] In this randomized controlled trial, there was a 19% increase in the density of the trabecular bone of the lumbar spine after twelve months' treatment with pamidronate, in comparison with a 9% decrease in those receiving placebo. There were smaller but statistically significant benefits in the cortical bone mass of the metacarpals. In those patients proceeding to a second year of therapy, the gains in bone density were maintained, whereas there was progressive loss in the placebo group. Oral pamidronate is not widely available, but three monthly intravenous infusions in a dose of 30 mg given over 30 mins in 250 ml normal saline appear to be comparably effective.[14,15]

Etidronate

There are a number of studies showing that cyclic etidronate is an effective therapy in steroid-treated subjects, and this treatment has high patient acceptability, since medication is only taken for two weeks every three months (400 mg daily for 2 weeks followed by calcium citrate 500 mg daily for 11 weeks). A large randomized controlled trial of etidronate has now been reported[16] and has demonstrated prevention of bone loss in both the lumbar spine and proximal femur in patients recently started on steroid treatment (Figure 11.3). Furthermore, it suggested that etidronate reduced fracture rates by 50% and that height loss was also diminished.

Alendronate

A similar trial of alendronate has recently been reported (Figure 11.4).[17] This study included those already long established on steroid treatment as well as those just commencing therapy, and again demonstrated beneficial effects on bone density throughout the skeleton for doses of 5 mg/day and 10 mg/day, though the higher dose tended to be more effective. Benefit was seen in men, premenopausal women, and post-menopausal women, whether or not receiving

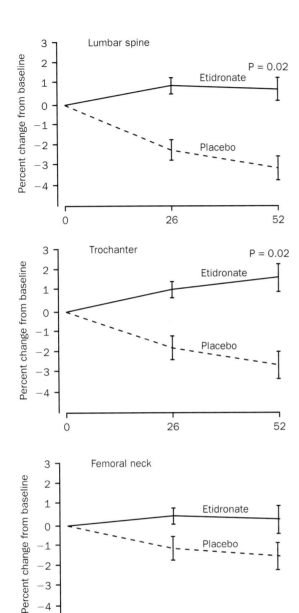

Figure 11.3 Effects of cyclical etidronate or placebo on bone density of subjects recently having begun glucocorticoid treatment. *P* values indicate significance of differences between treatment groups. From Adachi et al. (1997), *New Engl J Med 337*: 382,[16] used with permission.

hormone replacement therapy. Gain in bone mass occurred irrespective of the duration of previous steroid use. Vertebral fracture rates were reduced by about half in those on alendronate, though this was only statistically significant among the postmenopausal women. Two further studies have demonstrated the effectiveness of alendronate in steroid-treated patients with sarcoidosis[18] and in patients with Cushing's syndrome.[19]

All bisphosphonates are very insoluble, and therefore have a low oral bioavailability. To achieve benefit from oral dosing, they must be taken fasting with water at least 30 minutes before food, and separated by some hours from the ingestion of mineral supplements (such as calcium or iron) or antacids. Rarely, they cause gastrointestinal irritation, alendronate being associated with oesophageal erosions (in those with gastro-oesophageal reflux) and etidronate with diarrhoea. Of the various agents investigated to date, the bisphosphonates have produced the most consistently positive results on bone density in steroid-treated subjects, and the only evidence of reduced fracture rates.

Sex hormones

Oestrogen and testosterone are not thought to interfere specifically with the actions of glucocorticoids. Thus, their use is not advocated as glucocorticoid antagonists, but rather as a treatment for any co-existing sex hormone deficiency, with a view to correcting this additional risk factor for bone loss (Chapter 8). In premenopausal women menstruating regularly, sex hormone replacement does not have a place. In postmenopausal women on steroids, the increases in bone density following the institution of conventional hormone replacement therapy are at least as large as those that occur in other postmenopausal women.[20,21] Thus increases in lumbar spine bone density of more than 5% are seen in the first year of treatment. These changes are at least as great as those seen with potent bisphosphonates in postmenopausal women. There is also some evidence that sex hormone replacement improves control of rheumatoid arthritis,[21] one of the conditions for which glucocorticoids are commonly prescribed.

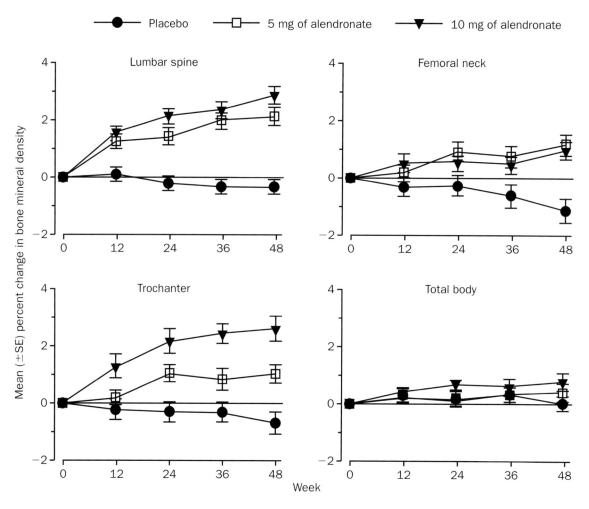

Figure 11.4 Effects of alendronate or placebo on bone density in steroid-treated subjects. Both active therapy groups were significantly different from placebo at 48 weeks at all sites except the total body, where only those receiving 10 mg/day showed significant benefit. From Saag et al. (1998), *New Engl J Med 339*: 292,[17] used with permission.

In steroid-treated men, circulating testosterone levels are reduced by almost one-half, a factor likely to contribute to the development of osteopenia. We have recently shown that testosterone replacement (250 mg testosterone esters per month) produces a 5% increase in lumbar spine bone mineral density after 12 months, as well as reversing the accumulation of body fat and loss of lean tissue that accompany steroid therapy.[22] In this study, mean serum testosterone concentrations had returned to baseline at the end of the one month inter-dose interval, suggesting that greater benefits may be possible with a more sustained normalization of circulating sex hormone levels. This might be achieved by administration of these depot preparations at 2–3 week intervals, or by the use of transdermal delivery systems. In some steroid-treated men, testosterone replacement is associated with a significant increase in well-being.

Anabolic steroids, which are androgens modified to reduce their virilizing effects, have also been used for treating steroid-induced osteoporosis. They would seem to have little place in the management of men, in whom they are likely to reduce testosterone levels further and in whom testosterone itself can be used if deficiency is demonstrable. Their use in women is associated with beneficial effects on bone mass but also with virilizing side-effects in almost one-half of treated patients. Of these adverse effects, deepening of the voice is of particular concern, since it is often irreversible.

A novel use of sex hormones in the treatment of steroid osteoporosis has been proposed by Grecu,[23] who utilized the ability of proges-terone to block the binding of glucocorticoids to their receptor. He showed that bone mass increased in steroid-treated men given medroxyprogesterone acetate. However, the use of such a non-specific glucocorticoid antag-onist would be expected to interfere with the therapeutic action of the glucocorticoid, thus defeating the purpose of giving the treatment in the first place. Continuous progestogen therapy should not be given to premenopausal women with steroid osteoporosis, since it results in oestrogen deficiency and bone loss.[24]

Fluoride
Fluoride ion is a potent osteoblast mitogen capable of producing sustained gains in lumbar spine bone density when used long term. This unique beneficial effect is counter-balanced by its interference with the normal mineralization of bone when present in bone crystal at high concentrations. These opposing effects have made it difficult to translate fluoride's beneficial effects on bone mass into reduced fracture inci-dence in postmenopausal osteoporosis. Work is continuing in that condition to define the thera-peutic window for its effective use. It is, in theory, an attractive agent for use in steroid osteoporosis, because its greatest effects are on trabecular bone, the site of greatest bone loss in steroid-treated subjects. There is now clear

evidence that it can increase spinal bone den-sity[25–28] and increase trabecular bone volume of the iliac crest[29] in steroid-treated subjects. However, its anti-fracture efficacy in this con-text remains to be established, and it should not be used as a first-line agent in steroid osteo-porosis. Its cautious use may be appropriate as an adjunctive therapy in patients with severe bone loss. A recent study by Lems et al.[30] has shown significant benefit from the addition of fluoride to cyclical etidronate in the treatment of patients with steroid osteoporosis. Fracture rates were not different between the groups, as would be expected in a trial with a total of only 47 participants. This combination should be used with care, since both fluoride and etidronate have the potential to cause osteoma-lacia and bone biopsies were not performed in this study.

Doses of sodium fluoride of 40–50 mg/day for up to 3–4 years are probably satisfactory, and are equivalent to 15–20 mg/day of fluoride ion.

Calcitonin
Calcitonin acts via specific receptors on osteo-clasts, reducing bone resorption. It has been used in some countries for the management of postmenopausal osteoporosis, although its effectiveness is generally less than that of hor-mone replacement therapy or the bisphospho-nates. There have now been several controlled trials in steroid-treated subjects suggesting that it slows bone loss. Thus, Rizzato[31] found that injections of salmon calcitonin (100 IU every 1–2 days) prevented bone loss over a fifteen-month period, whereas vertebral bone mass declined by 14% in the control group. Using a similar regimen, Luengo[32] found more modest differences between treatment groups – an increase in spinal bone density of 4% in those receiving calcitonin versus a decrease of 2.5% in the control group over a twelve-month period. Similar results using intranasal calcitonin have been reported by Montemurro et al.[33] and by Adachi et al.[34] In the latter study, 31 patients starting steroids for polymyalgia rheumatica were randomized to receive intranasal calci-tonin 200 IU daily or placebo over a 12-month

period. Mean spinal bone density changed from 1.11 g/cm^2 to 1.08 g/cm^2 in the placebo group and from 1.06 g/cm^2 to 1.04 g/cm^2 in those on calcitonin. These results are statistically different, but their clinical significance must be marginal. In the proximal femur, the between-groups trends were of similar magnitude but in the opposite direction, and in the total body scans the two groups responded identically. Thus, the clinical utility of intranasal calcitonin (200 IU/day) must remain in doubt, while calcitonin injections generally have a low acceptability to patients.

Thiazides

Thiazide diuretics have been advocated as therapy for both postmenopausal and steroid-induced osteoporosis. They clearly diminish urinary calcium loss in steroid-treated subjects,[35,36] and Yamada[37] has demonstrated that the addition of a thiazide to alphacalcidol and calcium leads to significantly more positive changes in bone mass in steroid-treated subjects. However, there are no other studies demonstrating a beneficial effect on bone density, and it is the present author's experience that thiazides frequently cause hypokalaemia in steroid-treated subjects, which means that their use requires close supervision, and sometimes the additional provision of potassium supplements.

Bone-sparing glucocorticoids

Deflazacort is a derivative of prednisone which has been suggested to exert less deleterious effects on calcium and bone metabolism than prednisone itself. Thus studies have demonstrated less marked hypercalciuria,[38,39] less effect on intestinal calcium absorption,[38] reduced bone loss[40–43] and less growth retardation in children treated with deflazacort.[44,45] However, all these studies were based on an assumption that the potency of prednisone relative to deflazacort was 1.2. Recently, there has been a re-examination of this question, with the finding that the relative potency is really 1.4 to 1.8.[46,47]

Thus much of the earlier literature may be invalid, because it has compared non-equivalent doses of the two agents. A recent study of bone density changes in patients with polymyalgia rheumatica in whom steroid doses were adjusted to produce symptom control also suggested that the glucocorticoid potency of deflazacort has been over-estimated in the past, and demonstrated no bone-sparing effect of this agent compared to prednisone when used in a therapeutically equivalent dose.[48]

CHOICE OF INTERVENTIONS

The above catalogue of available interventions should not produce the impression that there is a bewildering variety of therapeutic possibilities. Figure 11.5 sets out an approach to both the evaluation of a steroid-treated patient and the making of therapeutic decisions. Optimization of dietary and lifestyle variables is applicable to all subjects receiving steroids. In those whose bone density is at the lower end of the young normal range, intervention with a single agent is appropriate, usually sex hormone replacement (in those with demonstrable deficiency) or a bisphosphonate. Since the therapeutic efficacy of these agents is comparable, the choice is based on a consideration of the patient's other medical problems, possible side-effects, and cost. In a patient with marked bone loss, these agents can be combined with each other, and/or with other interventions such as calcitriol or fluoride. The use of such combination regimens results in substantial increases in bone density.

The availability of effective interventions in this condition places a responsibility on any prescriber of glucocorticoids to assess fracture risk and to provide prophylaxis against bone loss. The widespread adoption of this strategy will result in far fewer of those patients who are receiving glucocorticoids having to accept the morbidity of multiple fractures in addition to that of their other medical conditions.

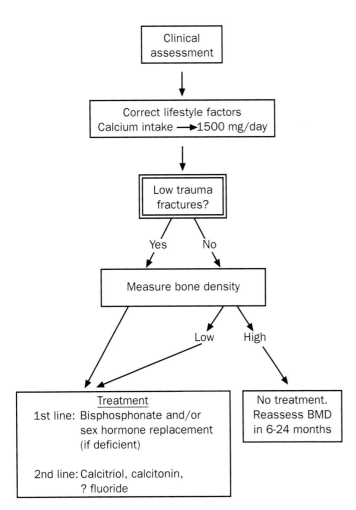

Figure 11.5 Flow chart for the evaluation and treatment of osteoporosis in patients receiving glucocorticoid therapy. Copyright © 1998 IR Reid, used with permission.

REFERENCES

1. Reid IR (1997). Glucocorticoid osteoporosis – mechanisms and management. *Eur J Endocrinol* 137: 209–217.
2. Laan RFJM, Vanriel PLCM, Vandeputte LBA et al. (1993). Low-dose prednisone induces rapid reversible axial bone loss in patients with rheumatoid arthritis – a randomized, controlled study. *Ann Intern Med* 119: 963–968.
3. Pearce G, Tabensky DA, Delmas PD et al. (1998). Corticosteroid-induced bone loss in men. *J Clin Endocrinol Metab 83*: 801–806.
4. Reid IR, King AR, Alexander CJ, Ibbertson HK (1988). Prevention of steroid-induced osteoporosis with (3-amino-1-hydroxypropylidene)-1,1-bisphosphonate (APD). *Lancet i*: 143–146.
5. Sambrook P, Birmingham J, Kelly P et al. (1993). Prevention of corticosteroid osteoporosis – a comparison of calcium, calcitriol, and calcitonin. *New Engl J Med 328*: 1747–1752.
6. Reid IR, Ibbertson HK (1986). Calcium supplements in the prevention of steroid-induced osteoporosis. *Am J Clin Nutr 44*: 287–290.
7. Nilsen KH, Jayson MIV, Dixon AStJ (1978). Microcrystalline calcium hydroxyapatite compound in corticosteroid-treated rheumatoid patients: a controlled study. *BMJ ii*: 1124.

8. Buckley LM, Leib ES, Cartularo KS et al. (1996). Calcium and vitamin D-3 supplementation prevents bone loss in the spine secondary to low-dose corticosteroids in patients with rheumatoid arthritis – a randomized, double-blind, placebo-controlled trial. *Ann Intern Med* 125: 961–968.

9. Hahn TJ, Hahn BH (1976). Osteopenia in patients with rheumatic diseases: principles of diagnosis and therapy. *Sem Arthritis Rheum* 6: 165–188.

10. Adachi JD, Bensen WG, Bianchi F et al. (1996). Vitamin D and calcium in the prevention of corticosteroid induced osteoporosis – a 3 year followup. *J Rheumatol* 23: 995–1000.

11. Hahn TJ, Halstead LR, Teitelbaum SL, Hahn BH (1979). Altered mineral metabolism in glucocorticoid-induced osteopenia. *J Clin Invest* 64: 655–665.

12. Di Munno O, Beghe F, Favini P et al. (1989). Prevention of glucocorticoid-induced osteopenia: effect of oral 25-hydroxyvitamin D and calcium. *Clin Rheumatol* 8: 202–207.

13. Dykman TR, Haralson KM, Gluck OS et al. (1984). Effect of oral 1,25-dihydroxy-vitamin D and calcium on glucocorticoid-induced osteopenia in patients with rheumatic diseases. *Arthritis Rheum* 27: 1336–1343.

14. Gallacher SJ, Fenner JAK, Anderson K et al. (1992). Intravenous pamidronate in the treatment of osteoporosis associated with corticosteroid dependent lung disease – an open pilot study. *Thorax* 47: 932–936.

15. Boutsen Y, Jamart J, Esselinckx W et al. (1997). Primary prevention of glucocorticoid-induced osteoporosis with intermittent intravenous pamidronate – a randomized trial. *Calcif Tissue Int* 61: 266–271.

16. Adachi JD, Bensen WG, Brown J et al. (1997). Intermittent etidronate therapy to prevent corticosteroid-induced osteoporosis. *New Engl J Med* 337: 382–387.

17. Saag KG for the Glucorticoid-induced Osteoporosis Intervention Study Group (1998). Alendronate for the prevention and treatment of glucocorticoid-induced osteoporosis. *New Engl J Med* 339: 292–299.

18. Gonnelli S, Rottoli P, Cepollaro C et al. (1997). Prevention of corticosteroid-induced osteoporosis with alendronate in sarcoid patients. *Calcif Tissue Int* 61: 382–385.

19. Di Somma C, Colao A, Pivonello R et al. (1998). Effectiveness of chronic treatment with alendronate in the osteoporosis of Cushing's disease. *Clin Endocrinol* 48: 655–662.

20. Grey AB, Cundy TF, Reid IR (1994). Continuous combined oestrogen/progestin therapy is well tolerated and increases bone density at the hip and spine in post-menopausal osteoporosis. *Clin Endocrinol* 40: 671–677.

21. MacDonald AG, Murphy EA, Capell HA et al. (1994). Effects of hormone replacement therapy in rheumatoid arthritis – a double blind placebo-controlled study. *Ann Rheum Dis* 53: 54–57.

22. Reid IR, Wattie DJ, Evans MC, Stapleton JP (1996). Testosterone therapy in glucocorticoid-treated men. *Arch Int Med* 156: 1173–1177.

23. Grecu EO, Weinshelbaum A, Simmons R (1990). Effective therapy of glucocorticoid-induced osteoporosis with medroxyprogesterone acetate. *Calcif Tissue Int* 46: 294–299.

24. Cundy T, Evans M, Roberts H et al. (1991). Reduced bone density in women using depot medroxyprogesterone acetate for contraception. *BMJ* 303: 13–16.

25. Bayley TA, Muller C, Harrison J (1990). The long-term treatment of steroid osteoporosis with fluoride. *J Bone Miner Res* 5(suppl 1): S157–S161.

26. Rizzoli R, Chevalley T, Slosman DO, Bonjour JP (1995). Sodium monofluorophosphate increases vertebral bone mineral density in patients with corticosteroid-induced osteoporosis. *Osteoporos Int* 5: 39–46.

27. Guaydier-Souquieres G, Kotzki PO, Sabatier JP et al. (1996). In corticosteroid-treated respiratory diseases, monofluorophosphate increases lumbar bone density – a double-masked randomized study. *Osteoporos Int* 6: 171–177.

28. Lems WF, Jacobs WG, Bijlsma JWJ et al. (1997). Effect of sodium fluoride on the prevention of corticosteroid-induced osteoporosis. *Osteoporos Int* 7: 575–582.

29. Meunier PJ, Briancon D, Chavassieux P et al. (1987). Treatment with fluoride: bone histomorphometric findings. In: *Osteoporosis 1987*, eds C Christiansen, JS Johansen, BJ Riis. Osteopress, Copenhagen.

30. Lems WF, Jacobs JWG, Bijlsma JWJ et al. (1997). Is addition of sodium fluoride to cyclical etidronate beneficial in the treatment of corticosteroid-induced osteoporosis? *Ann Rheum Dis* 56: 357–363.

31. Rizzato G, Tosi G, Schiraldi G et al. (1988). Bone protection with salmon calcitonin (sCT) in the long-term steroid therapy of chronic sarcoidosis. *Sarcoidosis* 5: 99–103.

32. Luengo M, Picado C, Del Rio L et al. (1990). Treatment of steroid-induced osteopenia with

calcitonin in corticosteroid-dependent asthma. A one-year follow-up study. *Am Rev Respir Dis 142*: 104–107.

33. Montemurro L, Schiraldi G, Fraioli P et al. (1991). Prevention of corticosteroid-induced osteoporosis with salmon calcitonin in sarcoid patients. *Calcif Tissue Int 49*: 71–76.

34. Adachi JD, Bensen WG, Bell MJ et al. (1997). Salmon calcitonin nasal spray in the prevention of corticosteroid-induced osteoporosis. *Br J Rheumatol 36*: 255–259.

35. Adams JS, Wahl TO, Lukert BP (1981). Effects of hydrochlorothiazide and dietary sodium restriction on calcium metabolism in corticosteroid-treated patients. *Metabolism 30*: 217–221.

36. Suzuki Y, Ichikawa Y, Saito E, Homma M (1983). Importance of increased urinary calcium excretion in the development of secondary hyperparathyroidism of patients under glucocorticoid therapy. *Metabolism 32*: 151–156.

37. Yamada H (1989). Long-term effect of 1 alpha-hydroxyvitamin D, calcium and thiazide administration on glucocorticoid-induced osteoporosis. *Nippon Naibunpi Gakkai Zasshi 65*: 603–614.

38. Caniggia A, Marchetti M, Gennari C et al. (1977). Effects of a new glucocorticoid, oxazacort, on some variables connected with bone metabolism in man: a comparison with prednisone. *Int J Clin Pharmacol 15*: 126–134.

39. Gray RE, Doherty SM, Galloway J et al. (1991). A double-blind study of deflazacort and prednisone in patients with chronic inflammatory disorders. *Arthritis Rheum 34*: 287–295.

40. Lo Cascio V, Bonnucci E, Imbimbo B et al. (1984). Bone loss after glucocorticoid therapy. *Calcif Tissue Int 36*: 435–438.

41. Gennari C, Imbimbo B (1985). Effects of prednisone and deflazacort on vertebral bone mass. *Calcif Tissue Int 37*: 592–593.

42. Loftus J, Allen R, Hesp J et al. (1991). Randomized, double-blind trial of deflazacort versus prednisone in juvenile chronic rheumatoid arthritis: a relatively bone-sparing effect of deflazacort. *Paediatrics 88*: 428–436.

43. Olgaard K, Storm T, Wowern NV et al. (1992). Glucocorticoid-induced osteoporosis in the lumbar spine, forearm and mandible of nephrotic patients. A double-blind study on the high-dose long-term effects of prednisone versus deflazacort. *Calcif Tissue Int 50*: 490–497.

44. Balsan S, Steru D, Bourdeau A et al. (1987). Effects of long-term maintenance therapy with a new glucocorticoid, deflazacort, on mineral metabolism and statural growth. *Calcif Tissue Int 40*: 303–309.

45. Aicardi G, Milani S, Imbimbo B et al. (1991). Comparison of growth-retarding effects induced by two different glucocorticoids in prepubertal sick children: an interim long-term analysis. *Calcif Tissue Int 48*: 283–287.

46. Dimunno O, Imbimbo B, Mazzantini M et al. (1995). Deflazacort versus methylprednisolone in polymyalgia rheumatica: clinical equivalence and relative antiinflammatory potency of different treatment regimens. *J Rheumatol 22*: 1492–1498.

47. Weisman MH (1993). Dose equivalency of deflazacort and prednisone in the treatment of steroid-dependent rheumatoid arthritis. In: *Proceedings of the 4th International Symposium on Osteoporosis*, eds C Christiansen, B Riis. 4th International Symposium on Osteoporosis, Copenhagen.

48. Krogsgaard MR, Thamsborg G, Lund B (1996). Changes in bone mass during low dose corticosteroid treatment in patients with polymyalgia rheumatica – a double blind, prospective comparison between prednisolone and deflazacort. *Ann Rheum Dis 55*: 143–146.

12

Osteoporosis in Men

Johann Ringe

Osteoporotic fractures in men • Diagnosis and classification • Prevention • Therapy
• Bone turnover modification

Osteoporosis has long been considered a disease of women. Only in the last few years has it become increasingly apparent that the incidence of osteoporosis in males has been significantly underestimated and that for them it is also an important public health issue.[1-5] There is no doubt however that the majority of clinical cases of osteoporosis will continue to present in females in the postmenopausal and senile phases of their life. In women oestrogen deficiency is the dominant pathogenetic mechanism, and in men hypogonadism is also important. However, a wide range of risk factors during childhood and adolescence may contribute to the development of low peak bone mass in both men and women, while others lead to increased bone loss during remodelling in adult life. It is recognized that the skeleton registers and sums up positive and negative influences on bone metabolism during our lifetime, and to some extent reflects the biography of an individual.[6]

On the basis of this multifactorial pathogenetic concept sex-hormone deficiency will be only *one* important risk factor. It has become clear that the proportion of secondary osteoporosis is much higher in men by comparison with women, with the consequence that important contributing risk factors may have been neglected because they have been overshadowed by the easy assumption of a dominant role for hypogonadism.

OSTEOPOROTIC FRACTURES IN MEN

The European Vertebral Osteoporosis Study (EVOS) has shown that 18% of males aged 50 and over has vertebral deformities. Although some of these may have been due to earlier occupational trauma it was estimated that about half the fractures might be osteoporosis-related.[3]

The sex ratio of hip fractures differs considerably between countries, and is influenced by ethnic and sociocultural factors.[7] In the industrialized countries men constitute 20 to 30% of the total hip fracture incidence.[4] There are no data available concerning the overall prevalence of symptomatic osteoporosis in males, but it is likely that it is of the order of about 10 to 15% of the total fracture population.

Several mechanisms have been proposed to explain the lower incidence of osteoporotic fractures in men.[5,8,9] As far as non-vertebral fractures in the elderly are concerned, the lower life expectancy of males compared to females is one important factor. Other mechanisms are related to differences in peak bone mass (PBM) and variations in the rate of bone remodelling in later life.

Men achieve a higher PBM in the appendicular skeleton, while the axial skeleton is not significantly different from that of females. On the other hand the larger size of the vertebrae and the larger cross-sectional area of the tubular bones contribute to a higher biomechanical strength.[9]

Another important factor is the lower rate of age-related bone loss as a percentage of PBM during remodelling. There is also evidence that the pattern of age-associated bone loss is different in males compared to females. Loss of trabecular bone in men occurs more as a result of thinning, rather than through perforation as occurs in women, with the result that connectivity is better preserved. Men appear to have a greater reduction in trabecular width with age, whereas women have a greater fall in the number of trabeculae. This may disproportionately reduce biomechanical strength in females.[10]

Cortical bone of men shows a lower rate of resorption with age, so that there is only a slight degree of intracortical porosity. Age-related endosteal resorption is also less in men, and with their lifelong periosteal bone apposition there is a continuously increasing bone diameter. There is therefore no reduction in tensile strength with age such as occurs in women.[4,11]

DIAGNOSIS AND CLASSIFICATION

Osteoporosis must be considered in the diagnosis of men with unexplained back pain, particularly if they have radiographic signs of low bone mass or risk factors for osteoporosis. The diagnosis may also be suspected in men with a history of fractures following apparently mild trauma who also show loss of height and kyphosis.

The clinical picture of established osteoporosis in men is not different from that in women, with kyphosis due to wedge-fractures of the thoracic vertebrae, protuberance of the abdomen and transverse skin folds over the dorsal trunk.

Figure 12.1 shows these typical changes in body shape in a 57-year-old man with severe established osteoporosis due to primary hypogonadism. He had lost both testes as a consequence of a war injury, and for 35 years had not been supplemented with androgens. The lateral radiograph of this patient (Figure 12.2)

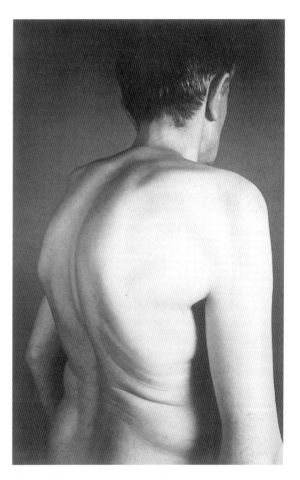

Figure 12.1 Kyphosis, loss of height and typical transverse skin folds in a 57-year-old man with established secondary osteoporosis due to hypogonadism.

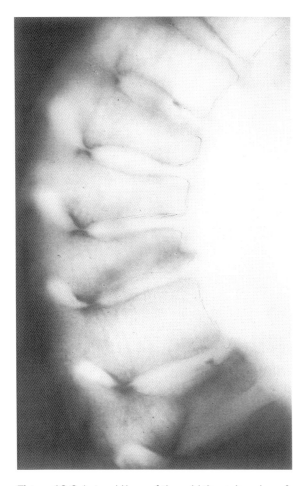

Figure 12.2 Lateral X-ray of the mid-thoracic spine of the patient in Figure 12.1. Advanced loss of cortical and trabecular bone with wedge fractures of T6, 7, 8 and 10.

shows an advanced loss of trabecular and cortical bone, with wedge-shape fractures of T6–8 and T10. In a study of 63 males with symptomatic vertebral fractures it was clearly shown that there is a considerable morbidity associated with this type of osteoporosis.[12]

In each case of suspected osteoporosis a thorough history and clinical examination, including routine radiology and laboratory tests, are indicated to exclude other localized or generalized bone pathology and to establish the diagnosis. Figure 12.3 gives a scheme for the diagnosis and pathogenetic classification of osteoporosis in men. Measurement of bone mineral density (BMD) is the next important step. A normal BMD excludes osteoporosis, and may lead to the diagnosis of an alternative focal bone disease. If a low BMD is detected then a review of the history, physical examination, specialist laboratory tests, and in most cases further radiography are required. In this way the various forms of primary and secondary osteoporosis can be identified and other types of osteopenic metabolic bone disease can be excluded.

As a guideline for practical management four diagnostic steps are recommended:

1. exclusion of other osteopenic bone diseases (such as osteomalacia and hyperparathyroidism);
2. quantitation of the degree of osteopenia (if possible, measurement of BMD at different sites, such as the lumbar spine and the proximal femur);
3. determination of the clinical stage of osteoporosis (Table 12.1); and
4. classification into primary or secondary osteoporosis.

It is essential that appropriate reference ranges and fracture risk-thresholds for BMD are established for men in the near future. In the meantime the clinical stage of male osteoporosis can be determined according to Table 12.1 on the basis of the BMD value and the presence or absence of vertebral fractures. For this clinical classification the WHO criteria established specifically for the diagnosis of osteoporosis in Caucasian women have been used.[13]

In our own unpublished study of 500 consecutive men with a mean age of 55 years and osteoporosis (excluding patients with stage 0) we found 38% with stage 1, 38% with stage 2, and 24% with stage 3.

In terms of the pathogenetic classification of male osteoporosis about 50 to 60% will be found to have an identifiable cause.[14-16] Secondary osteoporosis may be due either to a single pathogenetic factor or sometimes to a combination of causes.[12,17] The increased risk of bone loss attributable to combinations of risk

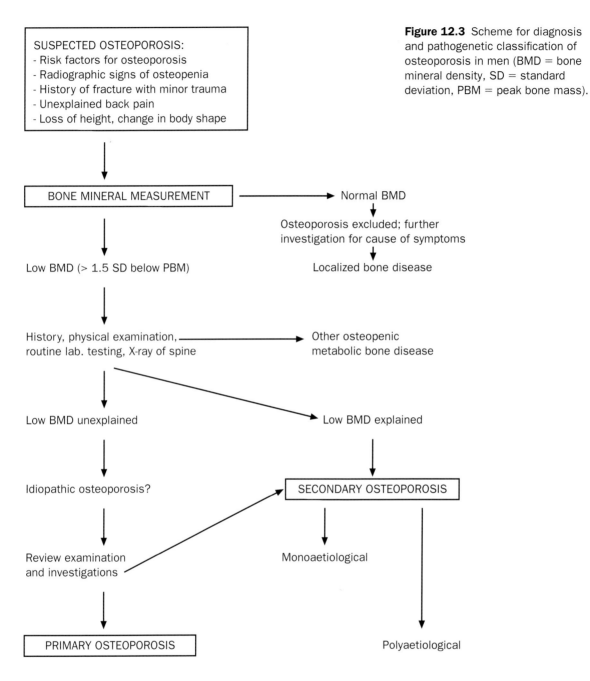

Figure 12.3 Scheme for diagnosis and pathogenetic classification of osteoporosis in men (BMD = bone mineral density, SD = standard deviation, PBM = peak bone mass).

factors is often neglected. For example, a Swedish group showed in a study of 129 partially gastrectomized men that low body mass index and smoking were major contributory risk factors for the low bone mass.[18]

In our own study of 500 males we found that 52% had primary and 48% secondary osteoporosis. Among the latter group we identified one subgroup of mono-aetiological ($n = 124$) and another of polyaetiological ($n = 116$) origin.

Table 12.1 Proposed stages for clinical classification of male osteoporosis (based on WHO densitometry thresholds).[13]

Clinical stage	Criteria
0 Osteopenia (preclinical disease)	— BMD T-score −1.0 to −2.5 SD — no vertebral fractures
1 Uncomplicated osteoporosis	— BMD T-score < −2.5 SD — no vertebral fractures
2 Osteoporosis	— BMD T-score < −2.5 SD — 1–3 vertebral fractures with minor trauma
3 Advanced osteoporosis	— multiple vertebral fractures — often non-vertebral fractures

In Table 12.2 the frequency of risk factors in the 240 males with secondary osteoporosis is shown in terms of mono- and polyaetiological subgroups. From this comparison it becomes obvious that some factors are 'strong' pathogenetic risks, leading to monoaetiological osteoporosis (for example, nos 1, 4, 5, 11, 15, and 21), while others are 'weak' risk factors that only cause osteoporosis when in combination (for example, nos 2, 3, 6–8, 10).

All these risk factors must be taken into consideration in the diagnosis and management of male osteoporosis. On the other hand BMD should be measured in men with one or more risk factors to achieve an early diagnosis and plan therapy.

PREVENTION

Emphasis must be placed on prevention of bone loss, because no therapeutic agent has yet been convincingly shown to be effective in preventing osteoporotic fractures in men (Table 12.3).[19] Early recognition of risk factors for osteoporosis is very important together with corresponding specific measures to counteract

or reduce the risk of bone loss. General preventive measures include regular exercise and maintenance of adequate calcium and vitamin D intake, with routine supplementation after the age of 70 years. This is based on a recent study which showed that supplementation with 1000 mg calcium and 800 IU vitamin D is capable of reducing the incidence of non-vertebral fractures in healthy men with a mean age of 70 years.[20]

Specific programmes for the prevention of falls and the selective use of hip protectors would be as likely to reduce the incidence of hip fractures in elderly men as they are in elderly women.

THERAPY

Most of the currently available studies of male osteoporosis have been of mixed male and female populations, and it is very difficult to disentangle the effects of the various treatments on men alone. Few trials have been performed in purely male populations, and those that are available have recruited rather small numbers of primary or secondary cases of male osteo-

Table 12.2 Frequency of risk factors in 240 males with secondary osteoporosis separated into mono- and polyaetiological subgroup (unpublished results from a total population of 500 males with osteoporosis).

Frequency of risk factors in 240 males with secondary osteoporosis	Total ($n = 240$)	Monoaetiological ($n = 123$)	Polyaetiological ($n = 117$)
1. Long-term GC-therapy	82	35	47
2. Chronic alcoholism	56	4	52
3. Heavy smoker	54	0	54
4. Hypogonadism	49	22	27
5. Idiopathic hypercalciuria	34	18	16
6. Chronic liver disease	19	1	18
7. Asthma (without GC)	17	1	16
8. Crohn's disease (without GC)	17	1	16
9. Gastric surgery	17	7	10
10. Anti-convulsant therapy	12	3	9
11. Multiple myeloma	11	10	1
12. Low calcium diet	10	1	9
13. Immobilization	10	1	9
14. Diabetes mellitus	7	0	7
15. Primary hyperparathyroidism	6	5	1
16. Thyrotoxicosis	4	0	4
17. Rheumatoid arthritis (without GC)	4	1	3
18. Thyroxine therapy	4	2	2
19. Heparin therapy	4	1	3
20. Familial osteoporosis	4	2	2
21. Mastocytosis	3	3	0
22. Hypophosphataemia	2	1	1
23. Lymphoproliferative disease	2	0	2
24. Cushing's disease	1	1	0
25. Cardiac transplantation	1	1	0
26. Bone marrow metastases	1	1	0
27. Osteogenesis imperfecta	1	1	0
28. Hypopituitarism	1	0	1
29. Coeliac disease	1	0	1

GC: Glucocorticoids.

Table 12.3 General measures for the prevention of osteoporotic fractures in men.

1. Long-term regular physical activity and exercise
2. Maintenance of adequate calcium and vitamin D intake throughout life by diet and/or supplementation (total intakes 1000–1500 mg calcium and 600–800 IU vitamin D)
3. Routine calcium/vitamin D supplementation after age 70 yrs
4. Limit alcohol intake and smoking
5. Recognize and treat testosterone deficiency
6. Identify other risk factors (Table 12.2) and consider specific prophylactic measures
7. Avoidance of falls and selective use of hip protection in elderly men

---

porosis by comparison with the large well-described studies in postmenopausal women.[21]

The current situation is that, unfortunately, therapy of osteoporosis in men is virtually unexplored.[22] This is reflected by the fact that in most countries there are no specific drugs approved for pharmacological intervention in male osteoporosis. Nevertheless, antiresorptive or other conventional therapy may be as useful in men as in women. Treatment specific to the underlying pathological condition may further stabilize or increase bone mass and reduce future fracture risk.

Practical management

A practical scheme for the treatment of male osteoporosis is summarized in Table 12.4. As in women, an optimal calcium and vitamin D intake is recommended as basic therapy and this should be achieved either through diet or supplementation to provide 1000–1500 mg calcium/day and 600–800 IU vitamin D/day. There is, however, no unequivocal evidence that calcium and vitamin D supplementation can reduce bone loss in men. In a three-year randomized study of healthy men, calcium and vitamin D did not alter the rate of bone loss at either the wrist or the spine.[23] In another recent

study of 176 men over the age of 65 years, however, supplementation with 500 mg calcium/day and 700 IU vitamin D/day for three years was followed by small increases of BMD at the lumbar spine and femoral neck (0.9% and 1.2% respectively) and a significant decrease in non-vertebral fractures.[20]

Another important aspect of basic therapy is to avoid lifestyle-related risk factors (poor nutrition or physical activity, and excessive alcohol or nicotine consumption).

In men with established osteoporosis complaining of back pain with a corresponding reduction in mobility, an individually tailored analgesic regimen is very important. The vicious cycle of pain, immobilization and osteopenia is an important mechanism leading to worsening of osteoporosis. Some physicians still prescribe several weeks of bed rest after a new osteoporotic fracture, as is usually the case after traumatic vertebral fractures with the risk of spinal cord damage. In osteoporosis this risk does not exist and patients should receive adequate doses of NSAIDs or centrally acting analgesics, together with a programme of physiotherapy and early mobilization.

The main aim of therapy is to avoid first fractures in stage 1 or further fractures in stages 2 and 3 osteoporosis (Table 12.1). To achieve this goal a specific long-term therapeutic strategy

---

Table 12.4 Practical management of osteoporosis in men: treatment options.

1. Correction of aetiological factors in secondary osteoporosis:
   — testosterone in hypogonadism
   — thiazides in hypercalciuria
   — reduction of glucocorticoid dosage

2. Assess activity of osteoporotic process:
   — clinical progression (bone pain, new fractures)
   — biochemical markers of bone turnover

3. Analgesia:
   — adequate pain relief
   — physiotherapy in symptomatic osteoporosis

4. Strategy:
   — quality of life, life expectancy
   — previous treatment: compliance, effectiveness, adverse events

5. Assess severity of osteoporosis:
   — bone mineral density
   — number and sites of fractures

6. Basic therapy:
   — calcium and vitamin D supplementation
   — measures to counteract identified risk factors

7. Modification of bone turnover
   — antiresorptive therapy (bisphosphonates, calcitonin, vitamin D-metabolites)
   — anabolic agents (fluoride, testosterone, parathyroid hormone)

---

has to be started to prevent further bone loss and increase bone mass. This scheme of treatment should be designed on the basis of incorporating all the risk factor and lifestyle information supplied by the patient (Table 12.4). In addition to basic therapy, analgesia, and, if possible, correction of aetiological factors, a choice has to be made between an antiresorptive and an anabolic agent.[6]

There are no controlled studies in the literature that have tested combinations of antiresorptive and anabolic drugs in men. In hypogonadal men with histologically proven low bone turnover, therapy based on the ADFR concept (Activate, Depress, Free, Repeat) that utilized inorganic phosphorus and salmon calcitonin showed dramatic increments in BMD over the 68-month period of therapy, without further fractures.[24] In a pilot study treating male patients with severe established osteoporosis, a cyclical regimen using a two-week course of etidronate (400 mg) followed by 76 days of 156 mg monofluorophosphate (MFP), with 1000 mg calcium and 800 IU vitamin D has shown very positive preliminary interim results (Ringe: unpublished). Results from a comparable study using combination treatment of etidronate, fluoride, calcium and vitamin D in men have only been reported in a German-language abstract.[25]

Treatment of the cause of secondary osteoporosis

Since about 50% of men have secondary osteoporosis it is very important to diagnose and treat the underlying cause whenever possible.

The most important aetiological therapy in male osteoporosis is testosterone replacement in proven primary or secondary hypogonadism. Testosterone therapy in hypogonadal men rapidly increases circulating 1,25-dihydroxyvitamin D and corrects calcium malabsorption leading to an improvement in calcium balance and an increase in bone formation.[26] In a histomorphometric case study it was shown that relative osteoid volume, total osteoid surface, linear bone apposition rate and bone mineralization are all increased by testosterone therapy,[27] confirming that androgens have a definite anabolic effect. In another case report of male hypogonadism, resorptive hypercalciuria and increased interleukin 1 concentrations were corrected with androgen therapy.[28] In two small trials, testosterone significantly increased spinal BMD in hypogonadal men over periods of 3–12 months.[29,30] The effect was most marked in younger men with open epiphyses compared to older men with closed epiphyses. This treatment is currently only appropriate for use in specialist centres. The most suitable preparations are either an injection of testosterone enanthate 250 mg every 2–3 weeks or application as testosterone patch (e.g. Andropatch, Androderm 2.5 mg/day).

Idiopathic hypercalciuria, another frequent cause of secondary male osteoporosis, should be treated with thiazide diuretics (e.g. bendrofluazide 2.5–5.0 mg daily), although data from controlled prospective trials are not available. However, a bone-sparing effect of long-term use of thiazides was documented in several studies in women.[31,32] In glucocorticoid-induced osteoporosis (GIOP) steroid withdrawal or dose reduction may be followed by a spontaneous increase in bone density,[33] particularly in younger patients. Depending on the response of BMD, specific treatment with bisphosphonates, active vitamin D metabolites or fluoride may be indicated in the individual case to increase BMD further. A recent prospective controlled study with etidronate in GIOP showed a significant increase in BMD with bisphosphonate treatment in a subgroup of 54 males.[34] A suitable treatment regimen would be cyclical etidronate 400 mg daily for 14 days followed by 76 days calcium citrate (500 mg daily).

For many types of secondary osteoporosis the potential efficacy of aetiological therapies is only known from isolated case reports. Interesting examples are the beneficial effect of interferon alpha-2b in a 33-year-old man with severe osteoporosis due to systemic mast cell disease[35] or the case of a 55-year-old man with Whipple's disease and decreased bone mass, which was reversible only by antibiotic treatment.[36]

After successful surgery for primary hyperparathyroidism a significant increase in BMD can be expected.[37] This is not always the case, and in a 49-year-old man who was not given specific medical treatment we found no significant change of BMD at the lumbar spine and proximal femur one year after parathyroidectomy. On the assumption that in this situation low bone turnover was present, therapy with MFP (152 mg/day – 20 mg fluoride ion) and 1000 mg calcium was commenced. Table 12.5 shows the change in BMD at the spine and hip over four years. Anabolic therapy was very effective in restoring bone mass despite the very low BMD at baseline. The patient had not suffered vertebral fractures (stage 1) and experienced no fractures during the study.

In most cases of secondary osteoporosis aetiological therapy alone will be insufficient to increase BMD above the fracture threshold. In this situation additional treatment to modify bone turnover is indicated. All the drugs and hormones used in women (except for oestrogen) can be used, and the choice should be made on the basis of individual aetiological factors (Table 12.2).

Table 12.5 Change in BMD at the lumbar spine and femoral neck in a 49-year-old man with secondary osteoporosis which was not improved by surgical correction of primary hyperparathyroidism. Response to therapy with monofluorophosphate (MFP) and calcium.

| | L2–4 | | Femoral neck | |
	g/cm	T-score	g/cm	T-score
Pre-operative	0.738	−4.27	0.785	−2.37
1 year post-operative	0.743	−4.22	0.796	−2.29
1 year after MFP/Ca	0.793	−3.79	0.845	−1.87
2 years after MFP/Ca	0.944	−2.47	0.875	−1.62
3 years after MFP/Ca	0.965	−2.29	0.935	−1.13
Total increase after 3 years of therapy	0.222	1.92	0.139	1.14

BONE TURNOVER MODIFICATION

Antiresorptive treatment

Calcitonin
Calcitonin, the classic antiresorptive drug, has not been studied in a purely male patient population. In a study of GIOP in which 40% of the patients were men, calcitonin (200 IU/day), given as a nasal spray, stabilized BMD over 2 years, resulting in a 1% increase compared with a 1.5% fall in a retrospective control group.[38] In a 1-year study of patients with osteoporosis after liver transplantation (10 men, 7 women) calcitonin injections (100 IU/day) or intermittent cyclical etidronate (400 mg daily for 14 days) produced similar increases in spinal BMD of 6.4% and 8.2% respectively.[39]

Bisphosphonates
With respect to the potent antiresorptive bisphosphonates, data in men are currently only available for etidronate. In an uncontrolled study of 42 men (mean age 60.5 years) with established idiopathic osteoporosis (stages 2

and 3) 14-day cycles of oral etidronate (400 mg daily) followed by 76 days of oral calcium (500 mg daily) were repeated over an average period of 31 months. This resulted in an average annual gain in BMD of 3.2% at the lumbar spine compared to baseline, with a small, non-significant improvement at the femoral neck.[40] Comparable results were obtained in a study from Belgium of 21 men with idiopathic osteoporosis.[41] After 2 years of treatment with intermittent cyclical etidronate (as above), increases of 7.3% at the spine and 2.4% at the femoral neck were observed. Both studies were too small to show any effect on the incidence of vertebral fractures.

In an interesting case report of a 68-year-old man with severe established osteoporosis associated with pernicious anaemia, a marked improvement was observed after combined therapy with vitamin B12 and cyclical etidronate.[42] Although vitamin B12 is important for osteoblastic function, the effect on bone density and fracture incidence of replacement of the vitamin in states of deficiency is unknown.

A large multicentre study examining the efficacy of alendronate (10 mg daily) in idiopathic male osteoporosis is currently in progress. Preliminary results from a prospective controlled study of 112 men with primary osteoporosis of our own already show very impressive increases in BMD at the lumbar spine (+7.7%) and proximal femur (+3.2%) at 12 months.

In GIOP, a study of 76 men and 156 women given alendronate 5 or 10 mg daily compared to placebo showed significant gains of BMD at the spine (+2.8%) and trochanter (+1.8%) for both sexes with the 10 mg dosage.[43] It seems likely that in the future the bisphosphonates will probably be the most important agents for the treatment of osteoporosis in men.

Anabolic treatment

Parathyroid and growth hormones

The use of parathyroid hormone (PTH) for osteoporosis remains controversial. The potential of this peptide significantly to increase trabecular bone volume appears to be similar in men and women,[44] but there is concern about possible loss of cortical bone. A small trial in men with idiopathic osteoporosis showed significant increases in trabecular bone density with the combination of PTH and 1,25-dihydroxyvitamin D.[45]

The use of growth hormone (GH) as an osteoanabolic agent is even more experimental at the present time. The hormone increases bone turnover in elderly men and women, as shown by rapid increases in biochemical markers.[46] In a randomized controlled study in elderly men, a six-months' course of GH raised IGF-1 levels to within the normal range for young men and led to a 1.6% gain in lumbar spine BMD.[47]

Fluoride

Fluoride is known to be a potent stimulator of new bone formation.[48] It is recognized that high doses (30 mg or more of fluoride ion per day) can induce a very rapid increase in axial bone density, but at the expense of peripheral bone, without increasing the mechanical strength of the vertebrae.[49,50] There is now increasing evidence that doses of NaF or MFP corresponding to 15–20 mg fluoride ion per day lead to moderate increases in BMD and a reduced fracture rate.[51,52]

In a randomized controlled study of 64 males with generalized idiopathic osteoporosis without prevalent vertebral fractures (stage 1) low-dose MFP resulted in a gain in BMD and a reduced fracture rate.[53] In a three-year study patients received either 114 mg MFP (15 mg fluoride ion) for 3 months on and 1 month off, plus 1000 mg calcium daily or 1000 mg calcium alone (control). The average changes in BMD at the lumbar spine, mid-radius, and femoral neck are shown in Figure 12.4. The mean annual changes in BMD at all six sites are shown in Table 12.6. The total increase of 9% at the lumbar spine at 3 years is small in comparison to other studies, where this gain was achieved within one year.[49] However, there was a highly significant reduction in the incidence of new vertebral fractures after three years, with 4 fractures in 3 patients in the MFP/Ca group and 17 fractures in 12 patients in the calcium-alone group. The findings indicate that intermittent low-dose MFP treatment combined with continuous calcium supplementation can significantly strengthen both cancellous and (to a lesser extent) cortical bone in men with early idiopathic osteoporosis. MFP can therefore reduce the risk of developing established disease, with its attendant increased risk of vertebral fracture.[49] A practical approach would be to give 15 mg bioavailable fluoride ion/day and continue for 3–4 years.

In several small studies on mixed patient groups with GIOP, fluoride produced positive effects on bone density.[48] In men after cardiac transplantation MFP/Ca therapy was also able to restore their low BMD to normal.[54]

Androgens

Androgens have both anabolic and antiresorptive effects.[26,27,29,55] The important role of testosterone replacement in the treatment of secondary osteoporosis in men has already been discussed. The possible role of androgen therapy in eugonadal men with idiopathic

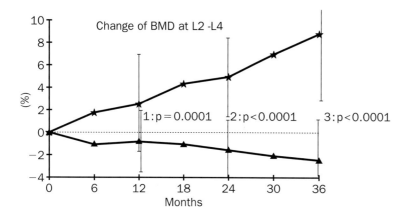

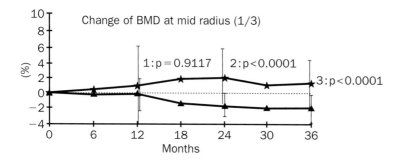

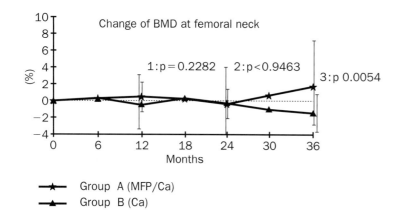

Figure 12.4 Mean (± SD) variations in the BMD of the lumbar spine, mid radius (1/3) and femoral neck during therapy with MFP/Ca or calcium alone.[53] Changes are expressed as percentages of baseline values, i.e.

1 : 12 months v baseline
2 : 24 months v baseline
3 : 36 months v baseline

osteoporosis is at present being investigated in the UK.[21]

In an open pilot study of 23 men with established idiopathic osteoporosis (all having at least one vertebral fracture) the use of intra-muscular injections of 250 mg mixed testosterone esters every 2 weeks for six months was investigated.[55] No patient received additional calcium or vitamin D supplements. Spinal BMD increased significantly by 5% over this period,

Table 12.6 Mean annual rates of change in BMDs observed during fluoride therapy.

	Change in BMD from baseline (% pa)	
	MFP/Ca	Calcium
L2–L4	+3.0	−0.8
Femur: neck:	+0.6	−0.5
Wards triangle	+1.6	−1.5
Trochanter	+0.6	−0.5
Radius: distal 1/3	+0.4	−0.7
Ultradistal	+2.6	−1.7

Adapted from Reference 52.

while no changes were seen at the femoral neck. Gains in BMD correlated better with serum oestrogen levels than with testosterone, indicating that conversion of androgens to oestrogens may be an important feature of the therapeutic effect. No significant adverse effects on cardiovascular risk were observed. Biochemical markers showed a reduction of both formation and resorption, suggesting that, at least in the short term, testosterone treatment of eugonadal men increases spinal BMD by reducing bone turnover.[56]

It therefore appears that testosterone therapy may be beneficial in eugonadal men with osteoporosis, but confirmation is required that the benefit in terms of a reduction in fracture risk can be achieved without long-term adverse effects. This approach should not be used outside specialist centres until the trial results are known.

Testosterone has also been studied in males with GIOP, some of whom were hypogonadal, and resulted in a significant increase in spinal BMD.[57]

Combined therapies

Future options for the treatment of osteoporosis in men may include combined anabolic–antiresorptive regimens.

In women with osteoporosis treated with combined HRT/MFP there was a substantial gain in BMD.[58] This suggests that it might also be of interest to study the efficacy of the combination of androgen and fluoride in men.

The positive effect in male osteoporosis of the combination of the anabolic hormone PTH with the mainly antiresorptive 1,25-dihydroxyvitamin D3 has already been mentioned.[45]

There are only very preliminary results describing the interesting possibility of combining fluoride and bisphosphonates. In a study on 9 men and 23 women with osteoporosis, a continuous oral combined regimen of 150 mg pamidronate and 152 mg MFP daily produced significant progressive increases in lumbar spine BMD over two years.[59]

In another recent Dutch study 14 men and 33 women with established GIOP were treated with either etidronate alone or etidronate plus NaF. The effect of the combination on spine BMD was significantly superior to that of the bisphosphonate alone.[60]

REFERENCES

1. Niewoehner C (1993). Osteoporosis in men: is it more common than we think? *Postgrad Med 93*: 59–68.
2. Seeman E (1993). Osteoporosis in men: epidemiology, pathophysiology, and treatment possibilities. *Am J Med 95*: 22S–28S.
3. O'Neil TW, Felsenberg D, Varlow J, Cooper C, Kanis JA, Silman AJ, the European Vertebral Osteoporosis Study Group (1996). The prevalence of vertebral deformity in European men and women: The European Vertebral Osteoporosis Study. *J Bone Miner Res 11*: 1010–1017.
4. Ringe JD (1996). Hip fractures in men. *Osteoporosis Int* Suppl 3: S48–S51.
5. Orwoll ES, Klein RF (1996). Osteoporosis in men. Epidemiology, pathophysiology, and clinical characterization. In: *Osteoporosis*, eds R Marcus, D Feldman, J Kelsey. Academic Press, San Diego, New York and Toronto.
6. Ringe JD (1995). *Osteoporose. Postmenopausale Osteoporose – Senile Osteoporose – Sekundäre Osteoporose – Osteoporose des Mannes*. Georg Thieme Verlag, Stuttgart and New York.
7. Kanis JA (1993). The incidence of hip fractures in Europe. *Osteoporosis Int* Suppl 1: S10–S15.
8. Scane AC, Sutcliffe AM, Francis RM (1993). Osteoporosis in men. *Baillière's Clin Rheumatol 7*: 589–601.
9. Seeman E (1996). Advances in the study of osteoporosis in men. In: *Osteoporosis 1996*, eds SE Papopoulos et al., pp. 341–358. Elsevier, Amsterdam, Lausanne, New York, Oxford, Shannon and Tokyo.
10. Aaron JE, Makins NB, Sagreiya K (1987). The microanatomy of trabecular bone loss in normal aging men and women. *Clin Orthop 215*: 260–271.
11. Ruff CB, Hayes WC (1988). Sex differences in age-related remodeling of the femur and tibia. *J Orthop Res 6*: 886–896.
12. Scane AC, Sutcliffe AM, Francis R (1994). The sequelae of vertebral crush fractures in men. *Osteoporosis Int 4*: 89–92.
13. Kanis JA, Melton LJ, Christiansen C, Johnston CC, Khaltaev N (1994). Perspective. The diagnosis of osteoporosis. *J Bone Miner Res 9*: 1137–1141.
14. Francis RM, Peacock M, Marshall DH, Horsman A, Aaron JE (1988). Spinal osteoporosis in men. *Bone Miner 5*: 347–357.
15. Ringe JD, Dorst AJ (1994). Osteoporose bei Männern. *Dtsch med Wochenschr 119*: 943–947.
16. Peris P, Guanabens N, Monegral A et al. (1995). Aetiology and presenting symptoms in male osteoporosis. *Br J Rheumatol 34*: 936–941.
17. Ringe JD, Dorst AJ, Faber H (1997). Osteoporosis in men – clinical assessment of 400 patients and 205 controls by risk factor analysis, densitometry, and X-ray findings. *Osteologie 6*: 81–86.
18. Mellström D, Johansson C, Johnell O et al. (1993). Osteoporosis, metabolic aberrations, and increased risk for vertebral fractures after partial gastrectomy. *Calcif Tissue Int 53*: 370–377.
19. Jackson JA (1997). Osteoporosis in men. In: *Osteoporosis: fundamentals of clinical practice*, pp. 110–113. ASBMR-Publ., Lippincott–Raven, Philadelphia.
20. Dawson-Hughes B, Harris SS, Krall EA, Dallal GE (1997). Effect of calcium and vitamin D supplementation on bone density in men and women 65 years of age and older. *New Engl J Med 337*: 670–676.
21. Eastell R, Boyle IT, Compston J et al. (1998). Management of male osteoporosis: report of the UK Consensus Group. *Q J Med 91*: 71–92.
22. Orwoll ES, Klein RF (1997). Osteoporosis in men. Epidemiology, pathophysiology, and clinical characterization. In: *Osteoporosis*, eds R Marcus, D Feldman, J Kelsey, pp. 745–784. Academic Press, San Diego, New York, Boston and London.
23. Orwoll ES, Oviatt SK, McClung MR, Deftos LJ, Sexton G (1990). The rate of bone mineral loss in normal men and the effects of calcium and cholecalciferol supplementation. *Ann Intern Med 112*: 29–34.
24. Armamento-Villareal RC, Avioli LV (1992). Successful treatment of low bone turnover osteoporosis resulting from prolonged reserpine therapy with intermittent calcitonin and phosphate therapy. *Calcif Tissue Int 51*: 282–284.
25. Keck E, Spicher ID, Werner G, Körner K-H (1997). Therapie der primären Osteoporose des Mannes. *Osteologie 6*(suppl 1): 46.
26. Francis RM, Peacock M, Aaron JE et al. (1981). Osteoporosis in hypogonadal men: role of decreased plasma 1,25-dihydroxyvitamin D, calcium malabsorption, and low bone formation. *Bone 7*: 61–68.
27. Baran DT, Bergfeld MA, Teitelbaum SL, Avioli LV (1978). Effect of testosterone therapy on bone formation in an osteoporotic hypogonadal man. *Calcif Tissue Res 26*: 103–106.
28. Axelrod DW, Lachman LB, Judge D, Mallette LE, Gagel RF (1989). Resorptive hypercalciuria and

increased interleukin 1 in a young male with hypogonadism and osteoporosis: reversal with androgen treatment. *Clin Res 37*: 21A.

29. Finkelstein JS, Klibanski A, Neer RM et al. (1989). Increases in bone density during treatment of men with idiopathic hypogonadotropic hypogonadism. *J Clin Endocrinol Metab 69*: 776–783.

30. Isaia G, Mussetta M, Pecchio F, Sciolla A, di Stefano M, Molinatti GM (1992). Effect of testosterone on bone in hypogonadal males. *Maturitas 15*: 47–51.

31. Transbol I, Christensen MS, Jensen GF, Christiansen C (1982). Thiazide for the postponement of postmenopausal bone loss. *Metabolism 31*: 383–386.

32. Wasnich RD, Benfante RJ, Yano K, Heilbrun L (1983). Thiazide effect on the mineral content of bone. *New Engl J Med 309*: 344–347.

33. Rizzato G, Montemurro L (1993). Reversibility of exogenous corticoid-induced bone loss. *Eur Respir J 6*: 116–119.

34. Adachi JD, Bensen WG, Brown J et al. (1997). Intermittent etidronate therapy to prevent corticosteroid-induced osteoporosis. *New Engl J Med 337*: 382–387.

35. Lehmann T, Beyeler C, Lämmle B et al. (1996). Severe osteoporosis due to systemic mast cell disease: successful treatment with interferon alpha-2B. *Br J Rheumatol 35*: 898–900.

36. Carnevale V, Minisola S, Romagnoli E, Rosso R, Marcheggiano A, Iannoni C, Mazzuoli G (1996). Case report: reversal of decreased bone mass by antibiotic treatment in a patient with Whipple's disease. *Am J Med Sci 311*: 145–147.

37. Ringe JD, Kruse HP, Kuhlencordt F (1980). Increase of bone mineral content after surgical treatment of primary hyperparathyroidism. In: *Proceedings of the 4th International Conference on Bone Mineral Measurement*, ed. RB Mazess. NIH Publ. No 80-1938, May.

38. Montemurro L, Schiraldi G, Fraioli P, Tosi G, Riboldi A, Rizzato G (1991). Prevention of corticoid-induced osteoporosis with salmon calcitonin in sarcoid patients. *Calcif Tissue Int 49*: 71–76.

39. Valero A, Loinaz C, Larrodera L, Leon M, Moreno E, Hawkins F (1995). Calcitonin and bisphosphonates treatment in bone loss after liver transplantation. *Calcif Tissue Int 57*: 15–19.

40. Anderson FH, Francis RM, Bishop DJ, Rawlings D (1997). Effect of intermittent cyclical disodium etidronate therapy on bone mineral density in

men with vertebral fractures. *Age Ageing 156*: 359–365.

41. Geusens P, Vanhoof J, Raus J, Dequeker J, Nijs J, Joly J (1997). Treatment with etidronate for men with idiopathic osteoporosis. *Ann Rheum Dis 56*: 280.

42. Melton ME, Kochman ML (1994). Reversal of severe osteoporosis with vitamin B_{12} and etidronate therapy in a patient with pernicious anemia. *Metabolism 43*: 468–469.

43. Saag K, Emkey R, Gruber B et al. (1997). Alendronate for the management of glucocorticoid-induced osteoporosis: results of the multicenter US study. *Am Coll Rheumatol 40*: Suppl, abstr. 630.

44. Reeve J, Meunier PJ, Parsons JA et al. (1980). Anabolic effect of human parathyroid hormone fragment on trabecular bone in involutional osteoporosis: a multicenter trial. *BMJ 2*: 340–344.

45. Slovik DM, Rosenthal DI, Doppelt SH, Potts jr JT, Daly MA, Campbell JA, Neer RM (1986). Restoration of spinal bone in osteoporotic men by treatment with human parathyroid hormone (1-34) and 1,25-dihydroxyvitamin D. *J Bone Miner Res 1*: 377–381.

46. Marcus R, Butterfield G, Holloway L, Gilliland L, Baylink DJ, Hintz RL, Sherman BM (1990). Effects of short term administration of recombinant human growth hormone to elderly people. *J Clin Endocrinol Metab 70*: 519–527.

47. Rudman D, Feller AG, Nagraj HS et al. (1990). Effects of human growth hormone in men over 60 years old. *New Engl J Med 323*: 1–6.

48. Ringe JD, Meunier PJ (1995). What is the future for fluoride in the treatment of osteoporosis? *Osteoporosis Int 5*: 71–74.

49. Riggs BL, Hodgson SF, O'Fallow WM et al. (1990). Effect of fluoride treatment on the fracture rate in postmenopausal women with osteoporosis. *New Engl J Med 322*: 802–809.

50. Kleerekoper M, Peterson EL, Nelson DA, Philips E, Schork MA, Tilley BC, Parfitt AM (1991). A randomized trial of sodium fluoride as a treatment for postmenopausal osteoporosis. *Osteoporosis Int 1*: 155–161.

51. Reginster JY, Meurmans L, Zegels B et al. (1998). The effect of sodium monofluorophosphate plus calcium on vertebral fracture rate in women with moderate postmenopausal osteoporosis: a randomised controlled trial. *Ann Intern Med 125*: 1–8.

52. Ringe JD, Kipshoven C, Cöster A, Umbach R (1999). Therapy of established postmenopausal

osteoporosis with monofluorophosphate plus calcium: dose-related effects on bone density and fracture rate. *Osteoporosis Int 9*: 171–178.

53. Ringe JD, Dorst A, Kipshoven C, Rovati LC, Setnikar I (1998). Avoidance of vertebral fractures in men with idiopathic osteoporosis by a three year therapy with calcium and low-dose intermittent monofluorophosphate. *Osteoporosis Int 8*: 47–52.

54. Meys E, Terraux-Duvert F, Beaume-Six T, Dureau G, Meunier PJ (1993). Bone loss after cardiac transplantation: effects of calcium, calcidiol and monofluorophosphate. *Osteoporosis Int 3*: 1–8.

55. Anderson FH, Francis RM, Faulkner K (1996). Androgen supplementation in eugonadal men with osteoporosis – effects of 6 months of treatment on bone mineral density and cardiovascular risk factors. *Bone 18*: 171–177.

56. Anderson FH, Francis RM, Peaston RT, Wastell HJ (1997). Androgen supplementation in eugonadal men – effects of 6 months of treatment on markers of bone formation and resorption. *J Bone Miner Res 12*: 472–478.

57. Reid IR, Wattie DJ, Evans MC, Stapleton JP (1996). Testosterone therapy in glucocorticoid treated men. *Arch Int Med 156*: 1173–1177.

58. Alexandersen P, Hassager C, Sandholt I, Riis B, Christiansen C (1997). Synergistic effect of hormone replacement therapy (HRT) combined with monofluorophosphate (MFP) on bone mass in late postmenopausal women. *J Bone Miner Res 12*(suppl 1): S104.

59. Bongers V, Raymakers JA, van Rijk PP, Duursma SA (1996). Effects of combination therapy with bisphosphonate and sodium monofluorophosphate on bone mass in osteoporosis. *Osteoporosis Int* Suppl 1: 144.

60. Lems WF, Jacobs JWG, Bijlsma JW et al. (1997). Is addition of sodium fluoride to cyclical etidronate beneficial in the treatment of corticosteroid induced osteoporosis? *Ann Rheum Dis 56*: 357–363.

13

Osteoporosis in Children

Nicholas Shaw

Aetiology • **Clinical presentation** • **History and examination** • **Diagnostic investigation**
• **Treatment**

Although osteoporosis is rare in children, when it does occur it can cause significant pain and long-term disability. The WHO definition of osteoporosis in adults is based on a bone mineral density measurement 2.5 standard deviations (SD) or more below the young adult mean.[1] This definition, which relates fracture risk to reduction in bone density, is based on several large epidemiological studies in adults. No such evidence exists in children and therefore the WHO definition of osteoporosis is inappropriate. In addition, because of the relationship between body size and bone density in children it is possible to misinterpret bone density scan results and inappropriately label children as having osteoporosis.

The definition of childhood osteoporosis should probably include the presence of low trauma fractures with evidence of a significant reduction (more than 2 SD below the age-matched mean) in bone density for age and body size. In practice bone density values in children with osteoporotic fractures are usually more than 3 SD below the mean. A pragmatic approach is to use the term 'osteopenia' for situations where bone density is 2 SD or more below the mean in the absence of fractures.

AETIOLOGY

Most cases of childhood osteoporosis are secondary to underlying diseases, particularly those inflammatory disorders such as juvenile arthritis or Crohn's disease that are treated with long-term systemic corticosteroids (Table 13.1). An increasing number of children are developing osteoporosis following organ transplantation, where the combination of the pre-existing disease and the immunosuppressive treatment compromises bone density. Osteogenesis imperfecta (OI) is the most important primary (genetic) cause of osteoporosis, and this has to be distinguished from idiopathic juvenile osteoporosis (IJO), which is one of the most important forms of acquired primary osteoporosis. The aetiology of IJO is currently unclear but this condition, which typically presents just before puberty, may undergo spontaneous remission.[2] Some of the features that may help in the discrimination between osteogenesis imperfecta and idiopathic juvenile osteoporosis are summarized in Table 13.2. Another rare form of osteoporosis is the osteoporosis-pseudoglioma syndrome, which is an autosomal recessive disorder characterized by severe

Table 13.1 Differential diagnosis of childhood osteoporosis.	
Primary	
Idiopathic juvenile osteoporosis	
Osteogenesis imperfecta	
Osteoporosis-pseudoglioma syndrome	
Secondary	
Endocrine:	Cushing's syndrome
Inflammatory:	Juvenile chronic arthritis
	Chrohn's disease
Immobilization:	Cerebral palsy
	Spinal cord injury
Haematological:	Leukaemia
	Thalassaemia
Metabolic disease:	Homocystinuria
Miscellaneous:	Corticosteroid therapy
	Post-transplantation

these conditions and to identify possible means of prevention. Aetiological factors include the effects of growth hormone and sex steroid deficiency, malnutrition and inflammatory cytokines.

CLINICAL PRESENTATION

There are three main presentations.

1. There may be obvious long bone fractures either at birth (as in some cases of osteogenesis imperfecta) or following trauma in later life.
2. Vertebral osteoporosis presents with back pain and difficulty walking which, with time, will lead to the development of kyphosis with evidence of disproportion and a reduced sitting height.
3. Alternatively low bone density may be identified as a result of a radiograph being taken for other reasons (following accidental trauma or for the determination of skeletal age).

HISTORY AND EXAMINATION

The assessment of a child presenting with osteoporosis should focus on trying to identify an underlying disorder. This may be obvious, as in a child with juvenile arthritis receiving corticosteroid therapy, or not immediately apparent, as may occur in inflammatory bowel disease.[5] Other considerations include a family history of fractures or osteoporosis suggestive of osteogenesis imperfecta, or concerns about the child's growth or pubertal development.

Examination should include looking for blue sclerae, abnormal dentition or hyperextensible joints such as may be seen in osteogenesis imperfecta. However, their absence does not exclude this diagnosis, as they are only seen in certain subtypes (see Chapter 14). Examination of the spine should attempt to identify any kyphosis or scoliosis and should include palpation of the vertebral bodies for local tenderness. In addition to examining for signs of chronic disease it is important to make accurate assessments of

childhood osteoporosis with congenital or juvenile-onset blindness.[3]

The mechanisms for the development of osteoporosis are varied, and include abnormalities of type I collagen synthesis as in osteogenesis imperfecta, prolonged immobilization with lack of weight-bearing exercise, and the effects of inflammatory cytokines and corticosteroids on bone turnover.

There are a variety of other chronic childhood conditions where reduced bone density has been identified but this may not be the presenting feature. The majority of these do not cause fractures in childhood, and therefore have been categorized as causing osteopenia (Table 13.3). They do however represent a significant risk of future osteoporotic fractures in adulthood that is now being increasingly recognized.[4] It is therefore important to understand the aetiology of the reduced bone density in

Table 13.2 Distinction between osteogenesis imperfecta and idiopathic juvenile osteoporosis.

	Osteogenesis imperfecta	Idiopathic juvenile osteoporosis
Family history:	Often present	Absent
Age at onset:	Birth	Late childhood/early adolescence
Clinical course:	Lifelong	1–4 yrs. May resolve spontaneously
Clinical features:*	Short stature Blue sclerae Multiple deformities Abnormal dentition Deafness Lax joints, hernias	Decreased upper segment height Dorsal kyphosis/back pain Abnormal gait May show spontaneous correction of vertebral deformity May have long-term disability and deformity
Biochemistry	Abnormal collagen Normal calcium homeostasis.	Calcium homeostasis usually normal Negative calcium balance and increased bone resorption during phase of evolution
Radiology	Pathological fractures (rarely metaphyseal) Wormian bones Narrow long bones	Vertebral fractures Metaphyseal fractures/consolidation Cortical thinning of long bones

* These features are not always present and vary according to the type of OI (see Chapter 14).

Table 13.3 Childhood conditions categorized as causing osteopenia.

Cystic fibrosis
Coeliac disease
Anorexia nervosa
Chronic liver disease
Renal failure
Burns
Growth hormone deficiency
Hypogonadism, e.g. Turner's syndrome, Klinefelter's syndrome

height, weight and pubertal status, since these are commonly reduced in many chronic diseases. This information is also important in the accurate interpretation of bone density results.

DIAGNOSTIC INVESTIGATION

Radiology

Radiography of the affected areas should include both antero-posterior (AP) and lateral films of the spine for evidence of vertebral compression. If idiopathic juvenile osteoporosis is suspected then radiographs of the ends of

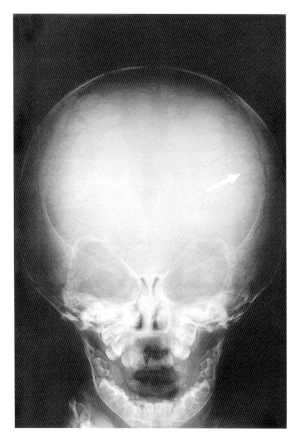

Figure 13.1 Skull X-ray to show wormian bones in a patient with osteogenesis imperfecta.

long bones, particularly of the legs, should be included to identify the characteristic metaphyseal compression fractures that may occur. Similarly, a skull radiograph may demonstrate the presence of wormian bones in some children with osteogenesis imperfecta (Figure 13.1).

Bone mineral density (BMD)

An accurate assessment of bone mineral density is essential not only to quantify the degree of demineralization but also to provide a baseline for the purpose of follow-up, particularly where medical treatment is being considered. Currently, assessment by dual energy X-ray absorptiometry (DXA) is likely to be the modality of choice owing to its ready availability, relative speed and low radiation dose. However, other techniques such as quantitative computed tomography, particularly at peripheral sites (pQCT), are also becoming available.[6] If DXA is performed it is useful to have measurements of both lumbar spine and whole body bone mineral density (BMD), since differences in the degree of demineralization between sites may often be seen, particularly with steroid-induced osteoporosis. Special paediatric software is required when assessing young children of less than 30 kg body weight.

It is extremely important that normative data for bone density in children should be available that are appropriate for the type of scanner being used; and ideally these should be based on studies of children from the same population. An additional important point that is often overlooked is that measurements of BMD using DXA reflect bone area rather than volume, and are therefore influenced by body size.[7] A child who is small for age will have a BMD value lower than normal, and hence might be inappropriately labelled as having osteoporosis. This is a particular problem in children with chronic disease, who are likely to be short and underweight and to have delayed puberty. A correction can be made to produce a value for volumetric bone density;[8] or alternatively a comparison can be made with the mean bone density expected for a child of the same body size. This is not helped by the fact that current reference data are related to age rather than body size.

Laboratory investigations

If there is no apparent cause for osteoporosis after examining the child then further investigation should be directed to a search for underlying disease (Table 13.4). This should include a full blood count and film, measurement of plasma viscosity or erythrocyte sedimentation rate (ESR), and assessment of kidney and liver function. If Cushing's syndrome is a possibility, then a 24-hour urine collection for urine-free cor-

Table 13.4 Investigation for underlying disease in childhood osteoporosis.
FBC* + film + ESR
Renal and liver function
Calcium, phosphate, alkaline phosphatase
Vitamin D and parathyroid hormone
Fasting urine calcium, creatinine
Skull radiography
Markers of bone turnover
Skin biopsy ⎫ where indicated
Bone biopsy ⎭

*Full blood count.

tisol is the best screening test. Measurements of plasma calcium, phosphate and alkaline phosphatase should be routinely performed, as well as plasma levels of vitamin D metabolites and serum parathyroid hormone. However, in most children with osteoporosis these measurements will be found to be normal. A urine calcium/creatinine ratio on a fasting morning urine will identify those children with hypercalciuria.

Some of the more recent biochemical markers of bone turnover should be considered, and these should include measures of bone formation (bone alkaline phosphatase or C terminal procollagen Type 1 peptide (P1CP) and resorption (urinary deoxypyridinoline or NTX). Low levels of P1CP have been observed in osteogenesis imperfecta[9] with high levels of bone resorption markers in some cases of idiopathic juvenile osteoporosis[10] and osteogenesis imperfecta.[11] Although these markers are often unhelpful in making a diagnosis, serial measurements are useful to document change in bone turnover, particularly after treatment.

Two additional investigations that should be considered in a child with idiopathic osteoporosis are biopsies of skin and bone. The skin biopsy is for the preparation of a fibroblast culture that can be analysed for abnormalities in synthesis of type I collagen, which, if present, would support a diagnosis of osteogenesis

imperfecta.[12] The bone biopsy is useful to demonstrate abnormalities of bone formation or resorption, and helps in distinguishing osteogenesis imperfecta from idiopathic juvenile osteoporosis. If bone biopsy specimens are obtained it is essential that these are prepared and examined in laboratories that regularly undertake bone histomorphometry.

TREATMENT

General measures

It is important to ensure adequate pain relief for a child with osteoporotic fractures. This is particularly true for vertebral compression fractures, where the pain is often severe and debilitating. Orthopaedic procedures may be required to fix long bone fractures internally or externally, while the placement of intramedullary rods to correct severe angular deformity may be needed in some cases of osteogenesis imperfecta. Bracing of the spine with an external support may be helpful where there is significant vertebral collapse. Appropriate rehabilitation will be required for many children. This should include physiotherapy to improve muscle strength and function, occupational therapy for the provision of walking aids and wheelchairs, with liaison with schools and the home which may both need appropriate adaptation.

Medical treatment

Unlike adult osteoporosis, where there are well-defined treatment options based on a substantial amount of clinical research evidence, the literature on the treatment of childhood osteoporosis is limited. The following section attempts to provide an overview of the current treatments that have been used in children; much of this is not evidence-based because of the lack of adequate data (Table 13.5).

Calcium and vitamin D
Although there is good evidence that calcium supplementation of the diet can improve bone

Table 13.5 Medical treatments for childhood osteoporosis
Calcium and vitamin D
Deflazacort
Growth hormone
Pubertal induction
Calcitonin
Bisphosphonates

mineral accretion in prepubertal children,[13] there is only limited evidence that it is of any value in established osteoporosis. One randomized cross-over study of 10 children with corticosteroid-treated rheumatic diseases[14] gave 400 units of vitamin D and 1 g of calcium daily for six months. There was a relative increase in spinal BMD of 11% during the period of supplementation compared to a six-month period without supplements. Calcitriol ($1,25(OH)_2D_3$) has also been used in some studies of idiopathic juvenile osteoporosis with improvement in symptoms, fracture frequency and bone mineral content.[15]

Although currently there is little evidence that calcium and vitamin D supplementation is of benefit in childhood osteoporosis, it is recommended that such children should receive an adequate calcium intake.[16] This can be achieved either by changes in diet or the addition of calcium supplements of 0.5 to 1.0 g daily.

Deflazacort

In children receiving long-term treatment with glucocorticoids such as prednisolone there is a significant risk of the development of vertebral osteoporosis. An alternative treatment option is the use of deflazacort, an oxazoline derivative of prednisolone that is reported to have similar anti-inflammatory effect when taken in equivalent dosage to prednisolone (prednisolone 5 mg equivalent to 6 mg deflazacort), but with the additional benefit of lower glucose intolerance, obesity and growth suppression.[17] Studies of the effect of deflazacort on bone density in children are very limited. One study described 31 children with juvenile arthritis[18] on maintenance glucocorticoid therapy who participated in a one-year randomized double blind study of deflazacort compared to prednisolone. The change in bone density accretion over this period was 13% greater in the deflazacort group when compared to those receiving prednisolone. Although these results are encouraging, there is clearly a need for more extensive studies of the effect of deflazacort on bone density in children. It is important to emphasize that this is not a treatment option in established osteoporosis, but a potential means of preventing its development or progression.

Growth hormone

Growth hormone is a powerful anabolic agent that is known to have important effects on bone formation and bone turnover. It is well established that children[19] and adults[20] with growth hormone deficiency have reduced bone mineral density that improves with growth hormone treatment. However, studies in adults with osteoporosis have shown no long-term beneficial effect on bone density, despite increasing bone turnover.[21] Studies in children with osteoporosis are limited. One study[22] examined growth hormone treatment in a group of 7 children with Type 1 osteogenesis imperfecta in a dose of 0.6 IU/kg per week over a one-year period. This showed not only an increase in growth velocity but also an increment in areal and volumetric bone density. Unfortunately, no data on changes in bone density in the untreated control group were reported and so it is difficult to be sure whether these beneficial responses were a genuine effect of growth hormone. The author has had experience of a patient with juvenile arthritis who developed vertebral osteoporotic fractures despite being on treatment with growth hormone for two years. Further studies need to be undertaken to assess whether growth hormone may be of potential benefit in the treatment of childhood osteoporosis.

Induction of puberty

In view of the known effect of hypogonadism on the production of reduced bone density and the beneficial effect of sex steroid replacement,[23,24] a potential treatment option for osteoporosis would be the induction of puberty. However, this would only be justified in a child who was of an appropriate age for puberty and had either delayed puberty[5] or either primary or secondary hypogonadism. Puberty could be induced in boys with the use of testosterone given orally or more effectively as intramuscular monthly injections. In girls induction would be either with ethinyloestradiol given orally or transdermal oestrogen patches.

There is a potential risk of too rapid epiphyseal maturation which would compromise adult height and such treatment should only be undertaken by a paediatric endocrinologist who has had regular experience in this area. Although there is extensive experience with such treatments in hypogonadal patients with osteopenia, there are few scientific data to support their use in established osteoporosis.

Calcitonin

Calcitonin is known to inhibit bone resorption by its effect on osteoclast function and therefore could be of potential benefit where osteoporosis is accompanied by increased bone resorption. Intranasal administration of salmon calcitonin in a dose of 100 units on alternate days given to five children with steroid-dependent nephrotic syndrome[25] preserved bone mineral content over 16 months, whilst four untreated children showed a continuing decline. There was also a significant reduction in urine calcium and hydroxyproline excretion in the calcitonin group. Another study of patients with thalassaemia,[26] which included some children, used 100 units of calcitonin in combination with 250 mg calcium given three times a week. After one year bone pain had disappeared and radiographic signs of osteoporosis had significantly improved in the treatment group when compared to the untreated controls. Neither of these studies reported significant side-effects although it is recognized that subcutaneous administration may produce episodes of flushing, nausea, vomiting and diarrhoea.

Bisphosphonates

These drugs, which are well established in the management of adult osteoporosis, have also been explored in the childhood disease. There have been several encouraging case reports of potential benefits in idiopathic juvenile osteoporosis, osteogenesis imperfecta (Table 13.6) and osteoporosis associated with juvenile arthritis and cerebral palsy (Figure 13.2).[27–30] There have not, as yet, been any randomized controlled trials of their use in children. There

Table 13.6 Change in bone density in a child with osteogenesis imperfecta treated with bisphosphonate (*Arch Dis Child* 1997; 77: 92–93 (ref. 28), with permission from the BMJ Publishing Group.)

Time (months)	Lumbar spine BMD (g/cm^2)	Z score	Whole body BMD (g/cm^2)	Z score
0	0.395	−4.0	0.731	−1.78
6	0.509	−2.83	0.791	−1.02
18	0.709	−1.51	0.895	−0.25

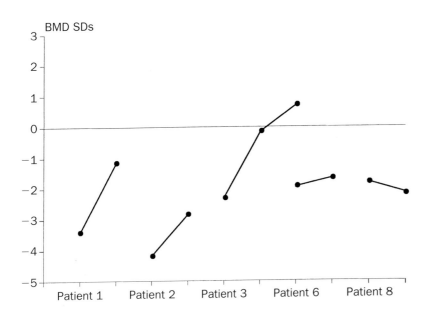

Figure 13.2 Changes in bone density standard deviation (SDs) score of lumbar spine in three children with cerebral palsy treated with bisphosphonates (Patients 1, 2 and 3) and two untreated children (Patients 6 and 8). (*Arch Dis Child* 1994; 71: 235–238 (ref. 30) with permission from the BMJ Publishing Group.)

have been a number of concerns expressed about potential adverse effects on the growing skeleton, particularly the fear that they may impair bone mineralization or compromise longitudinal bone growth. It is well known that following their administration they remain in the skeleton for many years and so these concerns are justified. However, apart from one report of the development of osteomalacia in a child with fibrous dysplasia[31] treated with etidronate, there appear to be few other long-term adverse effects; experience with these agents is still limited.

One unit has reported their experience of bisphosphonate use in twelve children with various types of osteoporosis over a follow-up period of 2.5 to 12 years.[32] These children received treatment for between two and eight years with either oral pamidronate in doses of 150–300 mg daily or oral olpadronate 10 mg daily. Two children received intravenous pamidronate prior to oral therapy. The mean bone mineral density (standard deviation score) improved from −3.8 to −1.9 over five years, with evidence of an early decline in bone resorption and a reduced fracture incidence in those patients with osteogenesis imperfecta. In addition, all children grew normally, and bone biopsies performed on six children showed the presence of normal lamellar bone.

The most comprehensive report to date presents the experience of repeated courses of intravenous pamidronate in a group of 30 children with severe osteogenesis imperfecta.[33] They received three consecutive daily infusions of pamidronate (1 mg/kg) given every four to six months for intervals ranging from 1.3 to 5.0 years. The mean annual increase in lumbar spine bone density was 41.9%, with the BMD standard deviation score improving from −5.3 to −3.4. The mean incidence of radiographically confirmed fractures fell by 1.7 per year. There were no adverse effects on fracture healing, growth rate or the appearance of the growth plates. In addition, mobility and ambulation improved in 16 of the children and they all reported relief of chronic pain and fatigue.

There does therefore appear to be increasing evidence that bisphosphonates are a treatment option in childhood osteoporosis; further research, particularly with randomized controlled studies, is required. In an attempt to record the potential benefits and adverse effects of bisphosphonates in children a database has been established to record all instances of their use in children and clinicians with experience are encouraged to report their cases.[34]

Spontaneous improvement

It is important to report that spontaneous improvement with no medical treatment can occur with childhood osteoporosis, as was reported by Smith in his series of twenty-one patients with idiopathic juvenile osteoporosis followed for up to 23 years.[35] Thus in some patients it may be appropriate to monitor their progress over time, particularly if they appear to have stopped fracturing.

Childhood osteoporosis is an uncommon condition, and as yet there are no clear treatment guidelines. It is therefore important that they are managed by a paediatrician with experience in metabolic bone disease or, in the absence of such by an adult metabolic bone physician in conjunction with a paediatrician. In addition, many of these children require the input of a multidisciplinary team that includes an orthopaedic surgeon, a physiotherapist and an occupational therapist.

Finally, it is important that families with children affected by osteoporosis are put in touch with appropriate organizations that can provide further information and support. In the United Kingdom such organizations are the National Osteoporosis Society (PO Box 10, Radstock, Bath, BA3 3YB) for all forms of osteoporosis and the Brittle Bone Society (30 Guthrie Street, Dundee, DD1 5BS) for osteogenesis imperfecta.

REFERENCES

1. *Assessment of fracture risk and its application to screening for postmenopausal osteoporosis: report of a WHO study group*, WHO Technical Report Series 843 (1994). WHO, Geneva.
2. Shaw NJ, Francis RM, Sutcliffe AM (1998). Idiopathic juvenile osteoporosis. In: *Paediatric Osteology, Prevention of Osteoporosis – a Paediatric Task?* eds E Schonau, V Matkovic, pp. 247–252. Elsevier Science, Singapore.
3. De Paepe A, Leroy JG, Nuytinck L, Meire F, Capoen J (1993). Osteoporosis-pseudoglioma syndrome. *Am J Med Genet 45*: 30–37.
4. Henderson RC, Specter BB (1994). Kyphosis and fractures in children and young adults with cystic fibrosis. *J Pediatr 125*: 208–212.
5. Cowan FJ, Parker DR, Jenkins HR (1995). Osteopenia in Crohn's disease. *Arch Dis Child 73*: 255–256.
6. Lettgen B (1996). Peripheral quantitative computed tomography: reference data and clinical experience in chronic diseases. In: *Paediatric Osteology, New Developments in Diagnosis and Therapy*, ed. E Schonau, pp. 123–133. Elsevier Science, Amsterdam.
7. Prentice A, Parsons TJ, Cole TJ (1994). Uncritical use of bone mineral density in absorptiometry may lead to size related artefacts in the identification of bone mineral determinants. *Am J Clin Nutr 60*: 837–842.
8. Kroger H, Kotaniemi A, Vainio P, Alhava E (1992). Bone densitometry of the spine and femur in children by dual-energy X-ray absorptiometry. *Bone Miner 17*: 75–85.
9. Proszynska K, Wieczorek E, Olszaniecka M, Lorenc RS (1996). Collagen peptides in osteogenesis imperfecta, idiopathic juvenile osteoporosis and Ehlers–Danlos syndrome. *Acta Paediatr 85*: 688–691.
10. Olszaniecka M, Lorenc RS, Lebiedoniski M, Marowska J, Matusik H (1998). Determination of bone mass in idiopathic juvenile osteoporosis. In: *Paediatric Osteology. Prevention of Osteoporosis – a Paediatric Task?* eds E Schonau, V Matkovic, pp. 237–246. Elsevier Science, Singapore.
11. Brenner RE, Vetter U, Bollen AM, Morike M, Eyre D (1994). Bone resorption assessed by immunoassay of urinary cross-linked collagen peptides in patients with osteogenesis imperfecta. *J Bone Miner Res 9*: 993–997.
12. Byers PH (1993). Osteogenesis imperfecta. In: *Connective Tissue and its Heritable Disorders*, eds PM Royce, B Steinmann, pp. 317–350. Wiley-Liss, New York.
13. Johnston CC, Miller JZ, Slemenda CW, Reister TK, Hui S, Christian JC, Peacock M (1992). Calcium supplementation and increases in bone mineral density in children. *New Engl J Med 327*: 82–87.
14. Warady BD, Lindsley CB, Robinson RG, Lukert BP (1994). Effects of nutritional supplementation on bone mineral status of children with

rheumatic diseases receiving corticosteroid therapy. *J Rheumatol 21*: 530–535.

15. Saggese G, Bertelloni S, Baroncelli GI, Perri G, Calderazzi A (1991). Mineral metabolism and calcitriol therapy in idiopathic juvenile osteoporosis. *Am J Dis Child 145*: 457–462.

16. Anonymous (1995). Optimal calcium intake, Sponsored by National Institutes of Health Continuing Medical Education. *Nutrition 11*: 409–417.

17. Ferraris JR, Pennisi P, Pasqualini T, Jasper H (1997). Effects of deflazacort immunosuppression on long term growth and growth factors after renal transplantation. *Pediatr Nephrol 11*: 322–324.

18. Loftus J, Allen R, Hesp R et al. (1991). Randomised double-blind trial of deflazacort versus prednisone in juvenile chronic (or rheumatoid) arthritis: a relatively bone sparing effect of deflazacort. *Pediatrics 88*: 428–436.

19. Saggese G, Baroncelli GI, Bertelloni S, Barsanti S (1996). The effect of long-term growth hormone (GH) treatment on bone mineral density in children with GH deficiency. Role of GH in the attainment of peak bone mass. *J Clin Endocrinol Metab 81*: 3077–3083.

20. Kaufman JM, Taelman P, Vermeulen A, Vandeweghe M (1992). Bone mineral status in growth hormone deficient males with isolated and multiple pituitary deficiencies of childhood onset. *J Clin Endocrinol Metab 74*: 118–123.

21. Clemmesen B, Overgaard K, Riis B, Christiansen C (1993). Human growth hormone and growth hormone releasing hormone: a double masked placebo-controlled study of their effects on bone metabolism in elderly women. *Osteop Int 3*: 330–336.

22. Antoniazzi F, Bertoldo F, Mottes M et al. (1996). Growth hormone treatment in osteogenesis imperfecta with quantitative defect of type 1 collagen synthesis. *J Pediatr 129*: 432–439.

23. Finkelstein JS, Klibanski A, Neer RM, Doppelt SH, Rosenthal DI, Segre GV, Crowley WF (1989). Increases in bone density during treatment of men with idiopathic hypogonadotrophic hypogonadism. *J Clin Endocrinol Metab 69*: 776–783.

24. Gulekli B, Davies MC, Jacobs HS (1994). Effect of treatment on established osteoporosis in young women with amenorrhoea. *Clin Endocrinol 41*: 275–281.

25. Nishioka T, Kurayama H, Yasuda T, Udagawa J, Matsumura C, Niimi H (1991). Nasal administration of salmon calcitonin for prevention of glucocorticoid induced osteoporosis in children with nephrosis. *J Pediatr 118*: 703–707.

26. Canatan D, Akar N, Arcasoy A (1995). Effect of calcitonin therapy on osteoporosis in patients with thalassemia. *Acta Haematol 93*: 20–24.

27. Hoekman K, Papapoulos SE, Peters AC, Bijvoet OL (1985). Characteristics and bisophosphonate treatment of a patient with juvenile osteoporosis. *J Clin Endocrinol Metab 61*: 952–956.

28. Shaw NJ (1997). Bisphosphonates in osteogenesis imperfecta. *Arch Dis Child 77*: 92–93.

29. Lepore L, Pennesi M, Barbi E, Pozzi R (1991). Treatment and prevention of osteoporosis in juvenile chronic arthritis with disodium clodronate. *Clin Exp Rheumatol 9* (suppl 6): 33–35.

30. Shaw NJ, White CP, Fraser WD, Rosenbloom L (1994). Osteopenia in cerebral palsy. *Arch Dis Child 71*: 235–238.

31. Liens D, Delmas PD, Meunier PJ (1994). Long term effects of intravenous pamidronate in fibrous dysplasia of bone. *Lancet 343*: 953–954.

32. Brumsen C, Hamdy NAT, Papapoulos SE (1997). Long term effects of bisphosphonates on the growing skeleton. *Medicine 76*: 266–283.

33. Glorieux FH, Bishop NJ, Plotkin H, Chabot G, Lanoue G, Travers RT (1998). Cyclic administration of pamidronate in children with severe osteogenesis imperfecta. *New Engl J Med 339*: 947–952.

34. Allgrove J (1998). Proposed database of children treated with bisphosphonates. In: *Paediatric Osteology, Prevention of Osteoporosis – a Paediatric Task?* eds E Schonau, V Matkovic, pp. 253–255. Elsevier Science, Singapore.

35. Smith R (1995). Idiopathic juvenile osteoporosis: experience of 21 patients. *Br J Rheumatol 34*: 68–77.

14

Osteogenesis Imperfecta and Other Heritable Conditions

Roger Smith

Introduction • Osteogenesis imperfecta • Osteopetrosis • Enzyme defects • Marfan's syndrome • Achondroplasia • Fibrodysplasia (myositis) ossificans progressiva (FOP) • Fibrous dysplasia

INTRODUCTION

Osteogenesis imperfecta (OI) is a syndrome of bone fragility due to mutations in the type I collagen gene.[1,2,3] It is the principal example of a metabolic bone disease resulting from a synthetic defect in collagen, the major component of the organic bone matrix. This chapter will deal largely with OI, but also briefly with rare disorders associated with defective osteoclast function (osteopetrosis), with enzyme deficiencies (hypophosphatasia, homocystinuria, alkaptonuria and the mucopolysaccharidoses), with defective function of other connective tissue components that affect the skeleton, such as fibrillin (Marfan's syndrome) and fibroblast growth factor receptors (achondroplasia), and with ectopic ossification (fibrodysplasia ossificans progressiva). Since the cause of fibrous dysplasia is now known and reports of its medical treatment exist, this disorder has also been included.

OSTEOGENESIS IMPERFECTA

Our understanding of this condition has increased considerably in the last 25 years, as a result of combined clinical, genetic and biochemical advances. It is important to recognize the wide phenotypic variability within this syndrome and hence the different aspects of its treatment.[2]

Classification

OI occurs in about 1 per 20 000 births. The current classification (Table 14.1) recognizes a mild dominantly inherited form with blue sclerae (Type I), a perinatal lethal form (Type II), a progressive deforming type (Type III) and a less severe variety (Type IV) in which the sclerae are often of a normal colour. Although many patients with OI do not fit easily into this classification, it has proved clinically very useful and correlates overall with the biochemical changes.

Cause

Type I collagen is the major structural member of the large collagen family, and is distributed through several tissues, including bone, skin, dentine and sclerae.[4] The collagen of bone is

Table 14.1 Sillence classification of osteogenesis imperfecta.

Type	Inheritance	Description
I	Autosomal-dominant	Mildest form of osteogenesis imperfecta
		Mild to moderate bone fragility without deformity
		Associated with blue sclerae, early hearing loss, easy bruising
		May have mild to moderate short stature
IA		Dentinogenesis imperfecta absent
IB		Dentinogenesis imperfecta present
II	Autosomal-dominant:	Perinatal lethal
	new mutation; autosomal-	Extreme fragility of connective tissue,
	recessive (rare)	multiple *in utero* fractures, usually intrauterine, growth retardation
		Soft, large cranium
IIA*		Long bones that are broad, crumpled; broad ribs with continuous beading
IIB*		Long bones that are broad, crumpled; ribs are discontinuous or lack beading
IIC*		Long bones that are thin, fractured; thin, beaded ribs
III	Autosomal-dominant: new	Progressive deforming phenotype
	mutation; autosomal-recessive	Severe fragility of bones, usually *in utero* fractures
	(rare)	Severe osteoporosis
		Relative macrocephaly with triangular facies
		Fractures heal with deformity and bowing
		Sometimes associated with white sclerae; extreme short stature, scoliosis
IV	Autosomal-dominant	Skeletal fragility and osteoporosis more severe than in Type I
		Bowing of long bones; light sclerae; with or without moderate short stature, with or without moderate joint hyperextensibility
IVA		Dentinogenesis imperfecta absent
IVB		Dentinogenesis imperfecta present

*Radiological subtype.

almost exclusively type I. This form of collagen has two alpha 1 chains and one alpha 2 chain wound together in a triple stranded helix. Each chain has a repetitive sequence represented as (GlyXY) 338, with glycine in every third posi- tion. This is essential for helix formation, with glycine in the centre of the helix. If a gene muta- tion causes glycine to be replaced by a larger amino acid, correct helix formation is not pos- sible. If the mutant chain is incorporated in the helix it prevents correct formation of the collagen molecule, and subsequent attempts to make a collagen fibril are thwarted. It appears that mild (Type I) OI results from a non-functional allele of type I collagen with a reduction in the RNA and type I collagen to 50% of normal. This contrasts with the situation in more severe forms of OI, particularly Type II, where an incorporated mutation leads to widespread failure of normal collagen formation.[5] The clinical effect of glycine substitutions depends on many factors, such as the replacing amino acid, its position in the chain, the number of cells affected (mosaicism), tissue expressivity and other factors not fully understood.[6] Knowledge of the different biochemical mechanisms underlying different forms of OI is important when we consider the possibilities for gene therapy (below).

Management

The management of OI depends largely on the type and the individual. It is especially in the severe forms that a multidisciplinary approach is essential.

In Type I the patient should remain as active as possible. Nutritional intake, including calcium, should be good. Fractures should be dealt with appropriately and in adult women hormone replacement therapy should be given at the menopause. Non-skeletal aspects, such as dentinogenesis imperfecta, early-onset deafness and valvular heart disease, should not be disregarded.

Since Type II causes perinatal death, little useful can be done. However, as in all forms of OI, the genetic situation should be explained to the parents and where necessary DNA sampling should be performed.

In contrast, in Type III, planned rehabilitation and surgery from the early years are very important. Recently, bisphosphonates have been used and gene therapy has been considered. Premature death from respiratory infections is common, and antibiotics should be given without delay.

In Type IV, the approach is much the same as in Type III, although the prognosis is better.

Surgical treatment
Skeletal aspects

Surgery currently offers more to the patient with OI than medical treatment. Correction of long bone deformity and the stabilization of fractures is a major application. Scoliosis and basilar impression may sometimes require surgery, although any improvement is often temporary.

In the infant or child with severe deformity and repeated fractures, the long bones can be stabilized by a variety of intramedullary pins or rods (which can be capable of lengthening with growth) (Figure 14.1). The aim of such operations is to reduce the number of fractures and to make it easier to deal with the child. It is not necessarily expected that such surgery will enable the infant to walk or even to stand unsupported.[7,8] Complications are frequent; different claims are made according to the enthusiasm and experience of the surgeon. The insertion of such rods is only one part of a rehabilitation programme. The operated limb may require external support, such as light splints or inflatable trousers. The outcome of intramedullary rodding will clearly depend on the type and severity of OI, the motor development before operation, and the experience of the operator. Most reported series are retrospective and deal with the use of expanding or overlapping rods. Clearly the outcome will be better in the less severe forms of OI. The likelihood of walking (supported or unsupported) after operation will be greater in those who have walked pre-operatively than in those who have not. Luhmann et al.[8] described the management of mild OI with operation at a mean age of 7.1 years; 8 of the 12 patients had walked with assistance before operation. In contrast, the subjects of Engelbert et al.[7] had severe Type III OI, and the average age of operation was 3.5 years. In these patients early rodding, performed only when there was unsupported sitting, improved neuromotor development. It is clear that complications are frequent, and re-operation is often necessary.

In severe OI progressive kyphoscoliosis often occurs, with considerable deformity and reduction in respiratory reserve. Reviews of the usefulness of corrective surgery differ in their

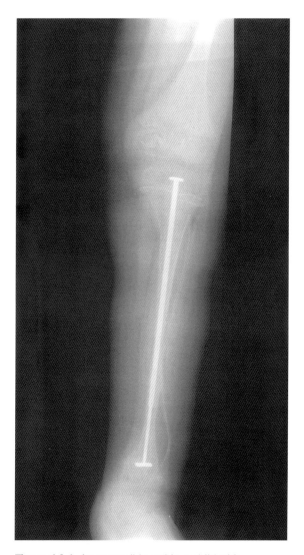

Figure 14.1 An extensible rod in a child with osteogenesis imperfecta.

conclusions.[9] Where spinal curvature can be partly corrected by traction and serial casts, this can be successfully followed by spinal surgery.[10] However, the combination of severe deformity and friable tissues (due to the collagen mutation) often prevents a successful outcome.

Basilar impression, in which the bone of the skull becomes deformed owing to the softness of the skeleton, may lead to ventricular obstruction and progressive long tract signs; this can be temporarily relieved by extensive surgery around the region of the odontoid process and foramen magnum.[11]

Extra-skeletal aspects

In the management of OI, it is important that extra-skeletal features are not neglected. Dentine, like bone, contains type I collagen exclusively, and dentinogenesis imperfecta (DI) is a common feature, especially of the more severe forms of OI. The fact that it is not constantly associated with brittle bones may be related to the different expression of the collagen gene mutation by osteoblasts and odontoblasts. In DI the teeth are translucent and misshapen and wear down rapidly. Milk and permanent teeth may be variably affected. Treatment requires specialist dentistry.

Valvular heart disease, particularly aortic incompetence, can occur in OI, and valve replacement may be required; but the friability of the tissues considerably increases the operative risk.[1]

Early-onset deafness, which is predominantly conductive, can be disabling. It may be due to fracture of the stapes, and is often confused with otosclerosis. Stapedectomy is not always effective, and progressive deafness is probably due to increasing sensorineural deficiency.[12]

Medical treatment

Since OI is due to a failure of bone matrix formation, it is logical to make attempts to correct this with growth hormone (GH) (also indicated because of short stature) or with gene therapy, which however is only in its infancy (see below). Failure of growth is a prominent feature of severe OI, and this led to investigation of the effectiveness of growth hormone. There is some evidence of a blunted insulin like growth factor (IGF-1) response to GH, but it is clear that the response to daily injections of GH in children with severe OI is not dramatic.[13] In Type I OI there was a significant increase in growth velocity and in measured and true bone density in seven children compared with an untreated group.[14] A controlled trial of sodium fluoride also failed to demonstrate a beneficial effect.[15]

The prevention of bone loss is an alternative approach. The skeleton should be used as much as possible (within the limits of its fragility). Early studies on the effect of injected calcitonin in children with OI demonstrated its side-effects more than its benefits.[16] In those with mild OI who reach the menopause, hormone replacement therapy should be strongly recommended, especially where the bone density is significantly reduced.

The main question is whether or not bisphosphonates should be given. In the postmenopausal woman with OI, the decision to give, for instance, etidronate or alendronate as well as HRT should depend on the same factors as in other forms of osteoporosis.

In children there is now accumulating experience with the use of bisphosphonates in severe forms of OI (Table 14.2), some of it anecdotal and only in abstract form.[17–24] Intermittent intravenous pamidronate (APD) appears to produce radiological and histological improvement and to reduce fracture rate; interestingly there is also considerable improvement in symptoms. There is considerable difficulty in assessing the usefulness of any form of treatment for OI because of the great variation in fracture rate with time and between individuals. Furthermore, the placebo response to intravenous treatment is likely to be significant. Ideally a placebo-controlled trial would be needed to assess the effect of bisphosphonates, but this would be very difficult to implement. A recent study[25] provides additional detailed information on 30 children with severe OI treated with pamidronate for up to five years. Clinical outcomes were improved, bone resorption decreased and bone density increased.

Because severe OI (particularly Type III) is such a catastrophic disease and because the molecular changes are now so well characterized, concerted attempts at gene therapy are now under way. There are two main approaches; bone marrow transplantation with stromal cell replacement, and antisense suppression of the mutant gene.[5] There is some evidence from animal studies that stromal cells from donor marrow may engraft to a limited extent in the recipient,[26] and preliminary work also exists in humans. It is theoretically possible to replace the abnormal Type III mutant cells by at least a small proportion of normal stromal cells with the production of normal collagen and normal bone.

Selective suppression of the mutant gene by targeted elimination of its RNA would (in theory) convert the situation of Type III OI to the mild form (Type I), where no mutant chains are incorporated into the collagen fibres and the amount of normal collagen is reduced by only 50%.[5]

Rehabilitation

The outcome of OI in many patients depends on their early care. Because the condition is rare, patients with OI are generally looked after badly and in a haphazard manner. It is important that a multidisciplinary approach is adopted. The paediatrician, physician, orthopaedic surgeon, rehabilitation expert, geneticist and many others should collaborate in constructing prospective care plans for individuals. The main problems are with Type III OI. Such infants may be born with fractures and deformity, or they may develop them in later infancy and childhood. A common feature of Type III OI is that the bone disease, and its complications, get worse, rather than better, with age. Dwarfing may be gross and deformity considerable. Such patients very rarely stand or walk, despite assistance and numerous operations.

The infant should be encouraged to use the skeleton as much as possible, and specialized physiotherapy and aids are necessary; decisions need to be made about surgery, and appropriate wheelchairs must be obtained.[27] Details are available from patient societies.

Differential diagnosis

Osteoporosis in infancy and childhood is rare (see Chapter 13). Apart from OI it may occur in corticosteroid excess (from Cushing's syndrome

Table 14.2 Bisphosphonates in osteogenesis imperfecta (OI).

Patient	Bisphosphonate	Route	Dose	Results	Reference
One girl 12 years old. Short stature, fractures, normal sclerae	Pamidronate	Oral	250 mg daily, 2 months on, 2 months off for a year	Spine BMC* increased, improved spine appearance, dense rings in metaphyses	Devogelaer et al.[22]
One boy 13 years old. Type I OI	Pamidronate	IV	15 mg single doses	Controlled hypercalcaemia due to immobilization	Williams et al.[17]
3 Type I and 1 Type III	Pamidronate Olpadronate	Oral Oral	Initially 300 mg daily 10–20 mg daily	Recovery spine shape Increase in BMD† Z score	Brumsen, Hamdy and Papapoulos[19]
3 boys Type III	Olpadronate	Oral	Continuous 5–7 years	Fractures down. Increased calcification in long bones. Improved vertebral shape	Landsmeer-Becker et al.[20]
8 children III/IV or IV	Pamidronate	IV	1 mg/kg per day for 3 days, at intervals 4–6 months, for up to 3 years	BMC and BMD up. Exercise tolerance up. Fatigue and pain down	Glorieux et al.[21]
3 children – severe phenotype	Pamidronate	IV	15–30 mg every 20 days up to 29 months	BMD up. Growth rate unaffected. Fractures down	Bembi et al.[24]
3 adolescent girls – severe OI – all in wheelchairs	Pamidronate	IV	10–30 mg/m² per month for 2–5 years	BMD up. Bone turnover down 2/3. Well-being up. Pain down in 2/3	Astrom and Soderhall[18]
5 children – 1 Type I, 4 Type III, mean age 6	Pamidronate	IV	0.6–1.2 mg/kg monthly up to 17 months	BMD up. Fractures down (non-significant). Linear growth rate unaltered	Fujiwara et al.[23]
30 children 9 type III, 9 type IV, 12 unclassified	Pamidronate	IV	1.5–3.0 mg/kg eash infusion cycle every 4–6 months	BMD up. Bone turnover down. Symptoms improved	Glorieux et al.[25]

*Bone mineral content.
†Bone mineral density.

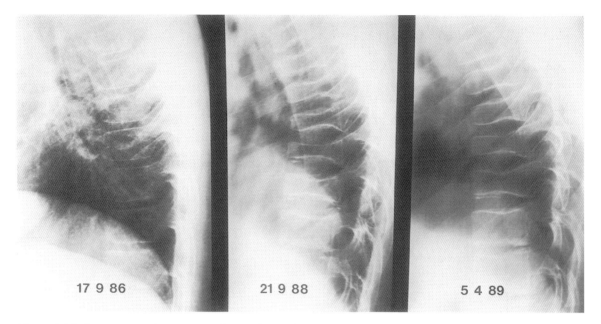

17 9 86   21 9 88   5 4 89

Figure 14.2 Spontaneous improvement in vertebral deformity in an adolescent with idiopathic juvenile osteoporosis. Symptoms began at the age of 11 in 1986; the vertebrae were biconcave by 1988; symptoms then spontaneously improved and the appearance of the vertebrae also improved (1989), and they were near normal by 1993 (from ref. 29).

or steroid treatment), coeliac disease, Turner's syndrome and other rare disorders. In practice, the main conditions to be distinguished from OI are idiopathic juvenile osteoporosis (IJO) and the osteoporosis pseudoglioma syndrome. The latter is an excessively rare bone disease associated with virtual blindness from infancy; it is recessively inherited on chromosome eleven, and there is no specific treatment.[28]

Idiopathic juvenile osteoporosis

IJO is a differential diagnosis that has its own specific features and therapeutic problems.[29] Pain in the back, failure to grow and difficulty in walking are associated with vertebral collapse and compression fractures of the long bones, particularly around the metaphyses. There is a severe reduction in bone density. Characteristically the disorder presents in late childhood or early adolescence, and in most cases it is self-limiting. Remarkable spontaneous correction of the deformed biconcave vertebrae may occur[29] (Figure 14.2). Since this disorder occurs in childhood, and since progressive deformity and fractures can occur, various attempts at treatment have been made. Unfortunately, it is not possible to predict which patients with IJO will improve without specific treatment. Early observations showed that intermittent bisphosphonates could produce corresponding lines of increased bone density in the long bones. It is not known what this implies about bone strength.[19]

OSTEOPETROSIS

In this rare condition (also known as marble-bones disease, or Albers–Schönberg disease) defects in osteoclast function lead to failure of

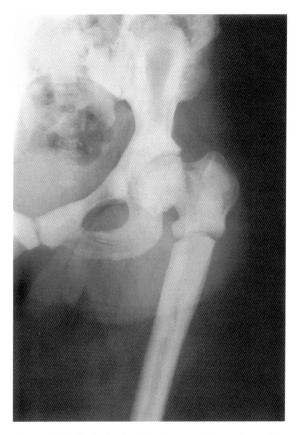

Figure 14.3 Pathological fracture and dense bone in marble bone disease.

bone resorption, and several causes are now described.[30] Clinically the main types are a severe recessively inherited disease that leads to death in childhood, associated with bony replacement of the marrow and haematopoietic failure; and a dominantly inherited mild form (itself subdivided) in which the dense bones are associated with increased fragility and fracture risk. In the severe form, bone marrow transplantation can lead to successful engraftment of normal donor haematopoietic cells from which osteoclasts are derived; but this result does not always follow.[31] Likewise clinical improvement can sometimes be produced by pharmacological doses of 1.25 dihydroxycholecalciferol, which appear to stimulate osteoclast activity. In the mild form, defective bone resorption can lead to nerve compression, which may require surgery (for instance, for relief of optic nerve compression). Fractures are particularly difficult to deal with because of the very dense bones (Figure 14.3), and there are similar difficulties with hip replacement.[32]

ENZYME DEFECTS

Hypophosphatasia

This condition, due to mutations in the tissue-non-specific alkaline phosphatase gene, may be clinically divided into a range of phenotypes, extending from the most severe, which causes perinatal death, to a mild form leading to fractures, chondrocalcinosis and ligamentous calcification in adult life.[33] Within this range various complications may require treatment; these include hypercalcaemia, craniosynostosis and fractures. Attempts have been made to produce improvement by transfusion of alkaline phosphatase-rich plasma, but without effect. It has been suggested that bone marrow transplantation has a role, if indeed mesenchymal cell engraftment can occur.

Homocystinuria

Patients with homocystinuria have skeletal abnormalities similar to those of Marfan's syndrome, especially scoliosis. Treatment of homocystinuria varies according to the degree of pyridoxine dependency.[34] There is no evidence that the skeletal abnormalities can be improved by medical means. If surgery is proposed, for example for spinal deformity, specialist advice should be taken to minimize the likelihood of extensive venous thrombosis.

Alkaptonuria

In this condition the absence of homogentisic acid oxidase is associated with widespread calcification of the intervertebral discs and early degenerative arthritis of the major joints, which may require replacement.[35] Reduction of the precursors before the metabolic block could in theory prevent complications; but there is no evidence that this is effective.

Mucopolysaccharidoses

The clinical features of the mucopolysaccharidoses and other lysomal storage diseases are due to defects in the enzymes responsible for the progressive breakdown of these large molecules.[36] The skeleton is often affected, but the serious complications such as progressive mental deterioration result from the accumulation of such molecules in extra-skeletal tissues. Enzyme replacement and bone marrow transplantation are potential forms of treatment.

MARFAN'S SYNDROME

Marfan's syndrome results from mutations in the fibrillin gene; fibrillin is a component of the elastin-associated micro-fibrillar system.[37] One important feature of Marfan's syndrome is skeletal disproportion, with excessively long limbs, arachnodactyly, high arched palate and deformity of the sternum. Correction of excessive height may require epiphyseodesis, or stapling of the epiphyses, to prevent further growth. Alternatively in girls, fusion of the epiphyses may be accelerated by the administration of oestrogen before growth ceases. Dilatation of the ascending aorta and its subsequent dissection may be slowed by the use of beta blockers,[38] although extensive vascular surgery is often necessary.

ACHONDROPLASIA

This is the most frequent form of chondrodysplasia, causing short-limb short stature. It is due to a mutation in the transmembrane region of fibroblast growth factor receptor 3.[39] It is not known how this mutation causes the achondroplasia phenotype. The treatment of achondroplasia is surgical, and is mainly concerned with decisions about leg lengthening. There is controversy about the wisdom of leg lengthening for symmetrical short stature. Individual advantages can be considerable but the procedure is prolonged and complications occur.[40]

FIBRODYSPLASIA (MYOSITIS) OSSIFICANS PROGRESSIVA (FOP)

In this very rare (less than one per million) condition, widespread endochondral ossification of the major striated muscles is associated with characteristic skeletal abnormalities – short monophalangic big toes, short thumbs, fusion of the cervical spine and wide femoral necks (Figure 14.4). It is an autosomal dominant disorder, and leads to severe disability, often by adolescence. Ectopic ossification is preceded by episodes of myositis, in which the muscles become painful, hard and inflamed. The cause is unknown, although it may be related to overactivity of bone morphogenic protein-4.[41]

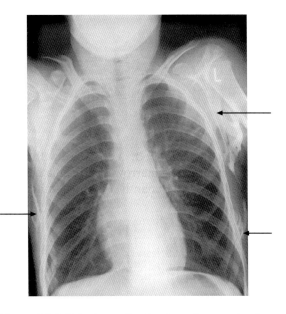

Figure 14.4 Ectopic ossification in major muscles in a boy with fibrodysplasia ossificans progressiva (arrowed).

Treatment is difficult; surgery is contra-indicated and specialized rehabilitation is necessary. Since ectopic mineralization occurs, etidronate has been given either after the removal of ectopic bone or in an attempt to prevent mineralization after myositis, but without significant improvement.[42] Since bisphosphonates, other than etidronate, are designed to prevent bone resorption without any effect on mineralization, their use in FOP is inappropriate. Recent reviews emphasize that the early myositis lesions in FOP can be mistaken for aggressive fibromatosis. This can lead to extensive, needless surgery or courses of chemotherapy.[43]

FIBROUS DYSPLASIA

Conventionally, fibrous dysplasia is divided into a monostotic form, which involves only one bone, and a polyostotic form. Polyostotic fibrous dysplasia may be associated with asymmetric

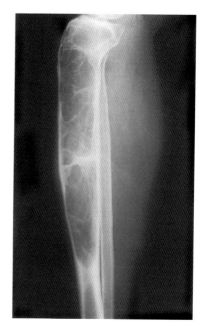

Figure 14.5 The appearance of the bones affected in extensive fibrous dysplasia.

Table 14.3 Bisphosphonates in fibrous dysplasia.

Patient	Bisphosphonate	Route	Dose	Results and comments
21 (2 monostotic, 18 polyostotic, 1 McCune–Albright)[46]	Pamidronate	IV	60 mg daily × 3 every 6 months up to 64 months	Pain reduced. Biochemical markers down. X-ray improvement in some
				Response variable. X-rays improved more in lower limbs
22-year-old female[47]	Pamidronate	IV	90 mg every 3–4 weeks	Pain down. BMD of right hip up
	Alendronate	Oral	10 mg daily	Expanding lesion right hip. Measured directly

pigmentation, precocious puberty (in females) and overactivity of other endocrine tissues such as the pituitary and adrenal cortex. This combination is referred to as the McCune–Albright syndrome.[44] It has now been established that all forms of fibrous dysplasia are due to activating mutations in the Gsα component of the G protein signalling system.[45] The bone lesions may be very extensive, and may lead to deformity, pain and fracture (Figure 14.5). Pamidronate is reported to cause considerable symptomatic improvement (Table 14.3).[46,47]

A rare complication of extensive fibrous dysplasia is hypophosphataemic osteomalacia. This may respond to oral phosphate and 1.25 dihydroxycholecalciferol.[48]

REFERENCES

1. Smith R (1986). Osteogenesis imperfecta. *Clin Rheum Dis 12*: 655–689.
2. Byers PH (1993). Osteogenesis imperfecta. In: *Connective Tissue and its Heritable Disorders*, 1st edn, eds PM Royce, B Steinmann, pp. 317–350. Wiley-Liss, New York.
3. Paterson CR (1997). Osteogenesis imperfecta and other heritable disorders of bone. *Ballière's Clin Endocrinol Metab 11*: 195–213.
4. Prockop DJ, Kivirikko KI (1995). Collagens: molecular biology, diseases and potentials for therapy. *Annu Rev Biochem 64*: 403–434.
5. Marini JC, Gerber NL (1997). Osteogenesis imperfecta. Rehabilitation and prospects for gene therapy. *JAMA 277*: 746–750.
6. Smith R (1994). Osteogenesis imperfecta. From phenotype to genotype and back again. *Int J Exp Pathol 75*: 223–241.
7. Engelbert RHH, Helders PJM, Keessen W et al. (1995). Intramedullary rodding in Type III osteogenesis imperfecta. *Acta Orthop Scand 66*: 361–364.
8. Luhmann SJ, Sheridan JJ, Capelli AM et al. (1998). Management of lower extremity deformities in osteogenesis imperfecta with extensible intramedullary rod technique; a 20 year experience. *J Pediatr Orthop 18*: 88–94.
9. Hanscom DA, Winter RB, Lutter L et al. (1992). Osteogenesis imperfecta. Radiographic classification, natural history and treatment of spinal deformities. *J Bone Joint Surg 74A*: 598–616.
10. Finidori G, Maroteaux P (1996). Orthopaedic management in osteogenesis imperfecta. In: *6th International Conference on Osteogenesis Imperfecta*, The Netherlands, September.
11. Harkey LH, Crockard A, Stevens JM et al. (1990). The operative management of basilar impression in osteogenesis imperfecta. *Neurosurgery 27*: 782–786.
12. Garretsen TJTM, Cremers CWRJ (1990). Ear surgery in osteogenesis imperfecta. *Arch Otolaryngol Head Neck Surg 116*: 317–323.
13. Marini JC, Hopkins E, Reing CM et al. (1996). Growth hormone treatment trial of children with Types III and IV osteogenesis imperfecta. In: *6th International Conference on Osteogenesis Imperfecta*, The Netherlands, September.
14. Antoniazzi F, Bertoldo F, Mottes et al. (1996). Growth hormone treatment in osteogenesis imperfecta with a quantitative defect of type I collagen synthesis. *J Pediatr 129*: 432–439.
15. Whyte MP, Schrank FW, McAlister WH (1996). Double blind placebo controlled sodium fluoride therapy for children with osteogenesis imperfecta. In: *6th International Conference on Osteogenesis Imperfecta*, The Netherlands, September.
16. Pederson U, Charles P, Hanson HH et al. (1985). Lack of effects of human calcitonin in osteogenesis imperfecta. *Acta Orthop Scand 56*: 260–264.
17. Williams CJ, Smith RA, Ball RJ et al. (1997). Hypercalcaemia in osteogenesis imperfecta treated with pamidronate. *Arch Dis Child 76*: 169–170.
18. Astrom E, Soderhall S (1998). Beneficial effect of bisphosphonate during five years of treatment of severe osteogenesis imperfecta. *Acta Paediatr 87*: 64–68.
19. Brumsen C, Hamdy NAT, Papapoulos SE (1997). Long term effects of bisphosphonates on the growing skeleton. *Medicine 76*: 266–283.
20. Landsmeer-Beker EA, Massa GG, Maaswinkel-Moy PD et al. (1997). Treatment of osteogenesis imperfecta with the bisphosphonate olpadronate (dimethylaminohydroxypropilidene bisphosphonate). *Eur J Pediatr 156*: 792–794.
21. Glorieux FH, Bishop NJ, Lanoue G et al. (1996). The use of intermittent intravenous pamidronate in the treatment of children with severe osteogenesis imperfecta. In: *6th International Conference on Osteogenesis Imperfecta*, The Netherlands, September.
22. Devogelaer JP, Malghem J, Maldague B et al. (1987). Radiological manifestations of bisphosphonate treatment with APD in a child suffering from osteogenesis imperfecta. *Skeletal Radiol 16*:

360–363.

23. Fujiwara I, Ogawa E, Igarashi Y et al. (1998). Intravenous pamidronate treatment in osteogenesis imperfecta. *Eur J Pediatr 157*: 261–263.

24. Bembi B, Parma A, Bottega M et al. (1997). Intravenous pamidronate treatment in osteogenesis imperfecta. *J Pediatr 131*: 622–625.

25. Glorieux FH, Bishop NJ, Plotkin H et al. (1998). Cyclic administration of pamidronate in children with severe osteogenesis imperfecta. *New Engl J Med 339*: 947–952.

26. Pereira RF, O'Hara MD, Laptev AV et al. (1998). Marrow stromal cells as a source of progenitor cells for non hematopoietic tissues in transgenic mice with a phenotype of osteogenesis imperfecta. *Proc Natl Acad Sci USA 95*: 1142–1147.

27. Gerber LH, Binder H, Weintrob J et al. (1990). Rehabilitation of children and infants with osteogenesis imperfecta. *Clin Orthop 251*: 254–262.

28. Gong Y, Vikkula M, Boon L et al. (1996). Osteoporosis-pseudoglioma syndrome, a disorder affecting skeletal strength and vision, assigned to chromosome region 11q, 12–13. *Am J Hum Genet 59*: 146–151.

29. Smith R (1995). Idiopathic juvenile osteoporosis; experience of twenty one patients. *Br J Rheumatol 34*: 68–77.

30. Whyte MP (1995). Rare disorders of skeletal formation and homeostasis. In: *Principles and Practice of Endocrinology and Metabolism*, 2nd edn, ed. KL Becker, pp. 594–606. J Lippincott, Philadelphia.

31. Key LL, Ries WL (1996). Osteopetrosis. In: *Principles of Bone Biology*, eds JP Bilezikian, LG Raisz, GA Rodan, pp. 941–950. Academic Press, New York.

32. Ashby ME (1992). Total hip arthroplasty in osteopetrosis. *Clin Orthop Relat Res 276*: 214–221.

33. Whyte MP (1996). Hypophosphatasia. In: *Primer on the Metabolic Bone Diseases and Disorders of Mineral Metabolism*, 3rd edn, ed. MJ Favus, pp. 326–328. Lippincott-Raven, Philadelphia.

34. Skovby F (1993). The homocystinurias. Alcaptonuna in: *Connective Tissue and its Heritable Disorders*, eds PM Royce, B Steinmann, pp. 469–486. Wiley-Liss, New York.

35. Hazelmann BZ, Adebajo AO (1993). Alcaptonuria In: *Connective Tissue and its Heritable Disorders*, eds PM Royce, B Steinmann, pp. 591–602. Wiley-Liss, New York.

36. Leroy JG, Wiesmann U (1993). Disorders of lysosomal enzymes. In: *Connective Tissue and its Heritable Disorders*, eds PM Royce, B Steinmann, pp. 613–639. Wiley-Liss, New York.

37. De Paepe A, Devereux RB, Dietz HC et al. (1996). Revised diagnostic criteria for the Marfan syndrome. *Am J Med Genet 62*: 417–426.

38. Shores J, Berger KR, Murphy EA et al. (1994). Progression of aortic dilatation and the benefit of long term B adrenergic blockade in Marfan's syndrome. *New Engl J Med 330*: 1335–1341.

39. Horton WA (1996). Molecular genetic basis of the human chondrodysplasias. *Endocrinol Metab Clin North Am 25*: 683–697.

40. Bell DF, Boyer MI, Armstrong PF (1992). The use of the Ilizarov technique in the correction of limb deformation associated with skeletal dysplasia. *J Pediatr Orthop 12*: 283–290.

41. Shafritz AB, Shore EM, Gannon FH et al. (1996). Overexpression of an osteogenic morphogen in fibrodysplasia ossificans progressiva. *New Engl J Med 355*: 555–561.

42. Smith R, Russell RGG, Woods CG (1976). Myositis ossificans progressiva. Clinical features of eight patients and their response to treatment. *J Bone Joint Surg 58B*: 48–57.

43. Smith R (1998). Fibrodysplasia (myositis) ossificans progressiva. Clinical lessons from a rare disease. *Clin Orthop Relat Res 346*: 7–14.

44. Weinstein LS, Shenker A, Gejman PV et al. (1991). Activating mutations in the stimulatory G protein of the McCune–Albright syndrome. *New Engl J Med 325*: 1688–1695.

45. Weinstein LS (1996). Other skeletal diseases resulting from G protein defects – fibrous dysplasia and McCune–Albright syndrome. In: *Principles of Bone Biology*, eds JP Bilezikian, LG Raisz, GA Rodan, pp. 877–887. Academic Press, New York.

46. Chapurlat RD, Delmas P, Liens D et al. (1997). Long term effects of intravenous pamidronate in fibrous dysplasia of bone. *J Bone Miner Res 12*: 1746–1752.

47. Weinstein RS (1997). Long term aminobisphosphonate treatment of fibrous dysplasia: spectacular increase in bone density. *J Bone Miner Res 12*: 1314–1315.

48. Whyte MP (1996). Fibrous dysplasia. In: *Primer on the Metabolic Bone Diseases and Disorders of Mineral Metabolism*, 3rd edn, ed. MJ Favus, pp. 380–381. Lippincott-Raven, Philadelphia.

Appendix: Drugs used (see also Tables 14.2 and 14.3).			
Drug	Dose*	Route	Frequency
Pamidronate	Variable 15–30 mg	Oral Intravenous	Given in courses
Olpadronate	10–20 mg	Oral	Daily
Clodronate	520 mg	Oral	Twice daily
Alendronate	10 mg	Oral	Daily
Growth hormone	0.1 IU/kg	Subcutaneous	Daily 6 days a week
Sodium fluoride	1.0 mg/kg	Oral	Daily in 3 divided doses 5 months on, 5 months off

* The dose given varies widely and is less for infants.

Index